Pediatric Infectious Diseases case studies

54 Case Histories Related to Pediatric Infectious Diseases

By

THOMAS E. FROTHINGHAM, M.D.
Professor of Pediatrics and Community Health Sciences

LAURA T. GUTMAN, M.D.
Associate Professor of Pediatrics and
Assistant Professor of Pharmacology

ZIAD H. IDRISS, M.D.
Assistant Professor of Pediatrics and
Director, Graduate Training
Duke University Medical Center
Assistant Professor of Pediatrics
American University Medical Center
Beirut, Lebanon

DAVID J. LANG, M.D.
Professor of Pediatrics
Associate Professor of Virology and
Director, Division of Infectious Diseases

CATHERINE M. WILFERT, M.D.
Associate Professor of Pediatrics and
Associate Professor of Virology

Duke University Medical Center
Durham, North Carolina

 Medical Examination Publishing Co., Inc.
an Excerpta Medica company

969 Stewart Avenue • Garden City, New York 11530

Copyright © 1978 by
MEDICAL EXAMINATION
PUBLISHING CO. , INC.
an Excerpta Medica company

Library of Congress Card Number
78-59947

ISBN 0-87488-048-3

September, 1978

SIMULTANEOUSLY PUBLISHED IN:

Brazil   :   GUANABARA KOOGAN
                                   Rio de Janeiro, Brazil

Europe   :   HANS HUBER PUBLISHERS
                                   Bern, Switzerland

Japan   :   IGAKU SHOIN Ltd.
                                   Tokyo, Japan

Mexico,   :   EDITORIAL EL MANUAL MODERNO
Central America, and   Mexico City, Mexico
South America
(except Brazil)

South and East Asia   :   TOPPAN COMPANY (S) Pte. Ltd.
                                   Singapore

United Kingdom   :   HENRY KIMPTON PUBLISHERS
                                   London, England

FOREWORD

This collection of cases is intended for those who may wish, for any number of reasons, to sharpen their diagnostic acuity in the area of infectious diseases.

Five members of the Infectious Diseases Division of Duke University's Department of Pediatrics have collaborated in the selection and preparation of this collection of case studies. Their interests and talents are broad so that a full panorama of the field is covered. This includes infections due to viruses, chlamydia, mycoplasma, rickettsia, bacteria, fungi and parasites. Each example has been based on an actual patient seen in our clinics or inpatient units, so the reader is challenged by true clinical problems, not fictional examples. Because each of the authors possesses clinical experience as well as laboratory expertise, the two areas have been appropriately blended in an approach to problem solving. Rational therapy, where indicated, is an integral part of each case study.

The authors will be pleased to hear from the readers with comments on the cases or related experiences.

Samuel L. Katz, M. D.
Professor and Chairman of Pediatrics
Duke University Medical Center
Durham, North Carolina

PEDIATRIC INFECTIOUS DISEASES

CASE STUDIES

CONTENTS

PEDIATRIC INFECTIOUS DISEASES

CASE 1: FEVER, SWEATS, AND SHAKING CHILLS IN AN 8-YEAR-OLD BOY RECUPERATING FROM CARDIAC SURGERY

HISTORY: An 8-year-old black male who had undergone total repair of a ventricular septal defect six weeks previously was readmitted to hospital with spiking fevers, shaking chills, and sweats.

At the time of surgery he was afebrile and stable with respect to his cardiovascular condition. There had been no recent recognized respiratory infection and his immediate contacts were said to be in good health.

Open heart surgery was carried out to effect complete repair of the ventricular septal defect with a Teflon patch.

The surgical procedure, which employed a cardiopulmonary bypass pump primed with fresh heparinized blood, was completed without significant technical incident, although extensive oozing of the operative bed during and after the procedure increased the requirement for blood resulting in the ultimate administration of eight units of fresh whole blood and packed erythrocytes.

Postoperatively, a soft inconstant pericardial friction rub was audible for 2 days, and coincidentally there was a transient, mild elevation of temperature (maximum 38° C). Thereafter the patient's condition became stable and he was discharged afebrile on the 10th post-operative day.

About one month postoperatively, he was noted to become mildly anorexic and febrile. The family physician was consulted and, though he could find no specific abnormalities, placed the patient on oral ampicillin. The febrile episodes became more prominent and eventually were accompanied by frank shaking chills. He was referred back to the hospital having received his last dose of ampicillin (250 mg) that morning.

Between bouts of fever the patient was described as feeling quite well, although his appetite had subsided and he appeared easily fatigued. He was not cyanotic and he exhibited no signs of cardiac failure. There had been no rash or change in frequency, color, or character of his urine or stools. There was no cough and no coryza. During each febrile episode he was described as listless. He was occasionally chilly or had frank shaking chills after which he would become damp and sweaty.

PHYSICAL EXAMINATION: BP 110/70; P. 100 regular, R. 24, T. 37. 8°C. The skin was warm and dry without icterus, rash or petechiae. There were no Osler's nodes or Janeway spots. No splinter

hemorrhages were seen. There was moderate but not unusual adenopathy. The lungs were clear. A persistent systolic ejection murmur was present (unchanged). No friction rubs or thrills were detected. The liver edge was firm and felt 3 cm below the costal margin.
One observer thought he could palpate the tip of the spleen. The remainder of the examination was unremarkable.

LABORATORY DATA: Hb: 9. 2 gm% (it had been 11. 5 at the time of
discharge). WBC: 12000. Differential: 44% neutrophils, 55% lymphocytes (Several large immature lymphocytes were seen and 9% were described as "atypical") 1% monocytes. Reticulocytes: 3%. Erythrocyte
morphology: moderate hypochromia and anisocytosis. Liver function
tests: Both the SGOT (42) and the SGPT (38) were at or just above
the upper limits of normal. Bilirubin: 1. 2 mg%. Mono spot test -
negative. Hepatitis B surface antigen (HBsAg) negative by RIA. Urinalysis : 1+ protein, otherwise negative. Chest x-ray: unchanged.
No evidence of significant pericardial or pleural fluid and no pulmonary infiltrate.

QUESTIONS:

1. This postoperative condition is probably:
    A. Subacute bacterial endocarditis
    B. Post-perfusion mononucleosis-like syndrome
    C. Post-pericardiotomy syndrome
    D. Related to the presence of turbulence over an irregular
        Teflon patch

2. Additional appropriate laboratory tests will include which one
    or more of the following?
    A. Blood cultures, to be completed on the day of admission
    B. Liver-spleen scan
    C. Virus cultures of blood and urine
    D. Storage of serum sample for serology
    E. Blood cultures on day 2 and 3 after admission

3. The patient should be prepared for surgery to remove and re-
    place the defective, possibly infected, Teflon patch.
    A. True
    B. False

4. After appropriate cultures have been obtained, treatment should
    be initiated with:
    A. High dose penicillin (up to 20 million units/m^2/day to cover
        possibility of Streptococcus viridans) and streptomycin
        (1. 0 gram/m^2/day)
    B. Penicillin alone (12 million units/m^2/day)
    C. Methicillin (8 grams/m^2/day) (to cover staphylococcal in-
        fection) and kanamycin
    D. No antibiotics need be given at the moment
    E. Discretion of the physician

5. Virus cultures of the blood and urine taken on admission are
    most likely to be reported at 7 days as showing:
    A. Adenovirus, type to be determined
    B. Picornavirus, probably a Coxsackie B serotype
    C. Cytomegalovirus
    D. Hepatitis A

6. Now that an infectious agent has been isolated and identified,
    steroids should be administered to reduce the hemolysis and to
    relieve the mild persistent thrombocytopenia.
    A. True
    B. False

7. The source of this infection was probably:
    A. Postoperative contact at home
    B. Latent infection in the patient, congenitally acquired and
        probably responsible for the cardiac lesion, reactivated in
        connection with the operative procedure
    C. Blood administered during the surgery
    D. Intercurrent infection which was in the incubation phase at
        the time of surgery

8. When this patient is ultimately discharged he should be started
    on prolonged prophylactic antibiotic coverage.
    A. True
    B. False

ANSWERS:

1. (B)

Fever, chills, sweats, and the temporal relationship to open-heart
surgery all raised the suspicion that the patient had endocarditis -
probably subacute (SBE). However, between febrile episodes he appeared reasonably well and he manifested a peripheral lymphocytosis
with the presence of a significant number of "atypical" cells. There
is an absence of many features of endocarditis, such as petechiae
and hematuria, though this is not unusual in postcardiotomy endocarditis. [3]

The post-pericardiotomy syndrome is a condition of uncertain etiology associated with pericardial manipulation. It is characterized by
high fever, persistent pleural and/or pericardial friction rubs, as
well as malaise, prominent chest pain, and a leukocytosis with a
neutrophil predominance and a "shift to the left". Occasionally this
syndrome is accompanied by additional evidence of polyserositis -
such as arthritis. [4]

Turbulence at the site of a defective synthetic patch or artificial valve,
may result in the postoperative appearance of a high-grade hemolysis.

However, this is not accompanied by significant fevers, lymphocytosis, liver function abnormalities or other features which were prominent in this case.[5]

The pattern of illness manifested by this child best fits the descrip-
tion of a heterophile-negative mononucleosis. This clinical pattern
appearing 4-6 weeks after a cardiopulmonary bypass procedure has
been called the "post-perfusion syndrome" and is of virus etiology.
The febrile pattern of high spiking elevations accompanied by chills,
chilly sensations and sweats, as manifested in the present case, is
quite typical of this syndrome and causes considerable alarm because
of the suspicion of bacterial endocarditis. Patients with this post-
perfusion syndrome are described as appearing quite well between
febrile episodes though a bit tired and anorectic. These symptoms
are frequently accompanied by a moderate degree of hemolysis, mild
to moderate thrombocytopenia, and mild but definite abnormalities
of liver function.[6]

2. (C, D, E)

Although SBE is unlikely in this case, it is nevertheless essential to
obtain blood cultures to be certain that no treatable potentially serious condition is overlooked. The reason that Answer A has been
omitted is because the recent administration of ampicillin may con-
fuse blood cultures if only taken on the day of admission. It would be
proper to obtain cultures on the day of admission (perhaps with added
penicillinase) but cultures should be continued beyond, at least until
days 2-3 in order to assess the possible existence of a bacteremia.

Virus cultures of urine and blood must be sent in order to confirm
the diagnostic impression that this illness is indeed the post-perfusion syndrome associated with virus infection. If possible, these
virus cultures should be obtained with the knowledge and assistance
of the responsible virus diagnostic laboratory or State diagnostic
laboratory. The materials for tissue culture inoculation must be
obtained and sent promptly with minimal risk of bacterial contamination, and preferably maintained at the temperature of wet ice (4°C).
Virus cultures should always be accompanied by a serum sample for
serology. In most instances, it is advantageous or essential to obtain a second serum 1-2 weeks later for comparison.

A liver-spleen scan has no application to the present case.

3. (B)

There is absolutely no reason for this patient to undergo surgery for
exploration or operative revision. If a severe bacterial endocarditis
were in progress which involved a synthetic surface or an atypical
valve, surgical revision to remove and replace the artificial substance might become important. The treatment for an infected foreign

body is often analogous to the management of an abscess. The present illness however is a manifestation of a nonsuppurative infection.

4. (E)

This is a difficult question and one which must be resolved on the spot in each specific case. In this particular case, it does not seem that antimicrobial therapy is necessary. One could simply await the reports of the bacterial (blood) and viral cultures. The child does not appear dangerously ill and the presence of a lymphocytosis and "atypical" cells suggests that this is not a septic process. However, it can be argued, and quite reasonably, that the risks of even high dose penicillin and streptomycin (and this would be the proper choice of therapy) are less than the risks of waiting for the final results of cultures which might require many days.

5. (C)

The post-perfusion heterophile-negative mononucleosis-like syndrome has been associated with cytomegalovirus (CMV), a member of the herpesvirus group. A similar syndrome, often accompanied by a positive heterophile test, has been associated with Epstein-Barr Virus (EBV) infection. EBV, also a herpesvirus and closely related to CMV, has been associated with classical infectious mononucleosis. [2,6]

6. (B)

Therapy with corticosteroids is not indicated. This syndrome is self-limited and requires only symptomatic management. Steroids might contribute to the further dissemination of this virus. The hemolysis and thrombocytopenia will gradually subside, usually without the need for transfusions.

7. (C)

Epidemiologic evidence suggests that the source of CMV in these cases is transfused blood, and that symptomatic post-perfusion mononucleosis patients probably have experienced a primary CMV infection. Among the more numerous virus-positive asymptomatic patients, reactivation of latent CMV may have occurred in donor and/or recipient cells in the presence of pre-existing antibody. It has been hypothesized that the interaction of the antigenically dissimilar donor and recipient leukocytes is responsible for reactivation of latent virus.

An identical mononucleosis-like illness has been seen following multiple transfusions in the absence of extracorporeal perfusion. It has been suggested that a more appropriate descriptive name for the syndrome may be "post-transfusion mononucleosis." The identification of CMV carriers has thus far been largely unsuccessful. Although some cases may reflect activation of latent CMV in recipients, Answer B is inaccurate nevertheless since CMV has not been associated with congenital cardiac damage sufficiently to permit such an assumption. [8,9,10]

8. (B)

It is not warranted to treat VSD patients with continous prophylactic antibiotics, either before or after corrective surgery. However, in the presence of the synthetic patch, future dental manipulations should be covered by the administration of penicillin at least. The concurrent administration of an aminoglycoside antibiotic is a subject of controversy. The physician should be aware of the possibility that combined therapy for dental prophylaxis will become standard in the future.

REFERENCES

GENERAL:

1. Benzing, G. III, and Kaplan, S.: Late complications of cardiac surgery. Pediat. Clin. N. A. 18:1225-1242, 1971.

2. Lang, D. J.: Transfusion and perfusion-associated cytomegalovirus and Epstein-Barr virus infections: Current understanding and investigations. In: Transmissible Disease and Blood Transfusion, Greenwalt, T. J., and Jamieson, G. A. (eds.). Grune & Stratton, N. Y., 1974.

SPECIFIC:

3. Lerner, P. I., Weinstein, L.: Infective endocarditis in the antibiotic era. NEJM 274:199-206, 259-266, 323-331, and 388-393, 1966.

4. Ito, T., et. al.: Postpericardiotomy syndrome following surgery for nonrheumatic heart disease. Circulation 17:549-556, 1958.

5. Sigler, A. T., et. al.: Severe intravascular hemolysis following surgical repair of endocardial cushion defects. Am. J. Med. 35:467-480, 1963.

6. Kreel, I., et. al.: A syndrome following total body perfusion. Surg. Gynec. Obstet. III, 317-321, 1960.

7. Lang, D. J., et. al.: Association of cytomegalovirus infection with the post-perfusion syndrome. NEJM 278:1147-1149, 1968.

8. Lang, D. J., Hanshaw, J. B.: Cytomegalovirus infection and the post-perfusion syndrome: Recognition of primary infections in four patients. NEJM 280:1145-1149, 1969.

9. Klemola, E. , Kaariainen, L. : Cytomegalovirus as a possible
    cause of a disease resembling infectious mononucleosis. Brit.
    Med. J. 2:1099-1102, 1965.

10. Lang, D. J. : Cytomegalovirus infections in organ transplanta-
    tion and post-transfusion: An hypothesis. Arch. Ges. Virus-
    forsch 37:365-377, 1972.

:::

CASE 2: WRIGGLING WORMS IN THE DIAPER

CLINICAL FINDINGS: At 6:04 pm on November 19, 1976, MM, a
3-month-old white female, and her mother appeared in the emergency room of university hospital. Mrs. M declared that her baby
had eaten a flea and now had a tapeworm. This astonishing remark
received relatively little attention until three days later.

MM was born uneventfully after 35 weeks gestation. She weighed
2940 gm. The neonatal period was complicated by hyperbilirubine-
mia of uncertain cause that was treated with phototherapy and an
exchange transfusion. A systolic heart murmur was detected and
was thought to be due to a relatively insignificant degree of patency
of the ductus arteriosus. She went home weighing 2840 gm. at 1 week
of age, appeared to be thriving, and was feeding well at the breast.
No problems were identified at a clinic visit at one month of age,
but between one and two months there were ill-defined gastrointestinal problems that interfered with feeding. There was an associated
distinct slowing of linear growth and no weight gain during this
month. Supplementation with formula and some intensive discussions
of domestic problems seemed to help and normal growth resumed.

At $2\frac{1}{2}$ months the mother noticed motile worms in the diaper; she
phoned her physician who judged that the baby had pinworms. Pyr-
vinium was prescribed and taken by the whole family. The worms
continued to appear, so a week later, as mentioned above, mother
and baby visited the emergency room.

The infant was normal by physical examination. A "scotch tape test"
was negative for pinworm ova. The recorded differential diagnosis
was "ascaris vs. pinworms" and pyrantel was prescribed for the
whole family.

QUESTION:

1. The physician with whom the mother spoke on the telephone or
    encountered in the emergency room:
    A. Could have learned more with some relatively simple ques-
        tions and procedures
    B. Made a reasonable guess and prescribed appropriately

During the ensuing three days motile worms continued to be passed. A number of these were brought to the clinic and were identified as segments of a tapeworm. Two weeks later, after continued passage of increasing number of segments, 200 mg. of niclosamide (56 mg./ kg.) was administered orally in a single dose. Within a half hour approximately a dozen worms were passed. Subsequently, the mother has seen no segments; two months after treatment no parasites were found during laboratory examination of a stool specimen.

QUESTIONS:

2. What species of tapeworm infect man?

3. Man acquires tapeworms by:
   A. Going barefoot
   B. Using public toilets
   C. Eating larvae or ova
   D. "Messing around"

4. Infective worm larvae or eggs are in:
   A. Feces
   B. Meat and Fish
   C. Arthropods
   D. Fleas
   E. None of the above
   F. All of the above

5. Disease in man due to tapeworms is caused by:
   A. The adult worm
   B. The maturing worm
   C. The larval worm
   D. All of the above
   E. None of the above

6. You may get help in identifying suspected tapeworm segment(s) from:
   A. Pathologists
   B. Zoology teachers
   C. Veterinarians
   D. State laboratory
   E. Infectious disease specialists
   F. University parasitology department

7. In her remarks about fleas and tapeworms, the mother was:
   A. Misinformed
   B. Crazy
   C. Possibly correct

8. Which tapeworm did the baby have?

9. For each worm match the drug(s) of choice.
    A. Pinworm (Enterobius vermicularis)
    B. Roundworm (Ascaris lumbricoides)
    C. Strongyloides (Strongyloides stercoralis)
    D. Whipworm (Trichuris trichiura)
    E. Hookworm (Necator americanus, Ancylostoma duodenale)
    F. Tapeworm (Taenia spp. , Hymenolepis spp. , Dipylidium spp.)

    1. Thiabendazole
    2. Pyrvinium
    3. Mebendazole
    4. Piperazine
    5. Pyrantel
    6. None necessary in light infection
    7. Niclosamide

ANSWERS:

1. (A)

By far the most common worms or their eggs or larvae that are
passed in the feces of children in the United States are pinworms
(Enterobius vermicularis), ascaris (Ascaris lumbricoides), whipworms (Trichuris trichiura), strongyloides (Strongyloides stercor-
alis, and hookworms (Necator americanus and Ancylostoma duode-
nale). Hookworm eggs are identical; the latter species is rare in
the United States.

Of these only ascaris and pinworm are at all likely to be seen grossly
in the stool or in the diaper. Hookworms and whipworms and strongyloides are so attached to the mucosa as to preclude the likelihood of
their adults appearing in the stool. Ascaris are readily identified because of their earthworm-like appearance and lead pencil size. Pinworms, on the other hand, are short, like the lead that protrudes
from the end of the pencil, have a delicate diameter and taper to a
fine point. Both may be motile when passed. Pinworm eggs and/or
adults are more likely found on perianal skin than in feces.

Tapeworm segments are flat, often highly motile and vary in size
from a few millimeters to two centimeters. They often are passed
in chains made up of a number of segments. Bits of undigested vege-
table can mimic worms in size and shape and may even appear to
move as they curl or uncurl with drying.

Thus, a few simple questions regarding size and shape can by very
helpful, and if at all possible the worms should be brought in for identification prior to treatment, as there need be no rush to treat.

2. See Table 2.1 ⎫
3. (C)   ⎬ See Table 2.1 on Tapeworm Diseases, page 16.
4. (F)   ⎮
5. (D)   ⎭

TABLE 2-1: TAPEWORM DISEASES*

Agent	Definitive Host (mature worms in)	Intermediate Host (larval stages in)	Man Infected by Eating	Directly Communicable Man to Man	Eggs In Human Feces	Diseases in Man		
						Stage of Parasite Causing	Pathology	Specific Treatment (drugs listed in order of preference)
Taenia saginata	Man	Cattle	Beef containing larval worms	No	Yes	Adult	Intestinal irritation	Niclosamide Paromomycin Quinacrine
Taenia solium	Man	Hogs	Pork containing larval worms	Yes	Yes	Adult	Intestinal irritation	Quinacrine Paromomycin
		Man	Worm eggs from human feces	No	No	Larva (cysticercus)	Cysticercosis	Surgical removal
Diphyllobothrium latum	Man	Water, copepods, fish	Fish containing larval worms	No	Yes	Adult	Vitamin B12 deficiency, intestinal irritation	Niclosamide Paromomycin Quinacrine
Hymenolepis nana	Man, rodents	Man, rodents Arthropods	Worm eggs from human feces	Yes	Yes	Adult	Intestinal irritation	Niclosamide Paromomycin Quinacrine

Hymenol-epis diminuta	Rodents, man	Arthropods	Arthropods containing larval worms	No	Yes	Adult	Intestinal irritation	Niclosamide Paromomycin Quinacrine
Dipylidium caninum	Dog, cat, man	Fleas	Fleas containing larval worms	No	Yes	Adult	Intestinal irritation	Niclosamide Paromomycin Quinacrine
Echinococcus granulosus	Dogs, wolves	Domestic and wild herbivores, man	Worm eggs from canine feces	No	No	Larva (hydatid)	Circum-scribed "unilocular" hydatid disease	Surgical removal
Echinococcus multilocularis	Foxes, dogs	Field rodents, man	Worm eggs from canine feces	No	No	Larva (hydatid)	Invasive "multilocu-lar" hydatid disease	Surgical removal

*From: Report of the Committee on Infectious Diseases. American Academy of Pediatrics, 17th Ed., 1974. Reprinted with permission.

6. (F for sure; "maybe" for all the others)

Definitive identification often entails injection of a gravid segment with India ink in order to make the uterine pattern visible. Tapeworm segments are quite hardy and a day or two at refrigerator temperature in water or saline will not preclude this sort of examination. If a larger interval is anticipated before a resource person can be found, fix the specimen in standard 10% formalin that is available in any pathology laboratory.

7. (C)

Review of the history revealed the following additional information.

Upon leaving the hospital at one week of age the baby was taken to an empty house that her parents had recently purchased. There, the baby was left in a basket on the floor for one to two hours while the parents did some work in preparation for moving in. Large numbers of ravenous fleas were noticed, and it was recalled that the previous owners had a dog, and had quit the premises a week or two earlier. The baby had no further exposure to this house until after it had been "fumigated" in order to destroy the fleas.

8. Dipylidium caninum is a medium sized tapeworm that in its adult form lives in the intestinal tract of dogs, cats, related wild animals, and occasionally man. Eggs and segments are passed in the feces. Eggs then are ingested by scavenging, larval fleas. From the ingested eggs, larval stages of the tapeworm move to the body cavity of the flea where development may continue, so that by the time the adult flea emerges, infectious stages of the larval tapeworm may be present in the body cavity. Ingestion of the infected flea by a child can result in the development of adult tapeworm three weeks later. The patient's gastrointestinal symptoms occurred for a month's time beginning 3 weeks after the known heavy exposure to dog fleas and lasted until just prior to the appearance of tapeworm segments in the diaper. Considering the appropriateness of the temporal relationships and the unusually large number of worms finally expelled after niclosamide, it is conceivable that some of the baby's feeding problems may have been due to the maturing tapeworms.

How did Mrs. M know about these things? Concurrently, her neighbor had been to the veterinarian's office with a sick dog. While there she had read a pamphlet on Dipylidium caninum, and had transmitted this intelligence to Mrs. M during a discussion of the baby's worms.

9. A. 5, 3, 2   D. 3, 6
   B. 5, 3, 4   E. 5, 3, 6
   C. 1   F. 7

REFERENCES

STANDARD MEDICAL PARASITOLOGY TEXTS:

1. Markell, E. K. , Voge, M. : Medical Parasitology, 4th Ed. ,
    W. B. Saunders, Philadelphia, 1976.

2. Brown, H. W. : Basic Clinical Parasitology, 4th Ed. , Appleton-
    Century-Crofts, New York, 1975.

3. Faust, E. C. , et. al. : Clinical Parasitology, 8th Ed. , Lea and
    Febiger, Philadelphia, 1970.

4. Hunter, G. W. , et. al. : Tropical Medicine, 5th Ed. , W. B.
    Saunders, Philadelphia, 1976.

TREATMENT:

5. Report of the Committee on Infectious Diseases (Redbook).
    American Academy of Pediatrics, 18th Ed. , 1977.

6. The Medical Letter 20(4): 17-24, Feb. 24, 1978, issue 499.

CASE REPORTS:

7. Currier, R. W. II, et. al. : Dipylidium caninum infection in a
    14-month-old child. South Med. J. 66(9):1060-2, 1973.

8. Ratcliff, C. R. , Donaldson, L. : A human case of Hymenolepia-
    sis diminuta in Alabama. J. Parasitol. 51(5):808, 1965.

9. Anderson, O. W. : Dipylidium caninum infestation. Am. J. Dis.
    Child. 116(3):328-30, 1968.

10. Bartsocas, C. S. , et. al. : Dipylidium caninum in an infant. J.
    Pediat. 69(5):814-5, 1966.

::

CASE 3: PARASITES AND DIARRHEA

HISTORY: GW is the 5-year-old son of a U. S. embassy official in
Cairo, Egypt. He was well until July 4th, 1973, when he began to
have loose, bulky bowel movements numbering between 5 and 10 per
day. In addition, he experienced mid and lower abdominal discomfort from time to time and lost much of his appetite. There was
neither vomiting nor fever, but he lost one and a half pounds over
a three week period. The symptoms and signs fluctuated in their
intensity but continued in spite of several trips to a physician and

treatment regimens involving the usual nostrums and dietary manipulations that have found a respected place in the thinking of a cred-
ulous public and medical profession.

No one else in the family was sick and the history was otherwise
unremarkable.

PHYSICAL EXAMINATION: Revealed a petulent, smelly little boy.
Except for increased bowel sounds, physical examination was unremarkable.

LABORATORY: Hemoglobin, WBC, differential count, urinalysis
were all normal. Stool was soft, foul and greasy. There was no
blood. Stool culture for "pathogens" was negative. Examination of
several stools in the clinical laboratories at the local hospital failed
to reveal parasites. A stool submitted for examination to a laboratory known to be interested in parasitic diseases revealed Giardia
lamblia.

TREATMENT AND COURSE: The child was treated with conventional
doses of quinacrine with prompt cessation of symptoms. There were
no recurrences during the ensuing year.

QUESTIONS:

1. The diagnosis of Giardiasis calls for recognition of either the
    cyst or trophozoite form of the parasite in specimens from the
    gastrointestinal tract. In which of the following does one search?
    A. Feces
    B. Duodenal aspirate
    C. Jejunal biopsy specimen, fixed and stained section and mu-
        cous smear
    D. All of the above

2. Cultural and serological tests should also be part of establishing
    the diagnosis of Giardiasis.
    A. True
    B. False

3. Any competent clinical laboratory is able to properly examine
    a stool specimen for protozoa.
    A. True
    B. False

4. One can assess the competency of a clinical laboratory to pro-
    perly examine a stool sample for protozoan parasites with the
    following questions:
    A. Can you do a stool examination for parasites?
    B. What proportion of the fecal specimens that you examine
        are positive for protozoa?

C. Could I see some of your stained fecal films that show E.
    histolytica or Giardia lamblia?
D. How often do you encounter Dientamoeba fragilis?

5. Which of the following examinations are necessary in order to
    properly examine a stool specimen for parasites?
    A. A microscopic examination of a small (approximately 2 mg.)
        sample of stool mixed in a drop of saline and overlaid with
        a coverglass
    B. The same mixed with a drop of Lugol's iodine solution
    C. Examination of a concentrate of the stool prepared by either
        of the formalin-ether or hypertonic saline floatation methods
    D. The examination (and retention) of a permanently fixed and
        stained fecal film

6. Giardia lamblia is acquired:
    A. From contaminated drinking water
    B. From your best friend
    C. From canaries
    D. From infected food handlers
    E. From infected family contacts

7. The drug of choice in the treatment of Giardia lamblia is:
    A. Metronidazole
    B. Quinacrine
    C. Either

ANSWERS:

1. (D)

Giardia live and cause their mischief in the small bowel. They are
variably shed in the feces, so that it may be necessary to examine
several specimens before detecting the organisms. Fecal specimens
are obviously the easiest to obtain and are positive in at least half
of infected persons. Failure to detect the parasite in the stool of a
patient with chronic malabsorptive diarrhea should be followed with
examination of small bowel contents and tissue by methods of increasing complexity up to and including biopsy. One simple way of
sampling small bowel contents involves placement of a string from
the face to the duodenum by swallowing a capsule (Entero-test). Mu-
cus adherent to the string when it is pulled back out after a few
hours often contains parasites.

2. (B)

Giardia lamblia so far has defied all attempts at in vitro cultivation.

There are no serological tests. Immunoglobulin deficiency, however,
seems to be associated with an increased rate of infection of Giardiasis as well as with certain gastrointestinal enzyme deficiencies.

3. (B)

Most, otherwise competent, clinical laboratories are singularly
inept at examining feces for protozoa.

4. (B, C, D)

There should be a precise answer, in the range of 1 to 5 percent,
to question B. Protozoa, in contrast to ova, are small and require
practice, high, light-microscope magnification, and stained fecal
films for accurate diagnosis and for reference and external review.
If the laboratory cannot produce for your examination permanently
stained fecal films positive for the two pathogens named in (C), they
are grossly deficient in parasitic diagnostic procedure and cannot
be trusted.

Dientamoeba fragilis is a small, nonpathogenic protozoa that is found
in up to 1% of properly examined fecal specimens. Because of its
small size, its occasional recognition signifies competency.

5. (A, B, C, D)

"All of the above" for protozoa. Especially important is (D), for
without this permanent record there can be no check on such difficult
identifications as differentiating Entamoeba histolytica (pathogenic)
from Entamoeba coli (nonpathogenic).

6. (A)

Epidemiological data points to the drinking of contaminated water,
although the organism is rarely found in filtrates of large volumes
of suspected water supplies. Sophisticated urban and community
water supplies have been implicated as well as certain idyllic mountain streams. Normal chlorination is inadequate to kill Giardia as
well as E. histolytica cysts.

An unanswered question of obvious great importance is whether animal Giardia that are morphologically the same as Giardia from human feces are infective for man, thus making Giardiasis a zoonosis.

7. (C)

Quinacrine as used in treatment of Giardia can cause nausea and
vomiting. Metronidazole can cause similar gastrointestinal effects
and has shown oncogenic characteristics in the laboratory. Both
drugs rarely can cause CNS toxicity.

Treatment failures, as signified by recurrence of symptoms and
positive tests, occur with both. Quinacrine has been available longer
and therefore experience is greater. Each drug currently is considered the drug of choice by one or more authorities on the subject.

Dosages are:

Quinacrine hydrochloride 2 mg. /kg. /dose, 3 times per day, 5 days (maximal single dose 100 mg.).
Metronidazole 5 mg. /kg. /dose, 3 times per day, 10 days (maximal single dose 250 mg.).

GIARDIASIS REFERENCES

1. Barbour, A. G. , et. al. : An Outbreak of Giardiasis in a Group of Campers. Am. J. Trop. Med. and Hyg. 25:384-389, 1976.

2. Burke, J. A. : Giardiasis in Childhood. Am. J. Dis. Child. 129: 1304-1310, 1975.

3. Giardiasis - California, Colorado, Center for Disease Control, Morbidity and Mortality Weekly Report, 26:60, 1977. (See Errata 26:92, 1977).

4. Moore, G. T. , et. al. : Epidemic Giardiasis at a Ski Resort. NEJM 281:402-407, 1969.

5. Paine, T. F. , Gluch, F. W. : A Puzzling Case of Giardiasis. JAMA 236:2425-2426, 1976.

6. Schultz, M. G. : Giardiasis (editorial). JAMA 233:1383-1384, 1975.

7. Wolfe, M. S. : Giardiasis. JAMA 233:1362-1365, 1975.

:::

CASE 4: FEVER AND VOMITING IN AN INFANT WITH A VENTRICULOATRIAL CEREBROSPINAL FLUID SHUNT

HISTORY: A $6\frac{1}{2}$-month-old boy with communicating hydrocephalus and a ventriculoatrial CSF shunt inserted at the age of 4 months, was admitted because of fever, irritability, hypotonia and vomiting of 2 days duration. No history of cough, runny nose, or diarrhea.

PHYSICAL EXAMINATION: Temperature 39°C, respiratory rate 32/minute, blood pressure 90/70 mm Hg, weight 6.2 kg, head circumference 43 cms. The patient was irritable and hypotonic. The anterior fontanelle was flat and there was no nuchal rigidity. The lungs were clear, heart regular and the abdomen was soft. Fundi were normal and the remainder of the physical examination was unremarkable.

LABORATORY DATA: CBC: Hemoglobin, 10. 0 gm%, hematocrit 32%, leukocytes, 14,500/cu mm, PMN's 64%, lymphocytes 25%, monocytes 8%, and eosinophils 3%. Urinalysis: No RBC, WBC, casts or bacteria. Specific gravity = 1.026. Blood Chemistry: Normal BUN, sugar, electrolytes, calcium, phosphorus, and pH. Skull X-ray: Burr hole (shunt exit). No split sutures. Ventricular Tap: CSF pressure - 50 mm of CSF, cloudy, wbc - 1000/cu mm, PMN's 85% and lymphocytes 15%, rbc - 100/cu mm (fresh), protein - 165 mg%, sugar 32 mg% with concomitant blood sugar of 90 mg%, Gram stain - no organisms, and culture - Staphylococcus epidermidis. Blood Cultures: Negative.

QUESTIONS:

1. The first diagnosis to consider is:
    A. Ventriculitis
    B. Infected ventriculoatrial CSF shunt
    C. Bacterial meningitis
    D. All of the above

2. Appropriate antimicrobial therapy prior to culture results must include:
    A. Ampicillin
    B. Methicillin
    C. Chloramphenicol
    D. Penicillin
    E. A and C
    F. B and either A or C

3. The organism isolated from the CSF was sensitive to all penicillins, chloramphenicol and gentamicin. Therefore, the appropriate antimicrobial regimen would be:
    A. Intravenous aqueous penicillin G
    B. Intravenous methicillin
    C. Intramuscular gentamicin plus intraventricular chloramphenicol
    D. Intravenous ampicillin plus intraventricular gentamicin
    E. A, plus intraventricular aqueous penicillin G

4. The patient responded to medical therapy with intravenous aqueous penicillin G and was discharged home. He was readmitted 3 weeks later with recurrent illness. Appropriate therapeutic decisions might include:
    A. Another course of intravenous and intraventricular penicillin G
    B. Replacement of the CSF shunt during therapy with intravenous penicillin G
    C. A and if it fails, treat as in B
    D. None of the above

5. CSF shunt infections are due to:
    A. Implantation of organisms at the time of surgery
    B. Transient bacteremia, which occurs during course of certain illnesses and secondary of infection of the shunt

C. Ascending infection via the catheter from infected thrombi within the heart or venous channels

D. All of the above

ANSWERS:

1. The best diagnosis is (D).

The patient had ventriculitis as defined by examination of the cloudy ventricular fluid which contained 1000 PMN's/cu mm, a low sugar, an elevated protein and growth of Staphylococcus epidermidis. This presumably represents an infection surrounding the shunt with this organism which is the commonest cause of this disease. Since the infant has communicating hydrocephalus, meningitis is probably present but examination of fluid from the subarachnoid space is necessary to establish this diagnosis.

2. Appropriate antimicrobial therapy prior to culture results must include (F).

Hemophilus influenzae is a common cause of bacterial meningitis in children older than 3 months of age and therefore ampicillin or chloramphenicol, which penetrate the blood-brain barrier, ought to be included in the initial antimicrobial regimen. Moreover, due to the presence of foreign body (CSF shunt) Staphylococcus epidermidis becomes the commonest identified pathogen. This organism may or may not be sensitive to penicillin G. Therefore, the use of a penicillinase resistant penicillin such as methicillin is necessary until sensitivity results are obtained.

3. The appropriate antimicrobial regimen is both intravenous and intraventricular aqueous penicillin G (E).

If the Staphylococcus epidermidis isolated is sensitive to all penicillins, aqueous penicillin G would be the drug of choice because of the high levels which can be attained in the serum and its ability to penetrate the blood-brain barrier in amounts adequate to sterilize the CSF. However, perhaps because the shunt and its valves represent a foreign body into which antibiotics may diffuse poorly, intraventricular administration of antibiotics in combination with systemic administration has given the highest rate of medical cures of infected shunts.

4. Appropriate therapeutic decisions might include (A, B).

The treatment of a recurrent or persistent CSF shunt infection must include another course of antimicrobial therapy (both intravenous and intraventricular) and the replacement of the CSF shunt while using intravenous antibiotics. Prompt shunt revision (plus medical therapy) is probably necessary after one documented failure of appropriate medical management.

Controversy concerning the mode of treatment of infected CSF shunts continues. In 1961 Cohen and Callaghan concluded that absolute cure could be achieved only by valve removal. Similar observations were reported by Bruce et al. in 1963 and by Nicholas in 1970. However, Schinke et al. in 1961 and McLaurin in 1973 reviewed several cases of shunt infection whose initial medical treatment was curative with one or more courses of both intravenous and intraventricular antibiotics. Once this mode of therapy fails, shunt removal with immediate replacement followed by a course of systemic and intraventricular antibiotics was advocated.

5.   CSF shunt infections are due to (D).

Ventricular shunts may become infected by organisms implanted at the time of surgery that remain dormant for weeks. Also, transient bacteremia may occur during the course of certain illnesses and consequently infect the shunt. Moreover, in the case of ventriculoatrial shunts, the distal end of the catheter may cause local trauma and formation of thrombi within the heart. These thrombi may become infected from transient bacteremia, and infection then results in an intravascular focus, constant bacteremia and septic emboli. Very infrequently, such infection of the distal portion of the shunt may ascend and involve the CNS.

REFERENCES

1.   Bruce, A. M., et al.: Persistent bacteremia following ventriculo-caval shunt operations for hydrocephalus in infants. Develop. Med. and Child Neurol. 2:461, 1963.

2.   Cohen, S. J., Callaghan, R. P.: A syndrome due to the bacterial colonization of Spitz-Holter valves. A review of 5 cases. Brit. Med. J. 2:677, 1961.

3.   Nicholas, J. L., et al.: Immediate shunt replacement in the treatment of bacterial colonization of Holter valves. Develop. Med. and Child Neurol. (Suppl.) 22:110, 1970.

4.   McLaurin, R. L.: Infected Cerebrospinal fluid shunts. Surg. Neurol. 1:191, 1973.

5.   Holt, R. J.: Bacteriological studies on colonized ventriculo-atrial shunts. Develop. Med. and Child Neurol. 22:83, 1970.

6.   Schimke, R. T., et al.: Indolent staphylococcus albus or aureus bacteremia after ventriculoatriostomy. Role of foreign body in its initiation and perpetuation. NEJM 264:264, 1961.

7.   Salmon, J. H.: Ventriculitis complicating meningitis. Amer. J. Dis. Child. 124:35, 1972.

CASE 5: FEVER, HEADACHE, SHAKING CHILLS, ABDOMINAL
CRAMPS AND DIARRHEA

HISTORY: A 12-year-old boy presented with delirium, fever, shaking chills, a nonproductive cough, dull continuous frontal headache, abdominal cramps, nausea, and diarrhea of one week duration. Two weeks prior to the present illness the patient visited Acapulco, Mexico where he was in excellent health and enjoyed the local food and beverages.

PHYSICAL EXAMINATION: Temp = 39. 7°C, pulse = 96/minute, resp. rate = 28/minute, blood pressure = 135/85 mm Hg. Patient appeared sick and apathetic, and complained of abdominal pain and headache. His cough was nonproductive and examination of the heart and lungs was unremarkable. The throat was injected and the abdomen was distended and moderately tender. The tip of the spleen was palpable below the left costal margin. Small papular spots that blanched on pressure were observed on the upper abdomen. There were no other skin lesions. The liver was not enlarged and neurologic exam was negative except for the headache and delirium. Fundi were normal.

LABORATORY DATA: CBC: Hgb. = 12.1, hct. = 37%, WBC = 12,100 cells/mm^3. PMN = 78%, lymphocytes = 20%, monocytes = 2%. Urinalysis: Essentially negative except for a mild proteinuria. Stools: (Routine and microscopy) = negative. Chest x-ray: Minimal infiltrates over the right middle lung field. Blood Chemistry: Normal sugar, BUN, and electrolytes. Cultures of Blood, Stools, and Throat: Taken on admission.

QUESTIONS:

1. The most likely diagnosis is:
    A. Mycoplasmal pneumonia
    B. Malaria
    C. Rocky Mountain spotted fever
    D. Typhoid fever
    E. Appendicitis

2. Definite diagnosis of typhoid fever may be made by:
    A. Elevated salmonella agglutinin titer (anti O and anti H)
    B. Blood culture and/or bone marrow culture
    C. Stool cultures
    D. History of contact
    E. B and/or C

3. Complications of typhoid fever include:
   A. Intestinal hemorrhage and/or perforation
   B. Acute cholecystitis
   C. Cerebral thrombosis and/or meningitis
   D. Pneumonia and/or osteomyelitis
   E. All of the above

4. The treatment of choice of typhoid fever is:
   A. Steroids and gentamicin
   B. Tetracycline
   C. Chloramphenicol or ampicillin
   D. Trimethoprim and sulfamethoxazole

5. Prevention of typhoid fever is achieved by:
   A. Prophylactic chloramphenicol
   B. Prophylactic ampicillin
   C. Proper immunization
   D. Treatment of chronic carriers
   E. Improved public sanitation

ANSWERS:

1. The most likely diagnosis is (D).

Fever, bronchitis, abdominal pain, toxicity and occasional rash are
signs and symptoms common to several disease entities such as
mycoplasma or viral pneumonia, malaria, Rocky Mountain spotted
fever, typhoid fever, and appendicitis. However, a history of travel
in areas endemic with typhoid fever or a prolonged febrile illness
with or without typical manifestations of typhoid should arouse suspicion. Typhoid fever remains a disease of major importance in
areas of the world that have not attained high standards of sanitation
and public health. This disease is caused by Salmonella typhi which
is excreted in feces, bile, or urine of patients with typhoid fever.
These bacilli can survive for weeks in water, ice, dust, and dried
sewage. Food or water contaminated directly or indirectly with human excreta is the usual source of infection. Oysters or other shell-
fish may be infected in polluted tidal waters and may be responsible
for infection of humans.

2. Definite diagnosis of typhoid fever is by (E).

Both blood and stool cultures of this patient were positive for Salmonella typhi. Isolation of the causative microorganism should be attempted for a definitive diagnosis of typhoid fever. An elevated salmonella agglutinin titer is insufficient without a fourfold or greater
increase in agglutinin titer, especially against the O antigen, in the
absence of recent immunization. In some instances of proven typhoid
fever, the agglutination titer does not rise or reach diagnostic levels.
The average laboratory does not possess the specific antigens and

standard antisera other than the O and H for S. typhi and S. paratyphi
A, B, and C. Related salmonellae may share antigens which may
lead to misinterpretation of agglutination titers. Prior vaccination
with TAB (typhoid, paratyphoid A and B) vaccine will result in production of anti-H agglutinins. Anti-O agglutinin may also rise following recent administration of vaccine. Vi agglutinins appear late in
the course of typhoid fever and usually disappear after the patient
recovers. Although they are not usually affected by typhoid vaccination, positive reactions without disease may occur thus minimizing
the usefulness of this test. Therefore, serologic tests for typhoid
fever are nonspecific, poorly standardized, often confusing and difficult to interpret.

3. Complications of typhoid fever include (E).

Intestinal hemorrhage and/or perforation may occur during the second or third week of illness. Severe bleeding occurs in about 2 percent of patients but a positive test for occult blood is even more common. Perforation usually occurs in the lower ileum in about 1 percent
of the patients. Typhoid of the gallbladder may result in acute cholecystitis, and pneumonia occurs in 2 to 3 percent of patients during
the second or third week of illness. Bacteremia with S. typhi may
result in osteomyelitis, meningitis, and endocarditis. Cerebral
thrombosis and thrombophlebitis, particularly of the femoral vein,
occur in a small portion of patients.

4. The treatment of choice of typhoid fever is (C or D).

Chloramphenicol, ampicillin, and trimethoprim-sulfamethoxazole
have been employed successfully in the management of typhoid fever.
Steroids may be considered only in patients with severe toxemia and
gastrointestinal hemorrhage. Fever persists longer in patients treated with ampicillin than with chloramphenicol, however, in a study
by Robertson et al. patients with salmonella enteric fever treated
with either ampicillin or ampicillin and chloramphenicol had fewer
relapses and carriers than patients treated with chloramphenicol
alone. In another study by Sardesai et al. it was concluded that the
combination of trimethoprim-sulfamethoxazole was superior to chloramphenicol in relief of toxemia and in prevention of relapse. Ampicillin remains the treatment of choice of typhoid carriers if there
is no evidence of gallbladder disease. Finally, Salmonella typhi resistant to chloramphenicol, ampicillin, and other antimicrobial agents
have been isolated in different areas of the world. This pattern of
resistance is associated with extrachromosomal DNA (R-factor)
transmitted between gram-negative enteric microorganisms of similar of different species. Those resistant strains are usually sensitive to aminoglycosides, however, the clinical response has been
unexpectedly poor.

5. Prevention of typhoid fever is achieved by (D, E).

In developed countries there are two main sources of typhoid fever. One is acquisition of disease during travel to an endemic area, as occurred in this case. The second is by exposure to a person who is a chronic carrier. For such exposure to result in transmission of disease, fecal-oral spread of organisms must occur. The contact is therefore usually a household member, and is frequently an older female household member. Prevention of disease in such an instance may be achieved by recognition and treatment of the chronic carrier. Such prevention will be imperfect since the chronic carrier status is usually asymptomatic. However, it is essential that persons with acute typhoid fever be examined after convalescence to ensure they are cured, to attempt eradication if they have become carriers, and to determine the source of their disease.

In underdeveloped countries typhoid is perpetuated through inadequate standards of water purification and through other forms of fecal-oral spread, such as use of night soil for fertilization. Although immunization may play a role in prevention of typhoid fever in these instances, the efficacy is marginal. Typhoid vaccines have shown protection rate ranging from 65 - 88% with the use of heat-killed-phenolized and acetone-killed vaccines respectively. Protection is evident only when relatively small numbers of S. typhi are used in inoculum. The protective effect of the vaccine does not correlate with the titer of agglutinins against O, H, or Vi antigens. Improvement of standards of public hygiene and consumption of fully cooked foods and beverages provide the primary methods for control of this classical scourge.

REFERENCES

1. Huckstep, R. L.: Typhoid fever and other salmonella infections. R. G. S. Livingston, Edinburgh and London, 1962, 334 pp.

2. Woodward, T. E., Smadel, J. E.: Management of typhoid fever and its complications. Ann. Intern. Med. 60:144, 1964.

3. Robertson, R. P., et al.: Evaluation of chloramphenicol and ampicillin in salmonella enteric fever. NEJM 278:171-176, 1968.

4. Sardesai, H. V., et al.: Comparative trial of Co-trimoxazole and chloramphenicol in typhoid fever. Brit. Med. J. 1:82-83, 1973.

5. Olarte, J., Galindo, E.: Salmonella typhi resistant to chloramphenicol, ampicillin, and other antimicrobial agents: Strains isolated during an extensive typhoid fever epidemic in Mexico. Antimic. Agts. & Chemoth. 4:597-601, 1973.

6. Schroeder, S.A.: Interpretation of serologic tests for typhoid
    fever. JAMA 206:839-840, 1968.

7. Ashcroft, M.T., et al.: A seven-year field trial of two typhoid
    vaccines in Gyana. Lancet II:1056-1060, 1967.

8. Phillips, W.E.: Treatment of chronic typhoid carriers with
    ampicillin. JAMA 217:913-915, 1971.

9. Wong, K.H., Feeley, J.C.: Adhesion of Vi antigen and toxicity
    in typhoid vaccines inactivated by acetone or heat and pheno.
    J. Infect. Dis. 129:501-506, 1974.

:::

CASE 6: WHEEZING, PNEUMONIA AND PROGRESSIVE
         RESPIRATORY FAILURE

HISTORY: This was the first hospital admission of a 7-month-old
male infant admitted with severe respiratory failure. He was well
until five days prior to admission at which time he developed rhinorrhea, cough, wheezing, fever, minimal vomiting and diarrhea.
The pediatrician on the army base where he lived examined the child
and prescribed oral ampicillin therapy. Progressive respiratory
distress necessitated a repeat visit to the physician at which time
parenteral ampicillin was initiated, but within 24 hours he was admitted to the hospital because of bilateral perihilar infiltrates which
were seen in association with the increasing severity of his symptoms. There was no recognizable outbreaks of respiratory illness
in the community.

PHYSICAL EXAMINATION: Pulse 150. Blood pressure 105/75. Respirations 60. This was a well-developed, well-nourished child in
obvious respiratory distress. The patient was lethargic and responsive only to painful stimuli. There was poor air exchange and scattered wheezes were present through both lung fields. Rales were
present intermittently and in varying locations. The abdomen was
soft with liver palpable 1-2 cm. below the right costal margin. Symmetrical peripheral pulses were present.

LABORATORY DATA: Hemoglobin, 9.0 grams. WBC, 9,200 with
82% polys, 1% band and 1% lymphocytes. Serum chemistries: BUN
4 mg%, Sodium 133 meq./L. Chloride 83 mg%, HCO_3 29 meq./L.
Potassium 5.3 meq./L. Endotracheal secretions contained neutrophils with no predominant bacterial flora visible on Gram stain and
were submitted for culture. Blood and cerebrospinal fluid were obtained for culture and were ultimately shown to be sterile for bacteria.

COURSE IN HOSPITAL: The patient required immediate endotracheal intubation with respiratory support. Chest x-rays showed extension of the pulmonary infiltrates (Fig. 6.1) and the patient

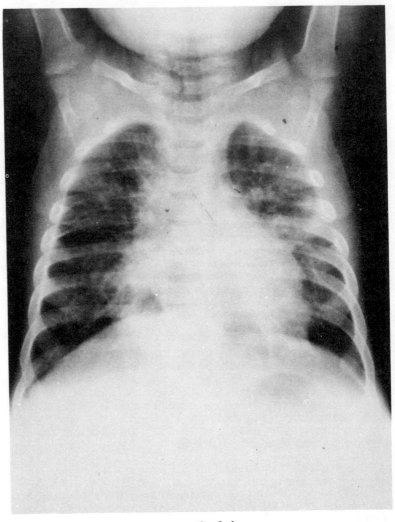

FIG. 6.1

evidenced increasing anoxia, tachycardia and enlarging heart, liver, and spleen during the first week in the hospital. Liver function was assessed with serum enzyme studies. The LDH reached 2234 IU, SGOT reached 273 IU, SGPT was normal and CPK reached 498 IU. Isoenzyme determinations showed evidence of hepatic, lung, and muscle damage. The patient developed remarkable peripheral edema and symmetrical peripheral cyanotic discoloration of the finger tips and toes during the second three weeks in the hospital. A platelet count of 72,000 was obtained at the time of the described discoloration of his extremities and simultaneously a normal prothrombin time, partial thromboplastin generation time and no elevation of fibrin split products were noted. The changes of the extremities resolved over the second month in the hospital with loss of the nails and skin of the digits. The patient became hypoproteinemic with extensive loss of muscle mass and subcutaneous tissue over the subsequent 2-4 months. Extensive therapy with bronchodilators, corticosteroids, respirator support, intravenous fluid and anticonvulsants, as well as digoxin and diuretics, were essential on chest film (Fig. 6. 2) and xenon studies showed areas of devascularized lung associated with no perfusion of the same areas. The patient expired with progressive pulmonary compromise at the end of six months of hospitalization.

QUESTIONS:

1. The best initial diagnosis for this patient would include:
   A. Acute bacterial pneumonia, probably staphylococcal
   B. Mycoplasma pneumoniae infection
   C. Respiratory syncytial virus infection
   D. Influenza virus infection
   E. Adenovirus infection

2. Which one of the viral agents associated with pneumonia in infants has been shown to produce disseminated infection with evidence of viral replication in other organs?
   A. Respiratory syncytial virus
   B. Influenza virus
   C. Adenovirus
   D. Parainfluenza viruses

3. The pathology of fatal adenovirus pneumonia includes:
   A. Necrosis of the bronchial epithelium
   B. Obliterative bronchiolitis
   C. Bronchiectasis
   D. Hemorrhagic pneumonia
   E. Abscess formation

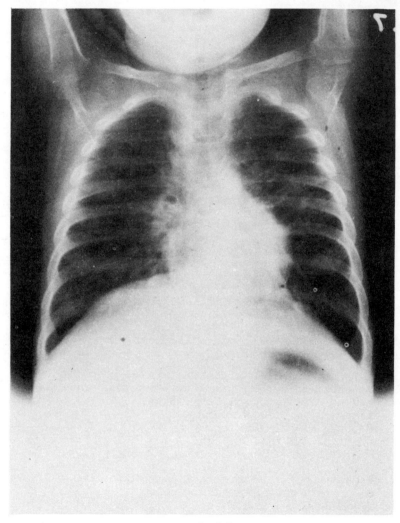

FIG. 6.2

4. Diagnosis of adenovirus infection may be confirmed by:
    A. Cultivation in vitro of the virus from respiratory tract
        secretions
    B. Cultivation of the virus from stool
    C. Cultivation of the virus from cerebrospinal fluid or urine
    D. A complement fixation antibody titer
    E. Microscopic demonstration of intranuclear inclusions in
        cells of the respiratory tract secretions or a tissue specimen

5. The outcome of this kind of infection is:
    A. Always benign
    B. Can cause significant mortality but survivors have normal
        lungs
    C. Can produce significant mortality and chronic pulmonary
        disease

ANSWERS:

1. (C, D, E) Respiratory syncytial virus, influenza virus, or adeno-
    virus infection.

Adenovirus infection is not unusual as surveillance studies would indicate that 2 to 7% of all respiratory tract infections in children may
be due to adenoviruses. [1,2] There are 33 serotypes of adenovirus, and
infants are usually encountering one of these agents for the first time.
Surveillance studies in various geographical areas implicate serotypes 1, 2 and 5 most frequently. There are more published reports
of devastating disease attributable to serotypes 3, 4, 7 and 21. [3,5]
The clinical illness of this patient is typical with upper respiratory
tract symptoms progressing over several days to rather severe
lower respiratory tract disease. The wheezing and dyspnea is commonly associated with fever. The majority of children with severe
disease are between the ages of 6 months and 3 years. This is in
contrast to respiratory syncytial virus, where the majority of these
severe infections occur in infants less than 6 months of age. Of additional significance is the patient's association with an army camp,
where adenoviruses are well-recognized as a course of epidemic illness among recruits, responsible for significant morbidity. In the
absence of recognizable influenzae illness in the community, it is
less likely to be causative in the sporadic case of illness in an infant
than an adenovirus, but is an initial consideration.

2. (C) Adenovirus

Respiratory syncytial virus, influenza virus, and the parainfluenza
viruses are almost always localized exclusively to the respiratory
tract. In contrast, children with severe adenovirus infection have
shown involvement of the central nervous system, the heart, the
kidneys and liver. They have evidenced also thrombocytopenia, leukopenia or leukocytosis. They also have had other hematological

manifestations of their disease including petechiae, anaphylactoid purpura and disseminated intravascular coagulation. This patient had adenovirus type 6 isolated from the respiratory tract in 3 specimens obtained during the first 3 days of hospitalization. Chemical evidence of hepatic involvement, findings consistent with anaphylactoid purpura at a time when he was thrombocytopenic, and possibly congestive heart failure were evident. The alteration in his state of consciousness could have been partially attributable to his seizure, to anoxia and/or invasion of the central nervous system by the virus. The absence of bacterial pathogens and the isolation of an adenovirus make this the best etiologic diagnosis.

3. (A) Necrosis of the bronchial epithelium, (B) obliterative bronchiolitis, (C) bronchiectasis

The pathology of the lungs shows dramatic destruction of the bronchial epithelium acutely. It may extend to the submucosa and intranuclear inclusions may be seen in the remaining epithelial cells. These inclusions are basophilic and tend to obscure the nuclear membrane. The bronchiolitis becomes obliterative with time. A diffuse interstitial pneumonitis characterized by mononuclear cell infiltrates and hyperplasia of the alveolar lining cells develops. Many of these cells also have intranuclear inclusions during the first weeks of illness. Alveolae appear edematous, contain fibrin, and in some areas may have erythrocytes.

4. (A-E) All of the answers with certain qualifications

Adenoviruses are isolated in cell culture systems from such materials as respiratory tract secretions, stool, urine, and rarely, cerebrospinal fluid. Adenoviruses are stable at refrigerator temperatures and are usually inoculated by the diagnostic laboratory into cell culture systems including human embryonic kidney. Virus has been isolated from postmortem materials including lung, lymph node, liver, kidney, and central nervous system. Virus is most frequently obtained from the lungs, and titers of 10^6 per gram of tissue have been obtained. Although antibody titers can be extremely useful, complement fixation studies are not sufficiently specific to identify serotypes of adenovirus. The complement fixation antibody study is not very sensitive and the absence of a rise in CF antibodies does not rule out the occurrence of an adenovirus infection. Where serological studies are available and virus neutralization antibody assays can be accomplished, they will be more sensitive and specific than complement fixation antibody titers. The microscopic demonstration of intranuclear inclusions is helpful but not specifically diagnostic of adenovirus infections. Reports have indicated that these changes can be seen in exfoliated cells from the respiratory tract as well as in tissues viewed at autopsy or biopsy. Virus has also been demonstrated by electron microscopy and can be morphologically identified as adenovirus. The confirmation rests with the isolation of virus by cell culture techniques. Serotyping is presently dependent upon isolation of the virus from the patient.

5. (C) Can produce significant mortality and chronic pulmonary
    disease

Patients have been described in several studies including those from
Scandinavia, Canada and New Zealand, [6, 8] indicating that patients
with severe adenovirus infections may have significant sequelae of
their illness. Of 69 patients examined in one study, 28 had bronchiectasis in follow-up periods ranging from 6 months to several years.
In these patients, the vascular bed was destroyed. Decreased pulmonary blood flow was demonstrated at a later point in time, both
by angiography and isotopic scan. Adenovirus pneumonia is certainly
one which causes severe pulmonary disease in a relatively small
number of infants but can leave a significant number of these infected
infants with long-term sequelae of their infection.

REFERENCES

1. Brandt, Carl D. , et al. : Infections in 18,000 infants and children
    in a control study of respiratory tract disease. I. Adenovirus
    pathogenicity in relationship to serologic type and illness and
    syndrome. Am. J. Epidem. 90:484-500, December 1969.

2. Brandt, Carl D. , et al. : Infections in 18,000 infants and children
    in a control study of respiratory tract disease. II. Variation in
    adenovirus infections by year and season. Am. J. Epidem. 95:
    218-227, 1972.

3. Dudding, Burton A. , et al. : Fatal pneumonia associated with
    adenovirus type VII in 3 military trainees. NEJM 286:1289, 1972.

4. Chaney, C. , et al. : Severe and fatal pneumonia in infants and
    young children associated with adenovirus infections. Am. J.
    Hyg. 67:367-378, 1958.

5. Angella, Joseph A. , Connor, James D. : Neonatal infection
    caused by adenovirus type VII. J. Pediat. 72:474-478, 1968.

6. Seppo Simila, et al. : Type VII adenovirus pneumonia. J. Pediat.
    79:605-611, 1971.

7. Lang, W. R. , et al. : Bronchopneumonia with serious sequelae
    in children with the adenovirus type 21 infection. Brit. Med. J.
    1:73-79, January 11, 1969.

8. Gold, R. , et al. : Adenoviral pneumonia and its complications
    in infancy and childhood. J. Canad. Assn. Radiol. 20:218-224,
    1969.

::

CASE 7: RECURRENT STAPHYLOCOCCAL INFECTIONS AND
         AN ABDOMINAL MASS

HISTORY: A nine-year-old, white male is admitted with a chief
complaint of abdominal mass which was first noted by the patient
two days prior to admission. This youth has a history of multiple
episodes of impetigo and an infection of an anal fistula requiring
surgery at the age of 18 months. He had multiple skin abscesses
requiring incision and drainage. A right upper lobe pneumonia at
the age of 4 was thought to be staphylococcal, and surgical removal
of the right upper lobe was accomplished in 1971. Five weeks prior
to the present admission, the patient began to experience episodic
vomiting occurring three to five times a week. He also developed
fever with temperature recorded as 38. 5 degrees C. occurring
three to four times weekly. Decreased activity and appetite were
observed. Two days prior to admission the patient noted a tender
mass in the upper abdomen, and he was referred to the hospital for
evaluation and admission. A weight loss of 5 pounds and a decrease
in hemoglobin from 11. 4 to 9. 8 grams % was observed over the
month prior to admission.

FAMILY HISTORY: Negative for increased infections. There are no
maternal brothers or uncles. The patient has one sibling, a sister
who is healthy.

PHYSICAL EXAMINATION: Reveals a thin, pale, chronically ill-
appearing youth in no acute distress. The temperature was 36. 8
degrees C. , pulse 88, respirations 20, blood pressure 100/70,
height 127 cm. Weight 22 kg. He had multiple, firm, small anterior
cervical lymph nodes palpable. The nose had mucopurulent drainage.
Examination of the chest showed the right thoracotomy scar. The
lung fields were felt to be clear to percussion and auscultation. Cardiac examination showed Grade II/VI systolic ejection murmur along
the left sternal border. The abdomen was soft with a moderately
tender, firm 5 x 5 cm. mass felt to be located within the liver. The
mass was palpable immediately below the xiphoid. The spleen was
palpable 4-5 cm. below the left costal margin. The liver was palpable 5 cm. below the right costal margin.

ACCESSORY LABORATORY INFORMATION OBTAINED AT THE
TIME OF ADMISSION: Hemoglobin 9. 7 grams %, hematocrit 29. 5%,
WBC 17,300 with 92% neutrophils, 5% lymphocytes, 3% monocytes
and adequate platelets. Urinalysis, chest x-ray and IVP were normal.

QUESTION:

1. Consideration of this patient's problem would now dictate that
    the following studies be obtained:
    A. Blood cultures
    B. A Tc-99m sulfur colloid liver-spleen scan
    C. Quantitative immunoglobulins

  D. NBT test
  E. Bone marrow aspiration
  F. Sweat test

The old record became available after admission and review of these admissions revealed the patient had a normal NBT test during the previous admission. Immunoglobulins in all classes were markedly elevated. Review of previous infections showed that staphylococci were always responsible for the cutaneous abscesses and draining lymph nodes. Pulmonary pathology from the previously removed segment of lung revealed Aspergillus species which was confirmed on culture as Aspergillus niger. Liver scan using Tc-99m sulfur colloid demonstrated multiple space occupying lesions within the liver. The largest was noted in the anterior projection in the mid-lateral right lobe of the liver (Fig. 7. 1).

QUESTION:

2. With the knowledge that this patient has had multiple pyogenic infections, the best course of action is to:
  A. Initiate antibiotic therapy for staphylococci (e. g. nafcillin 100 mg/kg/24 hours administered at 6 hourly intervals)
  B. Perform needle aspiration of the liver to determine the etiology of the filling defects observed on scan
  C. Obtain surgical consultation for planned exploration and drainage of the pyogenic abscesses of the liver

Two days after admission the patient was taken to the operating room where exploration and drainage of the liver abscesses were accomplished. Following the first procedure the patient developed pulmonary infiltrates with bilateral pleural effusions and a thoracentesis was done at that time. From the original liver abscess and from the thoracentesis fluid Staphylococcus aureus, coagulase positive, was grown with an MIC to penicillin of 1. 0 ugm/ml. Evaluation of the patient's antimicrobial therapy by serum Schlicters obtained after several days of therapy is revealed in Table 7-1.

TABLE 7-1: SERUM SCHLICTERS		
	SERUM DILUTION	
	Bacteriostatic level	Bactericidal level
Immediately Prior to The Dose of Nafcillin	1:2	1:1
1 hr After The Dose of Nafcillin	1:16	1:2

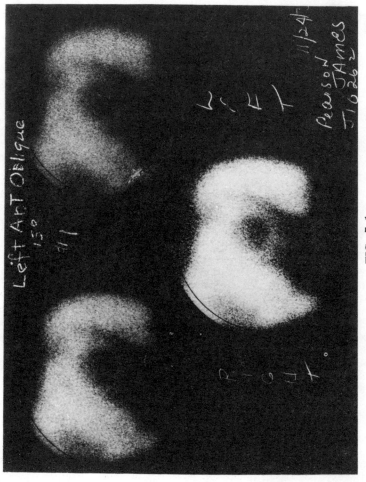

FIG. 7.1

QUESTION:

3. On the basis of this information:
   A. The patient's therapy should be changed from nafcillin to
      another penicillinase resistant penicillin
   B. Gentamicin should be added
   C. The nafcillin dosage should be increased
   D. Clindamycin should be substituted for nafcillin

Therapy was altered and a repeated determination of the MIC of the
patient's staphylococcus showed it to be sensitive to 1.25 units/ml
of penicillin and 1.56 ug/ml of methicillin. Serum Schlicters then
performed are shown in Table 7-2.

TABLE 7-2: SERUM SCHLICTERS		
	SERUM DILUTION	
	Bacteriostatic level	Bactericidal level
Immediately Prior to The Dose of Nafcillin	1:64	1:31
1 hr. After The Dose of Nafcillin	1:128	1:64

Fever continued and no new source of infection could be identified.
Laboratory reports now show an abnormal NBT test. The patient is
further evaluated.

QUESTION:

4. Which studies would confirm the diagnosis of chronic granulom-
   atous disease?
   A. Abnormal bacterial killing curves with patient's white blood
      cells
   B. Absence of increased oxygen consumption during in vitro
      phagocytosis
   C. Decreased hydrogen peroxide generation with phagocytosis
   D. Absence of chemiluminescence with phagocytosis
   E. All of the above

Fever and exudation from the drains continued. The patient underwent a second surgical procedure and further incision and drainage
of multiple liver abscesses was accomplished. The fever persisted
after his second operation and his condition deteriorated. Gentamicin
therapy was added for one week and during that week white blood cell
transfusions from a chronic myelogenous leukemic patient were administered on 3 consecutive days. During the 6th hospital week the
patient defervesced and was discharged at the end of 2 months
hospitalization.

QUESTION:

5. Which of the following statements are correct?
   A. Chronic granulomatous disease occurs only in males
   B. The white blood cells are abnormal in appearance in chronic granulomatous disease
   C. Monocytes, macrophages and neutrophils have demonstrable deficits
   D. The defect in the white blood cells is an ability to release enzymes from lysosomes
   E. These patients do not have unusual difficulties with alpha hemolytic streptococci, Group A beta hemolytic streptococci and pneumococci
   F. Commonly observed sites of infection include the skin, lymph nodes, lung, liver, spleen, and urinary tract

ANSWERS:

1. (A, B, C, D)

The presentation of an illness consistent with bacterial infection in this youngster, who has a history of multiple previous episodes of staphylococcal disease, dictates the necessity for blood cultures and justifies the hypothesis that the abdominal mass may be an abscess which should be defined as quickly as possible. An IVP was negative and liver-spleen scan are next in importance to attempt to locate the mass accurately. A 9-year-old child with this history also requires evaluation for possible host deficits. On the basis of the type of previous infections, agammaglobulinemia and chronic granulomatous disease are first in priority. Defining the underlying disease is essential in decisions concerning therapy. The NBT test is based upon the ability of normal white blood cells to reduce nitrotetrazolium blue from yellow to blue after ingestion of the dye. Cells of CGD patients cannot reduce dye normally. The test is sensitive and reproducible. Errors occasionally occur and often are a result of failure to standardize the number of white blood cells in the test.

2. (A, C)

The initial evaluation includes blood culture and, since disease has been demonstrated to be present in the liver with large filling defects, drainage will be essential in therapy. Initiation of therapy with antimicrobial agents effective against beta lactamase producing staphylococci is appropriate. Any penicillinase resistant drug administered by intravenous route is acceptable and the physician may choose the one of this group of drugs with which he is familiar. Nafcillin is an acceptable choice but methicillin or oxacillin are equally appropriate. Pyogenic abscesses of the liver require drainage for optimal therapeutic results. At the time of surgery, the liver can be thoroughly examined and visualization of other viscera is also

possible. Needle aspiration may be first choice in those situations
with no visible filling defects but with identified chemical abnormalities of liver function or palpable hepatic enlargement.

3. (C)

The organism is sensitive to nafcillin but the levels of inhibitory
activity demonstrated in the serum are inadequate. The dosage of
drug was increased to 200 mg/kg/24 hours. The serum Schlicters
have provided information that indicates therapy is not optimal, although the organism is sensitive to the drug employed.

4. (E)

The reproducible deficit in CGD is an inability of the patient's WBC
to kill ingested bacteria normally. In association with this deficit
there is no oxidative burst of metabolism during phagocytosis. Glucose utilization and H_2O_2 production are simply measurements of
this failure to normally increase glycolytic metabolism with phagocytosis. During the process of phagocytosis, normal leukocytes emit
a burst of luminescence that can be quantitated in a liquid scintillation spectrometer. This elaboration of luminescence is largely dependent upon generation of O_2^- (singlet oxygen). CGD cells do not
chemiluminesce normally. The present concept of phagocytosis and
bacterial killing hypothesizes the presence of an enzyme (oxidase)
in the cell surface and thus in a position to catalyze subsequent electron transfer to oxygen. CGD describes a syndrome with imperfect
bactericidal function. More than one specific enzymatic deficit altering the usual biochemical sequence will probably be identified in
subsequent years to give the same end result.

5. (C, E, F)

Patients with CGD have been observed whose mode of inheritance is
autosomal recessive. In that form of disease both males and females
may be affected. The parents have no demonstrable WBC deficits.
In contrast, the x-linked form of disease can be detected in female
carriers. The mother of an affected child has two populations of
cells. One is normal and one abnormal, so that bacterial killing
studies show values which are intermediate to those of normal and
those with disease. All phagocytic cells in an affected person are
defective but do not appear abnormal in light microscopy. Although
there are conflicting reports in the literature it seems that these
cells do degranulate (release enzymes from lysosomes) normally.
Organisms causing infection in patients with CGD include staphylococci and Serratia which are both catalase $\oplus$ organisms. The defective WBC can kill organisms which are catalase negative, e. g.
pneumococcus and group A beta streptococci. H_2O_2 generated by
bacteria continues to be available and is essential for participation
in bacterial killing. Catalase destroys H_2O_2 generated by bacteria

and these organisms are not killed normally by CGD cells. All of
the sites mentioned are frequent areas of infection as bacteria gain
entry at the usual portals and subsequently are able to multiply within the defective WBC, resulting in local suppuration. The prolonged
and complicated course is typical of these patients who cannot eradicate infection normally. WBC transfusions have been employed but
too little data is available to assess their efficacy.

REFERENCES

1. Johnston, Richard B. , Jr. : Screening test for the diagnosis of
   chronic granulomatous disease. Pediatrics 43:122-124, 1969.

2. Ochs, Hans D. , Igo, Robert P. : The NBT slide test: A simple
   screening method for detecting chronic granulomatous disease
   and female carriers. J. Pediat. 83:77-82, 1973.

3. Samuels, L. D. : Liver scan in chronic granulomatous disease
   of childhood. Pediatrics 48:41-50, 1971.

4. Webb, Lawrence S. , et al. : Inhibition of phagocytosis-asso-
   ciated chemiluminescence by supraoxide dismutase. Inf. and
   Imm. 9:1051-1056, 1974.

5. Stossel, Thomas P. : Phagocytosis. NEJM 290:717-723, 773-
   780, 833-839, 1974.

6. Baehner, Robert L. : Molecular basis for functional disorders
   for phagocytes. J. Pediat. 84:317-327, 1974.

7. De La Maza, Luis M. , et al. : The changing etiology of liver
   abscess, further observations. JAMA 227:161-163, 1974.

8. Rubin, Robert H. , et al. : Hepatic abscess: Changes in clinical
   bacteriologic and therapeutic aspects. Am. J. Med. 57:601-
   610, 1974.

9. Behner, Louis P. , Kissane, John M. : Pyogenic hepatic abscesses in infancy and childhood. J. Pediat. 74:763-773, 1969.

10. O'Mara, Robert E. , McAsee, John G. : Scintillation scanning
    in the diagnosis of hepatic abscess in children. J. Pediat.
    77:211-215, 1970.

11. Pitts, Henry A. , Zuidema, George D. : Factors influencing
    mortality and the treatment of pyogenic hepatic abscess. Gynec.
    and Obstet. 140:228-234, 1975.

CASE 8: FEVER, RASH, CONVULSIONS, AND COMA

HISTORY: This two-year-old girl was brought to the hospital in
North Carolina in May with a fever and rash of approximately 10
days duration. The child had diffuse muscle tenderness and ampicillin therapy was initiated for 2 days prior to her referral. The rash
became purpuric within three days, and although it originated on her
extremities it evolved so as to include her trunk. The child had a
major motor seizure originating with movements of the right upper
extremity. No one else in the family was ill and no known contact
with toxins or communicable illness could be identified. The family
had not traveled and no history of tick bite was elicited.

PHYSICAL EXAMINATION: Temperature 40. 5 degrees C. Pulse
170. Respirations 25. Blood pressure 110/70. Weight 12. 4 kilos.
The child was a comatose two-year-old with decerebrate posturing.
There was no evidence of trauma. She was capable of withdrawing
to pinprick. The patient had normal reflexes. Her skin showed a
petechial rash over the entire body including the palms and soles.
There was some oozing of blood from a venapuncture site. Her chest
was clear and there was no abnormality noted of the abdomen.

LABORATORY DATA: Hematocrit 32%. WBC 16,400, 77 segs, 2
bands, 17 lymphs, 4 monos, fibrin split product 16 ug/ml. Fibrin-
ogen 58 mg %. Partial thromboplastin time, 200 sec/58 sec. control.
Prothrombin time, 23 sec/11 sec. control. BUN 14 mg%. Na, 125
meq. /L. Glucose, 185 mg%. Potassium 4. 0 meq. /L. Bicarbonate
263 M osm/kg. Urinary specific gravity of 1. 013. pH 5.0, 2+ protein, rare red cells, 5-8 WBC, many coarse and finely granular
casts. Hepatic Profile: LDH 843 IU (Normal 26-186) CPK 591 IU
(Normal 0-130). SGOT 363 IU. SGPT 111 IU. Isoenzyme analysis
showed combined skeletal muscle, pulmonary and hepatic involvement. CSF: Protein, 05 mg%. ; Glucose, 60 mg%; 278, WBC. ; 98 rbc.
(55% poly, 45% lymphs). Weil-Felix titers: Ox 19 1:20, 1:40, 1:80
sequentially during 1 month of illness.

QUESTIONS:

1. The most likely diagnosis is:
    A. Meningococcemia
    B. Rocky Mountain spotted fever
    C. Mycoplasma pneumoniae
    D. Atypical measles
    E. Henoch-Schonlein purpura

2. Additional epidemiological information of potential value in-
   cludes:
   A. Exposure to ticks
   B. The state of residence
   C. Family resident on an army base
   D. Similar disease in the family
   E. Contact with dogs

3. Appropriate antimicrobial therapy would be:
   A. Penicillin
   B. Ampicillin
   C. Chloramphenicol
   D. Tetracycline
   E. Sulfonamides

4. The problems of management and the complications of this ill-
   ness include:
   A. Disseminated intravascular coagulation
   B. Hyponatremia
   C. Central nervous system symptoms
   D. Hematuria
   E. Azotemia
   F. Hepatic dysfunction

5. Supportive therapy most often requires which of the following?
   A. Normal saline
   B. Whole blood
   C. Plasma
   D. Albumin
   E. Heparin
   F. Steroids

6. Available serological means of diagnosis of this infection include
   which of the following?
   A. Widal agglutination
   B. The Weil-Felix agglutination
   C. Specific complement fixation reaction
   D. Microimmunofluorescence
   E. Passive hemagglutination

ANSWERS:

1. (B)

The presence of fever, a rash which becomes petechial, hyponatremia, and thrombocytopenia occurring in a small child in the summer
time in endemic areas should describe clearly the illness of Rocky
Mountain spotted fever. This disease is seen primarily in the southeastern United States and occurs in individuals exposed to infected
ticks. These patients almost invariably have fever and some malaise

which precedes the appearance of their typical eruption. Individuals who are old enough to describe headache will indicate this symptom as a prominent part of their illness. The appearance of the rash is quite characteristic and with some experience can usually be distinguished from that seen with meningococcal infection. There is usually a mixture of erythematous macules and petechiae. The rash involves the palms and soles. There may be characteristic periorbital edema and ankle edema of these patients. Myalgias are also a prominent characteristic of the disease.

2. (A, B, E)

Approximately one-half of all patients with Rocky Mountain spotted fever have a history of exposure to ticks or a documented tick bite. In the United States there are four indigenous species of Ixodid (hard) ticks related to the epidemiology of RMSF: Rocky Mountain wood tick (Dermacentor andersoni), American dog tick (D. variabilis), Lone Star tick (Amblyomma americanum) and the rabbit tick (Haemaphysalis leporuspalustris). Depending upon the weather and the environmental conditions, ticks become active and seek meals from available hosts. Rocky Mountain spotted fever has been identified in every month of the year in endemic areas, although it is usually far more common from May through August. The ticks need to feed before the rickettsiae are activated. Therefore, removal of attached ticks prior to engorgement is a reasonable preventive measure. Hosts of D. variabilis are primarily domesticated animals, including the dog, and thus infestation may be greater around areas of habitation. Persons removing ticks from dogs should use forceps to handle the ticks as these engorged ticks contain rickettsia in their gastrointestinal tracts and excrete the organisms in their salivary secretions and feces. Handling infected ticks may transmit rickettsiae to the skin of an additional person.

3. (C or D)

Both of these drugs are effective against the rickettsial organism, and chloramphenicol is effective against the majority of meningococcal strains. Early therapy with these drugs appears to alter the course of the infection. Severe rickettsial disease may produce measurable alterations in renal function and it may then be difficult to control the serum levels of tetracycline. None of the penicillins are effective against Rickettsia. Sulfonamides have been reported to exacerbate the severity of the illness.

4. (A-F)

The pathophysiology of rickettsial infection involves multiplication of the rickettsial organisms in endothelial cells lining small blood vessels. There is diffuse vascular damage throughout every tissue. The cutaneous rash, hepatomegaly and chemical alteration in liver

enzymes, azotemia and hematuria are evidence of involvement of
the skin, liver and kidneys respectively. The hyponatremia is a
commonly observed feature of this infection and probably represents
the results of a number of contributory factors. Vascular perme-
ability is greatly altered and the intravascular fluid and salt leak
into the extravascular space. This results in the visible peripheral
edema observed in many patients. In addition, it has been suggested
from observations on several patients that inappropriate ADH secretion contributes to the hyponatremia. Urinary sodiums have been
measured and found to be high. The diffuse endothelial damage of
small blood vessels may result in accumulation of fibrin and play
a role in initiation of intravascular coagulation. The central nervous
system effects of this infection vary from minimal involvement to
coma. The findings are more frequently of a diffuse nature and suggest encephalitis to the clinician. The cerebrospinal fluid may be
abnormal in at least one-fourth of the children with an elevation in
protein and pleocytosis. This,too, reflects involvement of multiple
small vessels and cerebral edema.

5. (B, C, D)

Supportive therapy is dictated by the severity of the illness. It is
frequently necessary to administer colloid of some type whether it
is albumin, plasma, or blood in an attempt to expand the intravascular volume. In addition to this, fluid maintenance can be accomplished with sodium containing fluids. Normal saline is not often
appropriate since the hyponatremia is not usually due to total body
losses of sodium. There are no studies to indicate that steroids
alter the course of disease but they have been utilized when cerebral edema appears to be a prominent part of the picture. In addition to treating the acute infection with appropriate antimicrobial
agents and supportive therapy, heparin has been utilized in the
therapy of disseminated intravascular coagulation. This is not done
routinely and is decided at the discretion of the responsible physician when the assessment for disseminated intravascular coagulation
is completed.

6. (B, C, D, E)

The Weil-Felix reaction or proteus agglutinations are utilized as
a practical means of approaching the diagnosis of RMSF. The rickettsial organism Rickettsia rickettsiae stimulates production of antibodies which are cross reactive with the capsular polysaccharides
of Proteus vulgaris. The proteus OX2 and OX19 strains are often
used as antigens for an agglutination test. The test is not specific
for R. rickettsiae of Rocky Mountain spotted fever and occasionally
remains negative in patients having this disease. It remains the
most readily available laboratory test for diagnosis. Specific complement fixation antibody tests are available from state laboratories
and research institutions. These antibodies appear at approximately
10 days to 2 weeks after the onset of symptoms and are a specific

means of diagnosis of infection. Research laboratories have developed immunofluorescent antibody and passive hemagglutination assays which appear to correlate well with the complement fixation antibody studies.

REFERENCES

1. Sexton, Daniel J.: Zinsser's Microbiology. 16th edition. Chapter 57, Rickettsiae. (In press)

2. Haynes, Ralph E., et al.: Rocky Mountain spotted fever in children. J. Pediat. 76:685-693, 1970.

3. Vianna, Nicholas J., Hinman, Alan R.: Rocky Mountain spotted fever on Long Island. Epidemiologic and clinical aspects. Am. J. Med. 51:725-730, 1971.

4. Hazard, Gerald W., et al.: Rocky Mountain spotted fever in the eastern United States. Thirteen cases from the Cape Cod area of Massachusetts. NEJM 280:57-62, 1969.

5. Rubeo, Tom, et al.: Thrombocytopenia in Rocky Mountain spotted fever. Am. J. Dis. Child. 116:88-96, 1968.

6. Sexton, Daniel J., et al.: Late appearance of skin rash and abnormal serum enzymes in Rocky Mountain spotted fever: A Case Report. J. Pediat. 87:580-582, 1975.

7. Dupon, H. L., et al.: Evaluation of chloramphenicol acid succinate therapy of induced typhoid fever and Rocky Mountain spotted fever. NEJM 282:53-58, 1970.

::

CASE 9: SWOLLEN, PAINFUL LEFT KNEE

HISTORY: This was the first hospital admission for a 5-month-old, white male infant admitted because of painful, swollen left knee. The patient developed fever, cough, and congestion one month prior to admission. He received penicillin therapy and did well with resolution of symptoms until 10 days prior to admission. At that time he developed fever of 38-40 degrees C, and received aspirin therapy. Eight days prior to admission the mother noted his swollen left knee which was tender to touch and painful when moved. The physician treated the patient with penicillin and noted some reduction in fever. Three days prior to admission the temperature again rose to 40 degrees C and the patient had shaking chills. One day prior to admission the mother noted swelling of the right upper arm and shoulder and discomfort associated with motion of the right upper extremity. There was no history of trauma or cutaneous infection.

The patient has 2 siblings, a sister age 4 and a brother age 3 who are well.

PHYSICAL EXAMINATION: Temperature 40 degrees C. Pulse 160. Respirations 55. Height 67 cm. Weight 8. 2 kilo. The physical examination was remarkable because of the irritability of the child and the dramatic findings in his extremities. The right elbow was enlarged and tender with restriction of flexion and rotation. The left knee was extremely tender, swollen and the tissues were indurated and warm. The patient refused to move this extremity. There were no cutaneous pustules, impetigo, ecchymoses or abrasions.

LABORATORY FINDINGS: Hematocrit, 30%. WBC. 29,000 with 80% segs, 17% lymphocytes, 3% monocytes. X-ray examination showed soft tissue swelling of both elbows and the left knee. Aspiration of the left knee was easily accomplished and viscous, purulent green fluid was obtained. Gram stain revealed polymorphonuclear leukocytes and small gram-negative rods.

QUESTIONS:

1. The differential diagnosis of arthritis in this child includes:
    A. Pyogenic arthritis due to Hemophilus influenzae B, Staphylococcus aureus, Streptococcus pneumoniae, Streptococcus agalactiae, and N. gonorrhea
    B. Tuberculosis
    C. Syphilis
    D. Trauma
    E. Hemarthrosis
    F. All of the above

2. The commonest etiologic agent observed in pyarthrosis in an infant 6 months to 2 years of age is:
    A. Staphylococcus aureus
    B. Streptococcus pneumoniae
    C. Hemophilus influenzae B
    D. Streptococcus algalactiae
    E. Neisseria gonorrhoeae

3. Culture of the joint fluid by the microbiology laboratory should include inoculation into:
    A. Supplemented thioglycolate broth cultures
    B. Chocolate blood agar in 5-6% CO_2 atmosphere
    C. MacConkey's agar or eosin-methylene blue (EMB)
    D. Bordet-Gengou agar
    E. Blood agar

4. Rapid laboratory diagnosis of the etiologic agent might be accomplished by antigen detection employing:
    A. Countercurrent-immunoelectrophoresis (CIE) of urine
    B. CIE of blood
    C. CIE of synovial fluid
    D. All of the above

5. Initial antimicrobial therapy for pyarthrosis in this 5-month-old child would be:
    A. Ampicillin
    B. Sulfonamide
    C. Penicillin
    D. Chloramphenicol
    E. Trimethoprim-sulfamethoxazole

6. Appropriate antimicrobial therapy eliminates the need for surgical drainage of the involved joint.
    A. True
    B. False

7. Pyarthrosis is frequently a result of osteomyelitis in infants less than one year of age, therefore:
    A. All patients require 4 weeks of parenteral antimicrobial therapy
    B. Evaluation by x-ray should be repeated of the involved joint and adjacent bones after the first week of therapy to look for detectable lesions of the bones
    C. Finding H. influenzae B as etiologic agent is helpful because this bacterium involves bone only in very rare situations

ANSWERS:

1. (F)

The febrile course of this patient and the acute onset of illness probably mitigate against both tuberculosis and syphilis. The administration of antibiotic therapy can alter and partially obscure symptoms of pyogenic infection if the organism is at all sensitive to the antimicrobial agents employed. A five-month-old infant would probably have syphilis acquired during gestation or delivery. It is usually manifest before this age but it is possible the more subtle manifestations of infection could have been missed by the mother/physician. Laboratory evaluation, that is, serological tests, is easy to perform and a decision can be made after examination of the joint fluid. Acquired tuberculosis certainly occurs in this age group as these infants cannot well control dissemination of this infection. Because of this, systemic manifestations of illness are usually detectable, i. e. , failure to grow appropriately and/or loss of weight. In addition, pulmonary disease and possibly central nervous system disease will be apparent at the time of dissemination of infection to an extremity

with evidence of clinical disease. Application of IPPD and a careful
history are indicated at the time of admission. Certainly trauma
must be considered, but in a five-month-old infant it is usually possible to identify the incident since they are not ambulatory. The infant may have sustained a fall or conceivably suffered as a result of
parentally inflicted trauma. Hemophilia may present with hemarthro-
sis, more often at the time of ambulation. Again aspiration of the
joint should allow this diagnosis to be made promptly. By far the
most urgent and commonest consideration is that of pyogenic infection. This possibility obligates the responsive physician to perform
needle aspiration of the afflicted joint and the subsequent therapy
will be determined by his findings.

2. (C)

In one series of patients evaluated at the University of Texas Southwestern Medical Center, 33 patients with Hemophilus influenzae type
B were identified at the same time that 6 patients with Staphylococcus aureus and 6 patients with streptococci (group A Streptococcus
pyogenes and group B Streptococcus agalactiae) were identified. N.
gonorrhea can be seen in septic arthritis in sporadic cases, especially in the newborn period. Other reports substantiate the finding
of Hemophilus influenzae type B as being the commonest etiologic
agent in this age group. The Gram stain of the joint fluid showing
small gram-negative rods occurring in a child this age can be assumed to be Hemophilus influenzae group B and appropriate therapy
initiated. Further questions will discuss other additional confirmation of the diagnosis.

3. (A, B, C, E)

Laboratories may differ in their choice of media to be used but those
outlined here are readily available. Blood agar is a general medium
for the growth and isolation of most pathogenic bacteria and some
yeast. It helps to define hemolytic properties of bacteria. Since
sheep blood contains a heat labile factor that inhibits Hemophilus
species, laboratories using this medium must also use chocolate
agar. Chocolate agar promotes the growth of fastidious organisms
especially those of the Neisseriaceae or Hemophilus species and incubation in 5-10% CO_2 will optimize growth. Chocolate agar is blood
agar, sometimes with added nutrients, that has been heated to the
point at which hemin is released in the red blood cells. This action
destroys the heat labile factors that may inhibit growth and make
certain nutrients more accessible to fastidious organisms. Thioglycolate broth is the general medium for the growth of most bacteria,
some yeasts, and fungi. In addition, it enhances the growth of obligate anaerobes. It is useful since the nutrients contained will support
the growth of many pathogens while thioglycolic acid produces a low
EH (oxidation-reduction potential) and a trace of agar reduces elec-
trical currents. This latter helps maintain reduced oxygen tension
and this aids the growth of obligate anerobes. MacConkey's agar or

EMB is a differential and selective medium for enteric and other hardy gram-negative bacteria. These organisms are all seen primarily in the newborn period. The growth of gram-positive organisms is inhibited while protein nutrients provide further growth of the Enterobacteriaceae, Pseudomonas sp. and other hardy gram-negative organisms. The organisms which utilize lactose will appear red, thereby separating the lactose negative colonies which are colorless from the lactose positive colonies which are red. Such selective medium can expedite identification of pathogen, although these organisms also grow on BA.

4. (D)

Countercurrent-immunoelectrophoresis utilizes a commercially available specific antiserum raised to the capsular substance of Hemophilus influenzae type B, that is, polyribose phosphate. This antiserum will form a visible precipitate with the capsular antigen of the bacteria. The use of electric current allows detection of very small quantities of polyribose phosphate by assisting in concentration of this material. The detection of antigen in joint fluid has the greatest significance for the patient with pyarthrosis, but antigen may also be detected in serum and/or urine. The advantage of this procedure is that the diagnosis can specifically be made in a matter of hours. The test itself is usually accomplished within 30 minutes.

5. (D or E)

Some strains of Hemophilus influenzae type B organisms are well documented to be resistant to ampicillin. These organisms produce a beta lactamase which is capable of destroying the antibiotic. For this reason, systemic infections due to Hemophilus influenzae type B organisms should be treated with chloramphenicol until the antimicrobial sensitivity testing of the organism is completed. These hemophilus organisms are also sensitive to trimethoprim-sulfamethoxazole, and although this combination of drugs is presently available only on an investigational basis it will probably prove to be a practical alternative form of therapy for many Hemophilus influenzae B infections.

6. (B)

Pyarthroses may require drainage. The pyarthroses due to N. gonococcus may require only a single needle aspiration at the time of diagnosis. These organisms are not very destructive to the articulating cartilage and the infection is rapidly treated with systemic penicillin therapy. On the other hand, organisms which are rapidly destructive of articulating cartilage include the S. aureus, the S. pneumoniae and a variety of gram-negative organisms. The patient management depends upon the findings at the time of aspiration, the duration of infection, and the response to therapy. All patients require at least one needle aspiration of the joint for diagnosis. The patient presented in this case required open drainage of all of his involved joints. The infection was established in the soft tissues adjacent to the joint and this type of drainage was essential in his management. The aim of drainage is to prevent destruction of the articulating cartilage as once this occurs regeneration is impossible. Other infections may require only repeated needle aspiration of the joint space.

7. (B, C)

Osteomyelitis in infants of this group may extend through the epiphyseal plate because of blood vessels which penetrate from the diaphysis to the epiphysis. Therefore, extension of the infection frequently perforates the epiphysis and involves the joint space in infants in this age group. If this has occurred, changes in the bone are usually apparent or become apparent as calcium is absorbed from the bone over the subsequent ten to fourteen days. For this reason evaluation of septic arthritis should include x-rays of contiguous bones evaluating for destructive lesions during the course of therapy. It is true, however, that Hemophilus influenzae only rarely involves the bone, and this allows the physician to concentrate on the therapy of the joint space. Other organisms such as Staphylococcus aureus frequently involve the bone, and it may be difficult to distinguish primary pyarthrosis from that which is secondary to osteomyelitis. Parenteral antimicrobial therapy of infected joints usually is given for a period of one week after the last fever, and the total duration of therapy is for 2-3 weeks. In this interval of time, if the patient has responded well to therapy, it is possible to evaluate for the presence of osteomyelitis. The presence of osteomyelitis usually obligates the physician to a course of therapy not shorter than four weeks and often for a period of six weeks. This is based on empirical observations that eradication of hematogenous osteomyelitis without relapse occurs more reproducibly with therapy administered for this period.

REFERENCES

1. Pittard, William B. , et al.: Neonatal septic arthritis: J. Pediat. 88:621-624, 1976.

2. Nelson, John D. , Koontz, Wayne C.: Septic arthritis in infants and children: A review of 117 cases. Pediatrics 38:966-971, 1966.

3. Nelson, John D.: Bacterial etiology and antibiotic management of septic arthritis in infants and children. Pediatrics 50:437-440, 1972.

4. Hutto, John H. , Ayoub, Eliam: Streptococcal osteomyelitis and arthritis in a neonate. Am. J. Dis. Child. 129:1449-1451, 1975.

5. Nelson, John D.: Antibiotic concentrations in septic joint effusions. NEJM 284:349-353, 1971.

6. Granoff, Dan M., Nankervis, George A.: Infectious arthritis in the neonate caused by Hemophilus influenzae. Am. J. Dis. Child. 129:730-733, 1975.

7. Khan, W., et al.: Hemophilus influenzae type B resistant to ampicillin: A report of two cases. JAMA 429:298-301, 1974.

8. Tomeh, M. Ousama, et al.: Ampicillin resistant Hemophilus influenzae type B infection. JAMA 229:295-297, 1974.

9. McGowan, John E., et al.: Susceptibility to Hemophilus influenzae isolates from blood and cerebral spinal fluid to ampicillin, chloramphenicol, and trimethoprim-sulfamethoxazole. Antimic. Agts. & Chemoth. 9:137-139, 1976.

::

CASE 10: CHICKENPOX WITH NECROTIC SKIN LESIONS

HISTORY: An 18-month-old, Indian boy was in good health until 5 days prior to admission when varicella lesions appeared on his trunk and spread to his extremities. Two brothers had just recovered from chickenpox. Three days before admission his mother had noticed a tender, red area on the left anterior thigh. His temperature rose to 39.5°C, and he became anorectic and lethargic. On the day before admission he was seen in an emergency room and given an intramuscular injection of penicillin for "infected varicella". On the following day, he was referred to a university medical center because of the induration and dusky blue color of the left thigh.

PHYSICAL EXAMINATION: Admission examination showed an 18-month-old boy who was alert and in no acute distress. Temperature was 38.0°C, pulse 135/min, respirations 45/min, height 83 cm., weight 19 kg. Crusted varicella lesions were distributed over the face and scalp and trunk. A 3 x 7 cm. area of necrotic tissue with a raised blue center and flat erythematous border was present on the left anterior thigh. Several 1 x 1 cm. femoral and inguinal nodes were present bilaterally. The circumference of the thigh 8 inches superior to the knee was 3 inches larger on the left than the right. A "strawberry tongue" was present.

LABORATORY VALUES: Hemoglobin, 13.3 grams%. Hematocrit, 40%. WBC. 38,400 with 85% neutrophils, 14% lymphocytes and 1% monocytes. Platelets, 312,500/cu. mm. Urinalysis was normal.

QUESTIONS:

1. The differential diagnosis of the necrotic skin lesions includes:
   A. Purpura fulminans
   B. Erysipelas
   C. Thrombocytopenic purpura
   D. Streptococcal gangrene

2. Additional diagnostic procedures should include:
   A. Gram stain and culture of the necrotic area
   B. Antiplatelet antibodies
   C. Prothrombin Time, Partial Thromboplastin Time, Fibrin Split Products
   D. ASO titer
   E. Blood culture

A Gram stain smear of the necrotic lesion showed gram-positive cocci. Cultures were obtained from the blood, wound, and throat, and nafcillin therapy 200 mg/kg/day was initiated by the intravenous route. Culture results showed group A beta hemolytic streptococci and alpha streptococci present in the wound. The blood culture was sterile. By the end of the first hospital day, a 3 cm. bulla formed in the center of the lesions which ruptured shortly afterwards draining seropurulent material. By the third hospital day the necrotic center had expanded to 6 cm. in diameter.

QUESTION:

3. Continued progression of the lesion on the left indicates that his present therapy should be re-evaluated. Which of the following decisions should be made?
   A. Change nafcillin therapy to clindamycin
   B. Change nafcillin therapy to kanamycin and ampicillin
   C. Continue watching the patient and institute no change in antimicrobial therapy
   D. Surgical debridement
   E. Change nafcillin to penicillin G

Cultures obtained at the time of surgery grew many colonies of group A beta hemolytic streptococci and a few colonies of Staphylococcus epidermidis, Candida sp. Escherichia coli and an anaerobic gram-positive cocci. The pathological analysis showed coagulation necrosis of the skin and subcutaneous adipose tissue with organized thrombosis of the subcutaneous vessels. Bacterial stains showed gram-positive cocci within the adventitia of the thrombosed vessels of the fibrous septae of adipose tissue.

QUESTION:

4. The presence of group A beta hemolytic streptococci in the tissues at the time of surgery indicates:

A. Resistance of the organisms to nafcillin therapy
B. That the organisms are not responsible for this infection
C. Antimicrobial therapy is frequently ineffective in devitalized
   tissue where the agent cannot reach the tissues

5. The cutaneous complications of varicella include:
   A. Abscess formation
   B. Lymphadenitis
   C. Cellulitis
   D. Erysipelas
   E. Gangrene

ANSWERS:

1. (A, D)

It is important to recognize group A beta hemolytic streptococcal
gangrene since other complications of varicella which may be similar in appearance warrant alternative therapy. The clinical picture
of streptococcal gangrene should allow differentiation from other
superficial complications of varicella. [2,3] Purpura fulminans is a
rapidly progressive condition that may also occur during the first
week of varicella exanthem. It usually starts as an ecchymotic area
on an extremity and is followed by other similar lesions on the same
or opposite limb. A frank hemorrhagic appearance ensues, causing
tenderness and swelling of the involved region. Bleeding of the mucous membranes and gastrointestinal or genitourinary tract may
occur. Laboratory studies may show thrombocytopenia, elevation
of fibrin split products and other parameters of disseminated intravascular coagulation. The color of streptococcal gangrene, with its
initial erythema which changes into dusky-blue on the second or
third day with no bleeding from other sites, differentiates it from
purpura fulminans. Bullae form and contain brown seropurulent
fluid. [12] Erysipelas has a raised border while the raised central
erythema of the streptococcal gangrene blends with the normal adjacent skin. Streptococcal cellulitis has a similar initial appearance
to early gangrene but fails to complete the characteristic progression. Thrombocytopenic purpura associated with varicella also characteristically occurs near the end of the period of time when the
exanthem is seen. This circumstance is unusual and the thrombocytopenia makes the evolution of many vesicular lesions into hemorrhagic lesions a diffuse process.

2. (A, D, E)

The procedure of most importance is that of the Gram stain and culture of the necrotic area. Visualization of gram-positive organisms
confirms the clinical impression of group A beta hemolytic streptococcal gangrene. Staphylococcus aureus may occasionally cause a clinical syndrome indistinguishable from streptococcal gangrene. [14,17]

If the Gram stain of the subcutaneous tissue aspirate reveals gram-positive cocci, it is suggested that parenteral therapy with penicillinase resistant penicillin in high doses be initiated. If group A beta hemolytic streptococci are reovered, then penicillin G is substituted as the drug of choice. The blood culture may be positive and further document the causative organism. An elevation of the ASO titer may also be supportive evidence of group A beta hemolytic streptococcal infection.

3. (D, E)

Surgical excision of the necrotic tissue down to the deep fascia remains the mainstay of therapy. [18] The only effective means of removing this involved tissue which serves as an excellent bacterial culture medium is by surgical extirpation. This also relieves congestion and edema of the surrounding area and assures better antibiotic penetration. As stated in answers #2 and 4, penicillin is optimal therapy for group A streptococcal infection and should be substituted for nafcillin.

4. (C)

Group A beta hemolytic streptococci remain uniformly sensitive to very small quantities of penicillin. The MIC of these organisms averages . 005 ug/ml against penicillin G and . 04 ug/ml to nafcillin. Parenteral administration of penicillinase resistant penicillins readily achieves adequate serum levels for therapy of group A beta hemolytic streptococcal infections, although the minimal inhibitory concentrations of semi-synthetic penicillins are somewhat higher. In contrast to this, occasional group A streptococcal strains which are resistant to antimicrobial agents such as erythromycin, clindamycin, and tetracycline have been reported. The failure to eradicate group A beta hemolytic streptococci from necrotic tissue is due to the inadequate vascularization and failure to penetration of the antimicrobials into the area of devitalized tissue.

5. (A-E)

Reports [1] indicate that any of these complications of group A beta streptococcal infections may occur. Abscesses, lymphadenitis and cellulitis are observed more frequently than erysipelas or gangrene. Careful hygiene of the child at the time of varicella is a useful means of trying to prevent superinfection of cutaneous lesions.

REFERENCES

1. Bullowa, J. G. M. , Wistrik, S. M.: Complications of varicella. Am. J. Dis. Child 49:923, 1935.

2. Stokes, W.: An eruptive disease of children. Dublin Med. Phys. Essays 1:146, 1807.

3. Hutchinson, J.: On gangrenous eruptions in connection with vaccination and chickenpox. Med. Chir. Trans. 65:1, 1882.

4. Barenberg, L. H., Lewis, J. M.: Gangrenous varicella. Arch. Pediat. 44:653, 1927.

5. Illinworth, R. S., Zachary, R. B.: Superficial gangrene of the skin in chickenpox. Arch. Dis. Child. 30:177, 1955.

6. Kieffer, C. F.: Varicella gangrenosa with report of a case. N Y Med. J. 82:1, 1905.

7. Leray, M.: Contributions a l'etude de la varicelle dite gangreneuse. Paris Theses, No. 139, 1922.

8. Joe, A.: A case of gangrenous chickenpox due to B. diphtheriae. Brit. J. Child. Dis. 25:112, 1928.

9. Banks, H. S., McCartney, J. E.: Varicella gangrenosa due to Streptococcus pyogenes. Lancet II:311, 1937.

10. Batch, J. W., Sepkowitz, S.: Varicella complicated by gangrene of the lower extremities. U. S. Armed Forces Med. J. 3:759, 1952.

11. Storrie, H. C.: Hemorrhagic and gangrenous varicella, with notes of two cases. Brit. J. Child. Dis. 11:62, 1914.

12. Meleney, F. L.: Hemolytic streptococcus gangrene. Arch. Surg. 9:317, 1924.

13. Wilson, B.: Necrotizing fasciitis. Am. Surg. 18:416, 1952.

14. Rea, W. J., Wyrick, W. J.: Necrotizing fasciitis. Ann. Surg. 172:957, 1970.

15. Paine, T. F., et al.: Fatal gangrene caused by Streptococcus pyogenes. Arch. Intern. Med. 112:936, 1963.

16. Collins, R. H., Nadel, M. S.: Gangrene due to hemolytic streptococcus: A rare but treatable disease. NEJM 272:578, 1965.

17. Weinberger, M., et al.: Necrotizing fasciitis in a neonate. Am. J. Dis. Child. 123:591, 1972.

18. Smith, Edward W. P., et al.: Varicella gangrenosa due to group A B-hemolytic streptococcus. Pediatrics 57:306-319, 1976.

CASE 11: VIRAL MENINGITIS IN A 5-MONTH-OLD INFANT

HISTORY: This was a first hospital admission for a 5-month-old, black male infant in good health until the day of admission (June 24) when he became increasingly irritable and vomited all feedings. Although the temperature was not taken, his mother felt that the child had a fever. There was no evidence of upper respiratory tract infection, diarrhea, or rash. One sibling was ill with a headache for one day but other symptoms, including fever and stiff neck, were not observed by the mother. No known tuberculosis was present in the family and no mumps infections were identified.

PHYSICAL EXAMINATION: Pulse 60. Respirations 20. Temperature 38. 5. Weight 9 kg. Head circumference 43 cm. He was a well-nourished, well-developed infant in no acute distress. There were no petechiae or rashes apparent. The anterior fontanelle was open and soft. Tympanic membranes were normal and the neck was supple. The examination of the heart and lungs showed no abnormalities. The abdomen was soft but the liver was palpable 2 cm. below the right costal margin. Normal bowel sounds were present and the abdomen was not distended. The neurological examination, with the exception of irritability, was within normal limits.

ACCESSORY LABORATORY FINDINGS: Hemoglobin, 12. 9 grams. Hematocrit, 30%. WBC 11,700 with 52% neutrophils, 48% lymphocytes. Screening test for sickle cell hemoglobin was negative. The urinalysis was normal. BUN, serum electrolytes and blood sugar were within normal limits. Blood culture was obtained and subsequently reported as sterile for bacterial growth. A lumbar puncture was performed (pressure did not appear increased) and the cerebrospinal fluid contained 352 cells, 100% of which were lymphocytes. Gram stain was negative. Sugar was 90 mg% and the protein was 36 mg%.

QUESTION:

1. The presumptive diagnosis of meningitis was entertained and the etiologic possibilities should include:
   A. Listeria monocytogenes
   B. Mycobacterium tuberculosis
   C. Hemophilus influenzae group B
   D. S. pneumoniae
   E. Viruses (Echo, Coxsackie, mumps)

The bacterial cultures of the blood and cerebrospinal fluid was negative for bacterial pathogens. The cerebrospinal fluid, nasopharyngeal and rectal swabs were submitted for attempted viral isolation on the day of admission. The inoculated specimens of cerebrospinal fluid, nasopharyngeal and rectal swabs showed cytopathic effect consistent with an enterovirus within 2 days of inoculation of the tissue culture systems.

QUESTION:

2. Cytopathic effect of enteroviruses consists of:
   A. Intranuclear inclusions
   B. Cytoplasmic inclusions
   C. Rounding up and distortion of cells with a decrease in the cell number
   D. Multinucleate giant cells

The enterovirus was subsequently identified as echovirus type 18. This serotype is infrequently identified and the observed features of infection with this virus do not allow clinical separation from other serotypes of echovirus.

QUESTIONS:

3. The pathogenesis of echovirus infections of the central nervous system includes the following:
   A. Colonization of the gastrointestinal tract
   B. Ascending infection from a distal site along a peripheral nerve to the central nervous system
   C. Viremia
   D. Direct access from the nasopharynx to the central nervous system

4. The outcome of viral meningitis is:
   A. Always benign
   B. Occasionally fatal
   C. May cause subtle intellectual deficits at a later time in life
   D. Inadequately evaluated in large numbers of small infants

ANSWERS:

1. (B-E)

It would be unusual for a previously healthy 5-month-old infant to acquire Listeria infection. These organisms are more frequently implicated in the newborn period and in immunocompromised hosts. M. tuberculosis can cause this picture in an infant and this child is in the age group which disseminates disease. The history and physical examination give no hint of preceding illness and no tuberculosis by history. The child should be tested with intradermal antigen but consideration of possible pyogenic disease is more urgent at the time of admission. H. influenzae type B and S. pneumoniae are the commonest pathogens, and appropriate cultures, Gram stain, and countercurrent immunoelectrophoresis (where available) should define the presence of these organisms. He had received no preceding antimicrobial therapy. His illness occurred in June and is an aseptic meningitis. Enteroviruses (Echo-Cox-Polio) are the commonest causes of such illness. Enterovirus disease is more prevalent in summer and early fall. This child represented one of many similar patients identified from June through September with the same echovirus infection.

2. (B, C)

The cellular destruction is nonspecific, but the time course of growth and the type of tissue where cytopathic effect (CPE) is apparent are frequently useful clues in the identification of enteroviruses in cell culture. The CPE must be transmissable to additional cultures and occasionally cytoplasmic inclusions are seen. The in vivo effects of enteroviruses are equally nonspecific, with mononuclear inflammatory responses but no pathogenic features, except poliomyelitis where anterior horn cell destruction is strongly suggestive of poliovirus infection.

3. (A, C)

Enteroviruses are excreted for days to weeks from the upper G. I. tract and for weeks to months from the lower G. I. tract. Epidemiology suggests that fecal to oral transmission and colonization of the G. I. tract precedes viremia and subsequent replication of virus in other tissues, e. g. the CNS.

The direct route of infection along peripheral nerve appears to be established for rabies, and the possible access of herpes simplex from the nasopharynx via olfactory cells penetrating the cribriform plate directly to CNS has been suspected. The majority of enterovirus meningitis seems to be a result of viremia.

4. (B-D)

Viral meningitis in young infants does not result in the excessive morbidity and mortality of pyogenic meningitis. Fatalities have been documented and recorded infrequently. Several recent studies suggest that careful longitudinal evaluation of infants demonstrate subtle deficits in CNS function, but all too few babies with this disease have the virus confirmed and even fewer are followed sequentially to observe their subsequent growth and development. Viral meningitis is not always benign.

REFERENCES

1. Lepow, Martha L. , et al. : A clinical epidemiologic and laboratory investigation of aseptic meningitis during the four-year period, 1955-1958. I. Observations Concerning Etiology and Epidemiology. NEJM 266:1181, 1962.

2. Lepow, Martha L. , et al. : A clinical epidemiologic and laboratory investigation of aseptic meningitis during the four-year period, 1955-1958. II. The Clinical Disease and Its Sequelae. NEJM 266:1188, 1962.

3. Farmer, Keitha, et al.: A follow-up study of 15 cases of neo-
    natal meningoencephalitis due to Coxsackie virus B5. J. Pediat.
    87:568, 1975.

4. Rantakallio, Paula, et al.: Coxsackie B5 outbreak in a newborn
    nursery with 17 cases of serous meningitis. Scand. J. Infect.
    Dis. 2:17-23, 1970.

5. Rantakallio, Paula, et al.: Follow-up study of 17 cases of neo-
    natal Coxsackie B5 meningitis and one with suspected myocar-
    ditis. Scand. J. Infect. Dis. 2:25-28, 1970.

6. Nogen, Alan G., Lepow, Martha L.: Enteroviral meningitis
    in very young infants. Pediatrics 40:617-626, 1967.

7. Sanders, Doris Y., Cramblett, Henry G.: Viral infections in
    hospitalized neonates. Amer. J. Dis. Child. 116:268, 1968.

8. Miller, David G., et al.: An epidemic of aseptic meningitis
    primarily among infants, caused by echovirus 11-prime.
    Pediatrics 41:77, 1968.

9. Marier, Robert, et al.: Coxsackievirus B5 infection and asep-
    tic meningitis in neonates and children. Am. J. Dis. Child.
    129:321, 1975.

10. Sells, Clifford, et al.: Sequelae of central nervous system en-
    terovirus infection. NEJM 293:1, 1975.

11. Wilfert, Catherine M., et al.: An epidemic of echovirus 18
    meningitis. J. Infect. Dis. 131:75, 1975.

:::

CASE 12: HIRSCHSPRUNG'S DISEASE, MALNUTRITION AND
          BACTEREMIA ASSOCIATED WITH TPN

HISTORY: This infant was a 5-pound, 15-ounce product of a full-
term gestation. He was delivered to a 15-year-old Para O, Gravida
O, Abortus O mother. The child began vomiting within the first 24
hours of life, was discharged home from the nursery at age 5 days,
but vomiting necessitated readmission after only 24 hours at home.
During his hospitalization, vomiting and diarrhea persisted and the
infant failed to gain weight. At the age of six weeks he was transferred to a tertiary care hospital after intermittent intravenous
fluids, multiple formula changes and contrast examinations of the
gastrointestinal tract had failed to reveal the etiology of his problems. At the time of admission his malnutrition was apparent and
his weight was less than his birth weight. During his hospitalization,
a barium enema was done which showed a flaccid terminal segment

of the rectosigmoid colon. The diagnosis of Hirschsprung's disease was entertained and a biopsy was performed which showed an aganglionic segment of bowel.

PHYSICAL EXAMINATION: Pulse 160. Respirations 80. Temperature 37. Weight 5-pounds, 6 ounces. Height 51 cm. This was an extremely emaciated red-haired infant with a distended abdomen and wizened facies. He had a short, early Grade II/VI systolic murmur, his abdomen was distended with decreased bowel sounds, and his liver was palpable 2 cm. below the right costal margin. The striking features of his physical examination were related to the severe emaciation with his skin which hung in folds from his body, and a maculo-papular rash over the face.

ACCESSORY LABORATORY INFORMATION: Hemoglobin 9. 9 grams, hematocrit 30%, white count 9,500/mm^3, neutrophils 57%, lymphocytes 21%, monocytes 1%, stabs 21%, and toxic granulation was described. Two nucleated red cells were seen/100 white cells and the platelet count was 65,000/mm^3. Erythrocyte sedimentation rate was 32 mm/hr. Urinalysis showed yellow, clear urine with a pH of 7. 5, and calcium oxylate crystals and positive ketone bodies. BUN, 15 mg/100 ml.; Sodium, 130 meq./L.; Potassium, 4. 3 meq./L.; Chloride, 106 meq./L.; CO_2, 20 mm/L.; Total Protein, 3. 3 gm/100 ml.; Albumin, 0. 6 gm./100 ml.; Calcium, 7. 6 mg./100 ml.; Phosphorous, 5. 3 mg/100 ml.; Bilirubin, 1. 0 mg./100 ml.

COURSE IN HOSPITAL: Malnutrition constituted his primary problem and the patient continued to have significant diarrhea and vomiting. Three days after admission a hyperalimentation catheter was inserted through the anterior branch of the facial vein into the internal jugular vein and into the right atrium. The catheter was burrowed through a subcutaneous tunnel for a distance of several cm. after its exit from the vein. Total peripheral nutrition was initiated and the infant did very well for the subsequent two weeks. At that time a perirectal abscess was observed. Incision and drainage was performed and Klebsiella sp, Proteus morganii and enterococci were identified by culture in the exudate. One day later the patient suddenly became pale, cyanotic and obtunded. It was apparent he was in shock with poor peripheral perfusion. Respirations increased to 70/min, the temperature varied between 36 and 37. 2 degrees, periods of tachycardia with a pulse rate of 200 to 240 were recorded, and systolic blood pressure was 35. Penicillin and gentamicin therapy was initiated. Cultures of the blood, CSF and Amigen hyperalimentation fluid were obtained. The perfusion set was changed. Within 24 hours the infant's status had stabilized. All of the preceding cultures grew Klebsiella sp sensitive to kanamycin, gentamicin, cephalosporin, carbenecillin and chloramphenicol. Blood cultures obtained over the subsequent two days continued to be positive for Klebsiella organisms. Four days after the episode of shock the hyperalimentation line was removed. After removal of the catheter, the patient's condition continued to stabilize, blood cultures were negative and another hyperalimentation line was inserted.

QUESTIONS:

1. Hyperalimentation fluid must contain a nitrogen source with essential and nonessential amino acids and sufficient non-protein calories to meet full caloric expenditure in the form of glucose or glucose plus fructose. The total osmolarity is about 1,700 mOsm/kg of water requiring continuous infusion. This hypertonic and acidic solution provides a growth medium which may be somewhat selective. Indicate which of the following statements are true:
    A. Candida albicans is capable of proliferating in D5W + protein hydrolyseate at 30^0 and 37^0
    B. If protein hydrolysate is contained in the solution, Candida sp can increase as rapidly as one log per 12 hours and three logs per 24 hours at room temperature
    C. E. coli, Seratia sp, Proteus sp and Enterobacter sp grow more slowly than Candida sp in hyperalimentation fluid with protein hydrodysate
    D. Candida sp proliferate less rapidly if the TPN solution is prepared with synthetic amino acid solution (freamine) and bacterial pathogens also show minimal growth

2. The following routes have proven useful for total peripheral alimentation:
    A. Peripheral scalp vein needles changed frequently
    B. Percutaneous insertion of a subclavian line as an operative procedure
    C. Venous cut down with tunneling of the external exit of the catheter and insertion of the catheter through the internal jugular vein into the right atrium
    D. Placement of the catheter without subcutaneous tunneling into internal jugular vein
    E. Placement of a catheter in the femoral vein

3. Appropriate care of the TPN line includes:
    A. Meticulous antisepsis of the skin with 2% iodine and 70% alcohol (or an iodofor) drying for 30 sec. and washing off with 70% alcohol
    B. Securing the cannula and regular inspection of the insertion site
    C. Careful recording of the date and time of insertion
    D. Mixing of all TPN components and additives by a trained member of the hospital staff using strict aseptic technique
    E. The TPN system should not be used to measure central venous pressure, administer blood products, other medications, or to obtain blood samples

4. Persistent bacteremia in this patient indicates that:
   A. The antimicrobial agents are ineffective against this organism and should be changed
   B. The dosage of antimicrobial agents should be increased
   C. The probability of an intravascular focus of infection, ie. the hyperalimentation line
   D. The need for prompt exploratory surgery with plans for a diverting colostomy

5. The bacterial contamination of the Amigen is:
   A. Of no importance because in-line filters protect patients
   B. Represents retrograde colonization from the infant
   C. Is probably the original source of his sepsis
   D. Is likely to have occurred during mixing of the solution

ANSWERS:

1. (A-D)

Chronic intractable diarrhea (whatever the etiology) leads to a state of malnutrition because of the malabsorption of nutrients. Losses are not replaced through oral intake and once malnutrition is established with deficiencies of either protein, calories, vitamins and/or iron, the gastrointestinal mucosa, flora, and/or motility are adversely affected. The diarrheal state is then perpetuated. Hyperalimentation is necessary. Administration of "broad spectrum antibiotics", steroids, or immunosuppressants appear to predispose patients to fungal septicemia. Candida sp. seem to proliferate more rapidly than the common bacterial pathogens in the TPN solutions although Klebsiellae sp proliferate more rapidly in D_5W. [6] Candida does grow well in vitro in a solution containing protein hydrolysate and D_5W at 30^0 and 37^0. The actual TPN solution contains D20 or D25, and with protein hydrolysate Candida proliferates easily (1 log/ 12 hrs and 3 logs/24 hrs) at room temperature. Under similar test conditions, Klebsiella and Staphylococci also grew extremely well and more rapidly than E. coli, Serratia sp, Proteus sp or Enterobacter sp. Candida sp grow less well in TPN solution containing synthetic aminoacid solution. The importance of fungal organisms is documented in retrospective as well as prospective studies of patients receiving hyperalimentation over a long period of time.

2. (A-D)

The use of peripheral scalp vein needles appears to reduce the risk of infection, but it is very difficult to sustain a patient with TPN for any period of time because of the necessity to frequently change the I.V. site. In small infants this certainly presents a significant problem. In skilled hands an intravenous catheter can be inserted into the suclavian vein via a percutaneous insertion. This procedure is performed in the operating room under aseptic conditions and has

been successful in very small infants as well as adult patients. The
procedure which has been utilized for the longest period of time is
the venous cut down, and thus more data has accumulated to date
with insertion of a catheter through the internal jugular vein into
the right atrium. This procedure must be accomplished with subcutaneous tunneling of the exit of the catheter, which seems to reduce the incidence of catheter related sepsis. This procedure also
requires strict asepsis and is considerably more complicated with
two cutaneous incisions for the catheter. Indwelling venous lines
are usually not inserted in the femoral vein. This area of the skin
is frequently contaminated with organisms from the stool and infection occurs more often.

3. (A-E)

Each of these measures is considered essential to maintain the hyperalimentation line safely with as little possibility of infection as
possible. In many hospitals, a trained group of nurses are responsible for the meticulous care of the hyperalimentation lines as well
as other I. V. lines. It has been demonstrated with peripheral intravenous infusions that trained personnel can conscientiously reduce
the associated rate of infections by limiting the duration of each
peripheral needle to 72 hours. The regular care and inspection of
the catheter and the trained personnel in the pharmacy are responsible for mixture of fluids. It should be clear that hyperalimentation is a team effort requiring the cooperation of physician, nurses,
and pharmacy personnel.

4. (C)

The patient's response to antibiotic therapy is dramatic. The inability to clear organisms from the blood is most likely an indication
of the intravascular foreign body and its colonization with these organisms. It is of course essential to do antimicrobial sensitivity
testing of the organisms obtained and to determine serum levels of
the appropriate antibiotic agent. However, it is frequently essential
to remove the hyperalimentation line. In some situations removal
of the line alone will cure the patient of their bacteremia or fungemia.

5. (C, D)

The detected colonization of the Amigen solution is probably indicative of fluid which became contaminated during mixing procedures.
It is quite likely that this original fluid represents the source of the
patient's infection. Although in-line filters are frequently used,
their efficacy remains to be established. In many situations the
pore size of the filter is sufficiently large so that bacteria might
pass through the filter. Small pore size filters tend to become oc-
cluded with protein materials from the hyperalimentation fluid and
require frequent changes. It should not be assumed that an in-line
filter will protect the patient.

REFERENCES

1. Ryan, John A. , Jr. , et al. : Catheter complications in total parenteral nutrition: A Prospective Study of 200 Consecutive Patients. NEJM 290:757-761, 1974.

2. Heird, William C. , Winter, Robert W. : Total parenteral nutrition. J. Pediat. 86:2-16, 1975.

3. Dillon, James D. , Jr. , et al. : Septicemia and total parenteral
   nutrition: JAMA 223:1341-1344, 1973.

4. Goldmann, Donald A. , et al. : Guidelines for infection control in
   intravenous therapy. Ann. Int. Med. 79:848-850, 1973.

5. Curry, Cynthia R. , Quie, Paul G. : Fungal septicemia in patients
   receiving parenteral hyperalimentation. NEJM 285:1221-1225,
   1971.

6. Goldmann, Donald A. , Maki, Dennis G. : Infection control in
   total parenteral nutrition. JAMA 223:1361-1364, 1973.

7. Deeb, Edward N. , Natsios, George A. : Contamination of intravenous fluids by bacteria and fungi during preparation and administration. Am. J. Hosp. Phar. 28:764-67, 1971.

8. Brennan, Murray F. , et al. : The growth of Candida albicans in
   nutritive solutions given parenterally. Arch. Surg. 103:705-708,
   1971.

:::

CASE 13: FEVER, SWOLLEN ANKLE, AND DYSPNEA

HISTORY: This is the first hospital admission of a 7-year-old, black
male admitted with fever of one week's duration. One week prior to
admission he was seen in the emergency room, and the diagnosis
of pneumonia was made. Penicillin therapy was administered but
because of persistent fever and progressive illness, he was again
seen six days later. He had begun to vomit and was observed to
have minimal right upper quadrant tenderness, and the urine was
reported to contain bile. He was advised to continue penicillin therapy. Two days later he returned acutely ill with continued fever and
a swollen, painful ankle. He had no history of rheumatic fever, heart
murmur or known heart disease. He was admitted to the hospital.
Abdominal examination was unremarkable. No jaundice was present.

PHYSICAL EXAMINATION: Blood pressure 100/65. Pulse 130. Respirations 30 with an expiratory grunt. T=103 degrees. (39.5C). The
patient appeared acutely ill. Examination of the chest revealed bilateral pleural rubs at the bases of both lungs. No rales or rhonchi

were heard. The left chest was dull posteriorly to percussion. Cardiovascular examination revealed massive cardiac enlargement with the left cardiac border at the AAL. A pericardial friction rub was audible at the middle and lower left sternal border. Apical heart sounds were felt to be diminished. Sinus tachycardia were present, no murmurs were heard. Examination of the abdomen revealed moderate right upper quadrant tenderness. The right groin was also tender and movement of both lower extremities produced pain at the hip joints. The right ankle was warm, edematous, tender, and an effusion was present. Abdominal examination was unremarkable. No jaundice was present.

LABORATORY STUDIES: Hemoglobin 10. 0 grams%. WBC count 21, 900 with 79 segs, 10 bands, 11 lymph. BUN 14 mg%, Na 129 meq./L. Potassium 4. 5 meq./L. CO_2 27 meq. /L. Chloride 88 meq. /L. Chest x-ray revealed cardiomegaly with no evidence of shunt to the lungs and no demonstrable pulmonary infiltrate (Fig. 13. 1). Sickle cell studies negative and all liver function tests were normal.

QUESTIONS:

1. Differential diagnosis for this child would include:
   A. Viral myocarditis
   B. Acute rheumatoid arthritis
   C. Acute rheumatic fever with pericarditis
   D. Bacterial sepsis with pericarditis and pyarthroses
   E. Tuberculosis

2. Essential diagnostic and therapeutic procedures would now include:
   A. Blood cultures
   B. Aspiration of the swollen ankle area and hip
   C. Penicillin and kanamycin therapy
   D. Consultation with a cardiologist concerning aspiration of pericardial sac

The above procedures were accomplished and purulent fluid containing numerous polyps was obtained after aspiration of the right ankle and pericardial sac. Gram-positive cocci were observed on Gram stain. Cultures of these materials were sent to the microbiology laboratory.

QUESTIONS:

3. Further therapeutic maneuvers would now include:
   A. Penicillin
   B. Gentamicin
   C. Methicillin or other penicillinase resistant penicillin
   D. Benemid

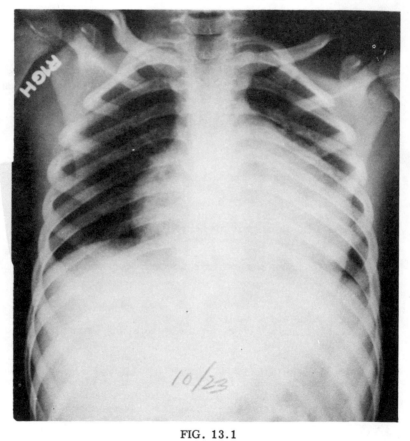

FIG. 13.1

4. Surgical drainage is necessary in the face of appropriate anti-
    microbial therapy.
    A. True
    B. False

The patient was taken to the operating room within 24 hours of admission and an arthrostomy of both hips and the right ankle was accomplished. Purulent material containing gram-positive cocci was
obtained from all three sites. At the same time, the pericardium
was explored. Thick, white, loculated material with the consistency
of coagulated protein was removed. This material contained gram-
positive cocci and a drain was inserted into the pericardial space.
Evaluation of the patient's organism revealed Staphylococcus aureus
coagulase positive in the pericardial fluid and the synovial fluid from
all three joints. The antibiotic sensitivities are reported as shown
in Table 13-1.

TABLE 13-1		
DRUG	(ugm/ml) Minimal inhibitory conc. (MIC)	(ugm/ml) Minimal bactericidal conc. (MBC)
Gentamicin	.312	1.25
Lincomycin	.039	1.56
Nafcillin	.039	.039

A serum Schlicter was also done which revealed:

	SERUM DILUTION	
	Bacteriostatic	Bactericidal
1 hr. before drug administration	1:8	1:8
2 hr. after drug administration	1:256	1:256

The patient received parenteral nafcillin therapy. The nafcillin was
administered intravenously every six hours with a total daily dose of
8 grams. Gentamicin therapy was initiated because of progression of
illness on the fourth hospital day in the dosage of 50 mg. q 12 hours
intravenously. The drug was administered for two days and discontinued prior to its initiation again at the same dosage for the subsequent two weeks. A decubitus ulcer had developed in the open hip
wound and was infected with Pseudomonas aeruginosa. The patient
remained febrile for 11 days and on the 12th day of antibiotic therapy
complained of left shoulder pain.

QUESTION:

5. An x-ray was taken (Fig. 13.2) and the x-ray film showed:

    _____.

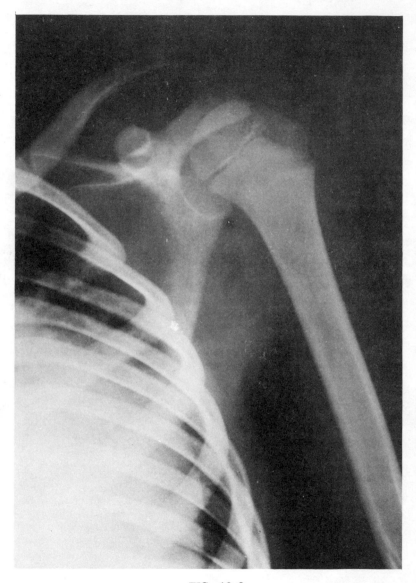

FIG. 13.2

This patient never had an elevation of BUN and received no diuretic therapy.

Initial hearing evaluation done at the end of his gentamicin therapy with conventional pure tone audiometry revealed mild sensorineural loss bilaterally. His 3 frequency averages were 23 dB and 30 dB in the right and left ear respectively. The loss was confirmed on a total of 3 evaluations, and at the time of his last testing, when his clinical illness has improved considerably, his average decrease in hearing acuity was 12 dB in the right ear and 15 dB in the left ear.

QUESTION:

6. This hearing loss as demonstrated by audiometry is:
    A. Unrelated to his present illness
    B. Probably caused by the staphylococcal bacteremia
    C. Related to nafcillin therapy
    D. Related to gentamicin therapy

ANSWERS:

1. (B, C, D)

The diagnostic considerations should place bacterial sepsis first in priority because of the urgency of the treatment and availability of antimicrobial agents specifically effective against the pathogenic bacteria likely to be responsible for his illness. The toxicity of this child, the presence of probable pericardial fluid and the possibility of impending tamponade are all signals for emergency action. Viral myocarditis would not be associated with arthritis. Cardiac involvement of this degree would probably be associated with significant myocardial involvement and congestive heart failure. Tuberculosis may involve the pericardium with acute primary involvement or constrictive disease which usually develops years after acquisition of tuberculosis. Fulminant onset of tuberculous disease of this type would be extremely rare in a 7-year-old child without involvement of the lungs or dissemination of M. tuberculosis to other sites, which occurs frequently.

2. (A, B, D)

Blood cultures must be obtained and examination of the buffy coat may prove a useful procedure in overwhelming sepsis. Bacterial counts of 10^5/ml will produce visible organisms in Gram stain of peripheral blood. The ankle joint is accessible and affords the possibility of obtaining a bacterial etiologic agent. The size of the heart, diminished heart tones, toxicity of the child and severity of illness dictate the necessity of attempted pericardiocentesis. These procedures can be accomplished quickly and any material obtained may show culpable organisms and guide specific antimicrobial therapy. Aspiration and drainage of pyarthrosis of the hip is an urgent therapeutic necessity to avoid compromise of blood supply of femoral head.

3. (C)

Penicillinase resistant penicillin therapy should be initiated as rapidly as possible. The child should be on therapy within the first hour of admission and an accurate diagnosis and treatment of the infection should take precedence over other aspects of the admission evaluation. Staphylococcal bacteremia, particularly with obvious areas of suppuration, may respond relatively slowly to therapy. It is not unusual to observe persistent evidence (eg. fever) of active infection for 3-7 days. However, the physician should not relax his vigilance and attention to additional complications of illness. Determining antimicrobial sensitivities of the organism and guiding therapy to achieve optimal therapeutic levels is of paramount importance for the child.

4. (A)

Adequate therapy will be impossible without drainage of sites named. Purulent pericarditis demands adequate drainage. There is data to indicate that methicillin resistant organisms are sensitive to gentamicin, and therefore while awaiting sensitivities additional therapy was added. [9]

5. Osteomyelitis of the left clavicle

The osteomyelitis has become apparent 12 days into the illness. The decalcification probably had been occurring during the previous several weeks of illness and this does not necessarily mean that the patient is inadequately treated. It must raise the questions of the necessity of drainage of purulent material or removal of necrotic bone. In addition, aspiration of the involved area would help to determine whether viable organisms were present or if this focus caused by bacteria other than staphylococci.

6. (D)

The incidence of recognized ototoxicity with gentamicin approaches 2%. 1/3 of the toxicity is decreased hearing and 2/3 is vestibular dysfunction. The hearing loss may improve and does not progress once therapy is discontinued. The loss is greatest in the high tone frequencies. The ototoxicity seen with gentamicin is best related to the serum levels attained during therapy. Serum concentrations in excess of 8 ugm/ml have been demonstrated more frequently in patients with ototoxicity than those with no toxicity, but this should not be construed as an absolute level at which toxicity occurs. In patients with normal renal function, ototoxicity was observed with mean dosages of 3. 4 mg/kg, and this seemed significantly different from mean

dosages of 2. 6 mg/kg in patients having no observed ototoxicity.
Two thirds of patients with ototoxicity have impaired renal function.
In the setting of decreased renal function, previous courses of potentially ototoxic drugs appear to enhance the risk to the patient.
Toxicity seems to be enhanced by furosemide, but this patient received no diuretics. The future use of potentially ototoxic drugs
should be avoided unless essential. He should receive counseling
and will require a front seat in class to help compensate for his
deficit.

REFERENCES

1. Bennett, Ivan L. , and Beeson, Paul: Bacteremia: A consideration of some experimental and clinical aspects. Yale J. Bio.
   Med. 26:241-262, 1954.

2. Van Reken, David, et al.: Infectious pericarditis in children.
   J. Pediat. 85:165-169, 1974.

3. Rubin, Robert H. , Moellering, Robert C. Jr.: Clinical, micro-
   biologic and therapeutic aspects of purulent pericarditis. Am. J.
   Med. 59:68-78, 1975.

4. Nadas, Alaxander S. , Levy, J. M.: Pericarditis in children.
   Am. J. Card. 7:109-117, 1961.

5. Boyle, James D. et al.: Purulent pericarditis: Review of the
   literature and report of 11 cases. Medicine 40:119-44, 1961.

6. Synbas, P. N. , et al.: Purulent pericarditis: A review of diagnostic and surgical principles. South Med. J. 67:46-48, 1974.

7. Tann, James S. , et al.: Antibiotic levels in pericardial fluid.
   J. Clin. Invest. 53:7-12, 1974.

8. Klastersky, Jean: Antibiotic suspectibility of oxicillin resistant
   staphylococci. Antimic. Agts. & Chemoth. 1:441-446, 1972.

9. Hoeprich, Paul B. , et al.: Susceptibility of methicillin: Resistant
   Staphylococcus aureus to 12 antimicrobial agents. Antimic. Agts.
   & Chemoth. pp. 104-110, 1969.

10. Echeverria, Peter, et al.: Age dependent dose response to gen-
    tamicin. J. Pediat. 87:805-808, 1975.

11. Jackson, George Gee, Archieri, George: Ototoxicity of gentami-
    cin in man: A survey and control analysis of clinical experience
    in the United States. J. Infect. Dis. 124 supplement:130-137,
    1971.

::

CASE 14:   WEAKNESS OF RIGHT LOWER EXTREMITY IN A
5-MONTH-OLD INFANT

HISTORY: This is the first hospital admission for a 5-month-old,
white male infant who lived in Greensboro, North Carolina and was
admitted for right lower extremity weakness of one month duration.
The infant was a six-pound product of an uncomplicated pregnancy
and delivery, and was considered to be a healthy child with normal
developmental motor milestones. On May 5, 1975 he received a
second diphtheria, pertussis and tetanus (DPT) immunization as well
as his second feeding of trivalent oral polio vaccine. Fever and irritability four weeks after the immunization led to the diagnosis of
otitis media, and he was treated with a single intramuscular injection of benzathine penicillin in right anterior thigh. His parents observed continued irritability and noted that 48 hours after the injection the patient failed to move his right lower extremity. Eleven
days later he was seen by a pediatrician and neurologist who noted
the flaccid paralysis, and the child was referred for further evaluation of suspected trauma secondary to an injection. There had been
no associated vomiting or diarrhea and no similar illness in the
family. There was no history of muscular weakness.

PHYSICAL EXAMINATION: Temperature 38. 3°C. Pulse 140. Respirations 40. Weight 6. 1 kg. Height 67 cm. Head circumference 42
cm. The anterior fontanelle was soft and the neck was supple. The
lungs were clear to percussion and auscultation and there were no
cardiac murmurs or organomegaly. No midline cutaneous dimples
or spinal abnormalities were observed. Rectal examination was
normal, good sphincter tone was present and no masses were felt.
The infant was alert, and cranial nerve function was intact. When
supine, the right lower extremity was maintained in abduction and
there was no movement of this extremity. In the prone position the
extremity could be moved with contraction of his gluteal muscles.
A right foot drop was apparent. The strength of his quadriceps and
hamstring muscles were graded as 2 with a possible maximum of 5.
There was a noticeable decrease in the motor tone of the right lower
extremity. Sensation was intact as tested by pin prick in all extremities. The deep tendon reflexes were symmetrical except for an absent right patellar reflex and ankle jerk.

LABORATORY DATA: Hemoglobin 12. 7 grams %, Hematocrit, 39%.
WBC 8, 500 with 46% neutrophils, 8% bands, 42% lymphocytes, 4%
monocytes and adequate platelets. The urinalysis was normal. The
spinal fluid showed no bacterial growth and the VDRL was negative.
CSF glucose was 41. 0 mg%. , protein was 49 mg. % and there were
210 mononuclear white cells. Serum electrophoresis showed normal
serum IgG and IgA, and an elevated IgM. He had normal numbers of
peripheral small lymphocytes and normal lymphocyte response to
mitogens (phytohemagglutinin and concanavallin A.).

QUESTIONS:

1. The presumptive diagnosis of illness in this child was peripheral
   nerve damage secondary to an injection of penicillin. Features
   of his illness which are atypical for this diagnosis include:
   A. Evidence of multiple nerve involvement
   B. Absence of pain with manipulation of the extremity
   C. Pleocytosis with mononuclear cells in CSF
   D. Normal conduction velocity of involved peripheral nerves

2. Poliomyelitis can occur following ingestion of attenuated virus
   vaccines. Indicate which of the following statements is correct.
   A. Onset of paralysis usually occurs within 30 days following
       vaccine exposure
   B. Such paralysis is due to wild type virus and not to attenuated
       virus
   C. Recovery from paralysis usually becomes apparent in less
       than 60 days after onset
   D. Paralytic disease occurs more frequently in immunologically
       compromised patients

3. Evaluation of this infant for the possibility of poliomyelitis included a stool culture. The stool contained poliovirus type 2
   during his hospitalization. Indicate whether each of these state-
   ments is true or false.
   A. The presence of poliovirus in the stool establishes the diag-
       nosis of poliomyelitis
   B. Characterization of this virus by antigenic markers is neces-
       sary to establish the diagnosis of paralytic poliomyelitis
   C. Serological evidence of infection with this virus could estab-
       lish the relationship of paralysis to this infection
   D. This baby is too young to have paralytic poliomyelitis

4. Poliomyelitis in the middle 1970's in the United States occurs:
   A. In unimmunized individuals as the result of isolated impor-
       tations from endemic countries
   B. In persons in contact with the vacinees
   C. In immunocompromised hosts
   D. Not at all

5. Inactivated poliovirus vaccines have been utilized in Scandinavia
   and have essentially eliminated poliovirus related disease from
   those countries. Indicate which of these statements is correct.
   A. Virus is still present in these countries and is detectable in
       sewage and from other sources
   B. Gastrointestinal excretion of virus appears to have been
       diminished substantially
   C. Inactivated virus does not produce lasting immunity and per-
       sons require continuous booster injections of antigen
   D. This vaccine could be utilized with equal effectiveness in the
       United States at the present time
   E. It is readily available from a number of manufacturers

ANSWERS:

1. (A-C)

This child had evidence of weakness in muscles innervated by scia-
tic, femoral and peroneal nerves. The diverse nature of this injury
with demonstrated normal nerve conduction mitigates against the
possibility of direct trauma to the nerve. The extensive loss of function of the right lower extremity prompted consideration of the involvement of the sacral plexus or spinal cord. A myelogram was
done and was normal. In addition, direct trauma to the nerve is usually associated with local inflammation and pain with manipulation of
the extremity. Local nerve damage should not cause an inflammatory
response in the cerebrospinal fluid. The presence of mononuclear
cells in the cerebrospinal fluid is consistent with meningeal inflammation from an undefined source. It is important to note that this
child had a febrile illness prompting his initial visit to the physician.
The diagnosis of otitis and the injection of penicillin was followed
2 days later by the observed loss of function of the right lower extremity. With this sequence of events it is not surprising that the
parents noted the temporal association of the injection of penicillin
and the occurrence of paralysis which then seemed casually related.

2. (A, C, D)

By arbitrary definition, vaccine associated poliomyelitis occurs within 30 days after exposure to vaccine virus. Exceptions to this may
occur particularly in immunocompromised patients when the onset
of paralysis may be further delayed. Poliovirus which has been recovered from those patients sustaining paralysis has been characterized as vaccine-like. This determination is accomplished by in-
tratypic serodifferentiation tests and growth at supraoptimal temperatures. At the present time, it is not possible to obtain primates
and perform tests for the neurovirulence of these strains. Therefore, these viruses conform to defined antigenic characteristics of
attenuated polioviruses, but the possibility of reversion to neuro-
virulent virus has not been totally excluded. At the time this child
was admitted to the hospital he was 2 months into his illness, and if
recovery of function was to occur some improvement should have
been noted. It is important to try to define the etiology of his difficulty as the prognosis is considerably better for recovery of function
after trauma to a peripheral nerve than with paralysis of this duration due to poliomyelitis. Fewer than 10 cases per year of paralytic
poliomyelitis are identified each year in the United States. It has
become clear the immunocompromised patients, including those with
isolated cellular or humoral deficits, as well as those with combined
immunodeficiency, are at increased risk from paralytic disease. Patients with these deficiencies may receive live poliovirus at a young
age prior to recognition of their immunological deficit. Prolonged
virus excretion from the G. I. tract has been documented in several

agammaglobulinemic patients. Several infants with combined immunodeficiency disease have succumbed to their poliovirus infections, and virus was detected in the CSF, which is most unusual for
polio infections. Virus isolated from several of these children has
also been defined as vaccine-like by antigenic markers. The increased risk of paralytic disease in these patients dictates that exposure to live vaccine be avoided.

3. All statements are false

This infant had received attenuated virus vaccine and would be expected to excrete virus for a number of weeks. The presence of
virus documents infection with poliomyelitis and suggests the very
strong possibility that he has indeed sustained paralytic illness due
to this agent, but does not prove this etiologic relationship. Characterization of the virus by antigenic markers as cited in answer
#2 is not necessary to establish the diagnosis of paralytic poliomye-
litis but rather characterizes the virus as vaccine-like or wild type.
A significant antibody rise in the serum as determined by neutralization studies would document the presence of infection temporally
related to the paralysis. Unfortunately, this infant was two months
into his illness and the antibody rise may have occurred prior to
his evaluation for paralysis. Once again, the infection would be substantiated by the antibody rise but the etiologic nature of the paralysis would not be proven. Persons of any age may have paralytic
poliomyelitis. Even infants born to mothers who sustain poliomyelitis during their pregnancy were seen with evidence of paralysis as
a result of intrauterine infection. It is also correct that a higher rate
of paralytic illness occurs in young adults than in young infants.

4. (A-C)

Reported paralytic poliomyelitis occurs in fewer than 10 persons
per year in the USA. Sporadic importations from Mexico, Central
and South America occur and unimmunized susceptibles may acquire
disease. In addition, attenuated virus has been associated with paralysis at an estimated frequency of $1:10^6$ vaccinees. This may occur
in the vaccinee or in an unimmunized (usually adult) contact of vaccinee. See answer #2 for discussion of disease in immunocompromised patients.

5. (B)

Although extensive surveys have not been reported, WHO studies
have indicated no detectable virus in the sewage of Scandinavian
countries. These changes have occurred at a time when < 10 cases
of polio/year have occurred in each country over the last 5 years.
In addition, it should be recognized that adjacent European countries
employ attenuated virus vaccines. It is true on the basis of additional
observations that in the Scandinavian countries as well as in the

United States in the late 1950's and early 1960's gastrointestinal
excretion of poliomyelitis was indeed diminished after immunization
with inactivated virus.

In the United States, inactivated viral antigens as presently manufactured can be obtained from only one manufacturer. This antigen
is sufficiently potent so that 3-5 injections would appear to produce
long-standing immunity. This objective has been achieved in the
Scandinavian countries where better than 90% of the population has
been immunized. Obligatory military service again provides the
opportunity for immunization of the male population. Within the
United States a significant number of children do not receive immunizations. With regard to poliomyelitis, the acquisition of attenuated
virus from contact with immunized persons probably extends the
protection achieved by attenuated viruses. It is doubtful that our
present health care delivery system would allow a comparable per-
centage of people to be immunized with inactivated vaccine.

REFERENCES

1. Wyatt, H. V.: Poliomyelitis in hypogammaglobulinemics. J.
   Infect. Dis. 128:802-806, 1973.

2. Oberhofer, Thomas R., et al.: Immunity to poliomyelitis in an
   American community. Am. J. Epidem. 101:333-339, 1975.

3. Katz, Michael, and Plotkin, Stanley A.: Oral polio immunization of the newborn infant; a possible method for overcoming interference by ingested antibodies. J. Pediat. 73:267-270, 1968.

4. Russeau, Wyatt E., et al.: Persistence of poliovirus neutralizing antibodies eight years after immunization with live attenuated
   virus vaccine. NEJM 289:1357-1359, 1973.

5. Linnemann, Calvin C., et al.: Poliovirus antibody in urban
   school children. J. Pediat. 84:404-406, 1974.

6. Witte, John J., et al.: Poliomyelitis immunity survey in Hills-
   boro County, Florida. South. Med. J. 66:696-699, 1973.

7. Ogra, Pearay L., Karzon, David T.: Distribution of poliovirus
   antibody in serum, nasopharynx and alimentary tract following
   segmental immunization of lower alimentary tract with polio
   vaccine. J. Imm. 102:1423-1430, 1969.

Case 15: FEVER, IRRITABILITY AND POOR FEEDING IN A
          NEONATE

HISTORY: The patient was a two-week-old black girl who was a
2200 gm. product of a term gestation complicated by preeclampsia.
The teenage mother had no prenatal care. The infant was discharged
on the fourth day after birth and did well until two days prior to admission when she was felt to be more sleepy than usual, developed
a fever, became irritable and was not taking her feedings well.
There had been no identified staphylococcal or streptococcal disease in the nursery during the preceding month.

PHYSICAL EXAMINATION: Temperature 39. 6°C, pulse 110/minute,
respiratory rate 36/minute with Cheyne-Stokes respirations, weight
2400 gm. The patient had a patent anterior fontanelle that was full but
not bulging. Skin examination revealed no rashes or pustules. Her cry
was vigorous. The left tympanic membrane was red and bulging. The
neck was supple. The lungs were clear. Heart regular rhythm without murmurs. Abdominal examination was normal and deep tendon
reflexes were hyperactive. The rest of the physical exam was essentially negative.

LABORATORY DATA: CBC: hemoglobin 17 gms%, hematocrit 50%,
white blood cell count 30, 000 cells/mm^3 with 17% polymorphonuclear leukocytes (2% stabs). Platelets were adequate. Serum
BUN, sugar, electrolytes were normal. Urinalysis and chest x-ray
were normal. Lumbar puncture revealed a CSF with a white blood
cell count of 16, 000 cells/mm^3 (80% polys), CSF sugar of 35 mg%
(blood sugar 137 mg%), CSF protein 120 mg%. Gram stain of the
CSF revealed gram-positive rods. Blood culture was obtained and
subsequently found to be negative. EEG was normal.

HOSPITAL COURSE: The patient was initially treated with parenteral
penicillin and kanamycin. This was changed on the second day to intravenous ampicillin, 200 mg/kg/24 hours which was continued for
a full three week period. Early during hospitalization the patient has
seizure-like activity in the extremities and was placed on phenobarbital for a short period of time. Lumbar puncture was repeated five
days after institution of therapy and revealed improvement with elevation of CSF sugar, decrease in the number of white blood cells,
and CSF protein. CSF culture was negative.

QUESTIONS:

1. The most likely etiologic agent of this infection is:
    A. Corynebacterium species
    B. Erysipelothrix species
    C. Listeria monocytogenes
    D. Streptococcus species
    E. E. coli
    F. Clostridia species

2. Infection of the baby occurs:
   A. Before birth
   B. During or after delivery
   C. A and/or B
   D. Through the respirator
   E. None of the above

3. The antibiotic of choice in the treatment of Listeria monocyto-
   genes is:
   A. Penicillin
   B. Chloramphenicol
   C. Sulfonamide
   D. Streptomycin
   E. A penicillin and an aminoglycoside

4. The host defenses against Listeria involve primarily:
   A. Cell mediated immune responses
   B. Humoral immunity
   C. The complement system
   D. B and C
   E. All of the above

ANSWERS:

1. The most likely agent is (C)

Listeria monocytogenes are gram-positive nonsporulating microaerophilic motile bacilli. Their motility, ability to reduce 2, 3,
5-triphenyltetrazolium chloride and their animal pathogenicity are
generally adequately different from the bacteria with which they
are often confused. These are Erysipelothrix species, Coryne-
bacterium species, Streptococcus species, and Clostridium species.
The incidence of listeriosis in the newborn is low when compared
with gram-negative coliform and group B streptococcal infections.
Listeria species are seriologically of seven major types on the basis
of somatic and flagellar antigens. Two distinct clinical syndromes
are seen in neonates: an early septicemic form and a delayed men-
ingitic form. The early onset form, which is predominantly septicemic, is characterized by prematurity, a history of obstetrical
complications, a higher frequency of maternal isolates, and an increased neonatal mortality. However, the late onset form, which
primarily involves the CNS, at 2-4 weeks of age, is characterized
by a normal birth weight, lower mortality, and the absence of obstetrical complications. These clinical features are similar to
those of group B streptococcal disease. In a recent report concerning the distribution of serotypes of Listeria monocytogenes isolated
from 40 infants with neonatal listeriosis, serotypes Ia, Ib, and IVb
were the predominant infecting serotypes in all cases of human
listeriosis in the United States. The distribution of these serotypes

differs between the early and late onset groups. Serotypes Ia and Ib
are mainly concerned with early onset while serotype IVb is mainly
concerned with late onset disease.

2. The correct answer is (C)

Infection of the offspring occurs either before birth (transplacentally),
during delivery or after delivery through contact with infected secretions. Listeriosis of the newborn is most often localized to the central nervous system and is manifested as meningitis. Meningeal localization is the commonest clinical form of listeriosis accounting
for about 75% of all bacteriologically proved infection. The pathology
of acute listerial meningitis does not differ from that of any other
pyogenic meningitis. Disseminated listeriosis may cause involvement of several organs such as the liver, spleen, lungs, GI tract,
skin, etc. resulting in abscesses or granulomas. Clinically, this
will be manifested by maculopapular skin lesions, hepatosplenomegaly, and may result in abortion, premature delivery, stillbirth,
or death within minutes to days following delivery.

3. The antibiotic of choice for treatment of Listeria monocytogenes
    is (E)

The minimal inhibitory concentration (MIC) of both ampicillin and
penicillin for all strains of Listeria is quite low (0. 5 and 0. 25 respectively). However, the minimal bactericidal concentration (MBC)
of both of these drugs seems to be much higher than the MIC. The
use of penicillin plus an aminoglycoside decreases the MBC but
relatively high concentrations of these antibiotics are necessary to
inhibit the growth of most strains of Listeria. Studies have shown
that the combinations of penicillin plus gentamicin, ampicillin plus
streptomycin, and ampicillin plus gentamicin produced enhanced
killing against all strains tested. No antagonism was observed when
ampicillin or penicillin was combined with streptomycin or gentamicin.

4. The host defenses against Listeria involve primarily (A)

T cell recognition by sensitized lymphocytes with subsequent mobil-
ization of effector responses, e. g. activated macrophages, has been
demonstrated to be the fundamental response to Listeria infections.
Stimulation of cell mediated immune responses by Listeria, as with
tuberculin antigens, has been shown to nonspecifically augment host
cellular immune responses. Interestingly, it has been postulated
that this adjuvant effect of Listeria infections on host immune reactions may upset the host-graft immunological balance and result
in an acute rejection episode. In a recent report of three renal transplant recipients in whom sepsis with Listeria monocytogenes developed, acute rejection episodes were observed a few days later.

REFERENCES

1. Albritton, W. L., et al.: Neonatal listeriosis: Distribution of serotypes in relation to age and onset of disease. J. Pediat. 88:481-483, 1976.

2. Center for Diseases Control: Zoonoses Surveillence, Listeriosis Annual Summary 1971, issued August, 1972.

3. Moellering, R. C., et al.: Antibiotic synergism against Listeria monocytogenes. Antimic. Agts. & Chemoth. 1:30-34, 1972.

4. Medoff, G., et al.: Listeria in humans: An evaluation. J. Infect. Dis. 123:247-250, 1971.

5. Finkelstein, F. O., et al.: Listeria sepsis immediately preceding renal transplant rejection. JAMA 235:844-845, 1976.

::

CASE 16: LOW GRADE FEVER, DECREASED APPETITE AND IRRITABILITY IN AN INFANT

HISTORY: A 9-month-old baby girl presented with low grade fever, decreased appetite and irritability of 2 weeks duration. She had occasional vomiting but no diarrhea or symptoms of upper respiratory tract infection. The mother had noticed that the patient had not been gaining weight over the past month. Patient smiled at 2 months, had no head lag at 4 months, and reached out for objects at 7 months of age. Past medical history is essentially negative.

PHYSICAL EXAMINATION: Temperature 39.8°C, Height 77 cms., Weight 7.5 kgm., Pulse 100/minute, Respirations 28/minute. The patient was quite irritable, with non-bulging anterior fontanelle, normal ear drums, no signs of an upper respiratory tract infection, clear lungs, regular sinus rhythm, soft abdomen without organomegaly or masses, normal neurologic examination and no vaginal discharge. External genitalia were normal and the kidneys were palpable bilaterally.

LABORATORY DATA: CBC: Hgb = 11.0 gm%. Hct = 34%, leukocytes = 9800/cu mm. PMN's 78%, lymphocytes = 20% and monocytes = 2%. Urinalysis: Color = turbid yellow, sp. gr. 1.005, sugar = +1, protein = +1, ketone = negative, rbc = 1/hpf, wbc = 10 - 15/hpf. Casts = absent, and gram-negative bacteria were seen on Gram stain of unspun urine. Blood chemistry: normal BUN, sugar and electrolytes. Lumbar puncture: normal CSF. Blood culture: no growth. Clean urine culture, colony count and sensitivity: E coli, 100,000 colonies/ml, sensitive to cephalothin, ampicillin, kanamycin, gentamicin, tetracycline and sulfonamide.

QUESTIONS:

1. The usual signs of urinary tract infection in infants are nonspecific and include:
   A. Urgency and frequency
   B. Burning on urination
   C. Failure to thrive and/or lethargy
   D. Unexplained fever and irritability
   E. Altered voiding pattern

2. Organisms accounting for most urinary tract infections in children are:
   A. Gram-positive organisms
   B. Gram-negative aerobic bacilla (Enterobacteriaceae)
   C. Anaerobic organisms
   D. All of the above

3. Females are more susceptible than males to urinary tract infection because:
   A. Boys have short urethra
   B. Females have shorter urethra and organisms from stool and perineum have ready access
   C. Males have less estrogenic hormones
   D. Females have smaller urinary bladder
   E. None of the above

4. Detection of significant bacteriuria rests primarily on:
   A. Symptoms of frequency and urgency
   B. Finding 5 - 10 PMN's/hpf in urine sediment
   C. Quantitative culture methods
   D. Seeing organism on Gram stain of unspun clean catch urine specimen
   E. C and D

5. Because urologic abnormalities may be associated with active urinary infection in children at the preschool and grade school age group, the following radiologic evaluation(s) should be done:
   A. Intravenous pyelography
   B. Voiding cystourethrography
   C. Cystoscopy and retrograde pyelography
   D. A and B
   E. All of the above

6. In dealing with first urinary tract infection not associated with an abnormal voiding mechanism, the medication of choice is:
   A. Short-acting sulfonamide
   B. Ampicillin
   C. Tetracycline
   D. Chloramphenicol
   E. Any of the above

7. Criteria and means for successful treatment of an acute urinary
   tract infection are by:
   A. Demonstration of a sterile urine culture 48 hours after
      initiating therapy and 1 week after completing therapy
   B. Administration of prolonged antimicrobial therapy irrespec-
      tive of whether the urine culture at 48 hours is sterile
   C. Suppressing organisms partially with anti-microbials and
      depending on local host defense mechanisms
   D. Administration of 10 - 14 days course with an appropriate
      drug
   E. A and D

8. Congenital anomalies of the urinary tract predisposing patients
   to UTI include:
   A. Vesicoureteral reflux
   B. Congenital hydronephorosis
   C. Megaloureters
   D. Vesical neck contracture
   E. Urethral valves
   F. All of the above

ANSWERS:

1. The nonspecific signs of urinary tract infection in infants are
   (C, D, E).

Unexplained fever, irritability, lethargy and/or failure to thrive are
the main signs of urinary tract infection (UTI) in infants, unlike the
classic signs of infection in some older children including dysuria
and/or urgency. In the newborn with UTI, abdominal distention may
be noted and the skin may be gray in color. On occasion, jaundice
and hepatomegaly may be associated with UTI in patients in this age
group. A great many UTI in infants are asymptomatic and the diagnosis will often be missed unless the possibility is considered in
any sick child. Among school-age girls with significant bacteriuria,
only about one third are symptomatic. Moreover, in about 50% of
asymptomatic cases, classic microscopic findings of at least 5 - 10
PMN/hpf in the urine sediment are absent.

2. Organisms accounting for most UTI in children are (B).

Gram-negative aerobic bacilli (Enterobacteriaceae) normally present
in the gut (namely Escherichia coli) are responsible for 75 - 80% of
first UTI. The Klebsiella-Enterobacter group account for 10 - 15%
and proteus, staphylococcus and pseudomonas species for the few
remaining cases. These patterns apply to UTI not associated with
anatomical abnormalities such as obstructive uropathy or defects of
the voiding mechanism. On the other hand, patients with anatomical
abnormalities who have received instrumentation or multiple courses
of antimicrobial therapy are more likely to be infected with Klebsiella, Enterobacter, Pseudomonas, or indole-positive Proteus species
or a mixture of organisms.

3. Females are more susceptible than males to UTI because (B).

UTI is more prevalent in females than males. Studies of school age
girls by Kunin et al. revealed a prevalence rate of UTI in 1 - 2% of
these girls as compared to 0. 03% in boys. Since most urinary tract
infections follow an ascending route, reaching the bladder more
readily via the short female urethra than through the longer passage
in the male, this alone may account for the marked difference in
susceptibility to UTI between the sexes. Thus the importance of
anatomical evaluation of males at any age with UTI.

4. Detection of significant bacteriuria rests primarily on (E).

Quantitative culture methods showing a bacterial colony count
$\geqslant 100,000$/ml of a single organism is essential for the diagnosis of
significant bacteriuria. Two consecutive positive cultures increase
the reliability of the diagnosis to more than 90%. Again, detecting
organisms on Gram stain of a clean catch unspun or on unstained
spun specimen of urine correlate with significant bacteriuria and
colony count of 100,000/ml or higher. Other situations with lower
colony count are indeed significant (e. g. specimens collected from
Foley catheter or nephrostomy tube). Gram-positive organisms such
as staphylococcus and enterococcus multiply less rapidly than gram-
negative organisms. Thus a repeat positive urine culture with these
organisms and a lower colony count may be significant. Aseptic collection methods (usually midstream clean-catch urine) and culturing
the specimen within an hour of voiding or within 48 hours if refrig-
erated are necessary to avoid false-positive results due to multiplication of contaminating bacteria. Prolonged refrigeration alters
formed elements. Any colony count on urine specimen obtained by a
suprapubic aspiration is significant. This method is performed
mostly on neonates who pass urine frequently, thus not allowing
enough time for bacterial multiplication in the bladder.

5. Radiologic evaluations that should be done to rule out urologic
    abnormalities are (D).

Intravenous pyelography (IVP) and voiding cystourethrography
(VCUG) are two sufficient radiologic procedures to examine the anat-
omy and function of the renal collecting system, localize renal cal-
culi, detect abnormalities in the bladder, its outlet, and to detect
reflux from the bladder into the ureter. If the above two procedures
are normal, little is to be gained by a cystoscopy and retrograde
pyelography. IVP and VCUG are indicated in any male developing
a UTI. Contrast studies in girls with UTI are frequently deferred to
the second episode. However, some authorities such as Kunin advocate that radiologic evaluation should be performed initially in
girls with UTI since the majority will have a recent infection. Recently developed techniques can be used to attempt to ascertain
whether the urinary infection is in the kidney or lower urinary tract.
Direct techniques such as renal biopsy, ureteral catheterization and

bladder washout are invasive and potentially hazardous. Indirect techniques such as examing the urine for antibody-coated bacteria and LDH isoenzyme assay (e. g. increased levels of isoenzymes are associated with pyelonephritis) are easier and safer.

6.   The medication of choice in an uncomplicated first UTI is (A, B).

In treating an initial episode of UTI, short acting sulfonamide or ampicillin can be used for a short-term. Both give good levels in the urine. Considering cost, effectiveness, and incidence of side effects - especially with first and second infections - sulfonamides are usually the best choice. Recent studies indicate that urinary concentration of an antimicrobial is more important in eradicating an infection than is its serum concentration. However, in the initial treatment of an acute pyelonephritis (as opposed to that for lower UTI), it may be more reasonable to choose a bactericidal drug that gives high serum levels (e. g. ampicillin) so as to better prevent rare but severe complications such as septicemia or perinephric abscesses.

7.   Criteria for successful treatment of an acute UTI are demonstrated by (E).

Having a sterile urine culture at 48 hours after initiating therapy and one week after therapy is completed are essential to make sure that the infection is sensitive to and has been eradicated by the drug used. A 10 - 14 day course with an appropriate drug is enough to treat an uncomplicated acute UTI. Prolonged therapy for about 3 - 6 months is used only for prophylaxis and/or suppression in patients with closely spaced episodes of recurrent infection or with persistent focus of infection. In such instances, nitrofurantoin is a good drug to use. Enteric bacteria tend to remain sensitive to nitrofurantoin after many courses of therapy, probably because very little of the drug appears in the stool.

8.   Congenital anomalies of the urinary tract include (F).

Many congenital anomalies of the urinary tract predispose the patient to UTI and, in addition, make eradication of the infection more difficult. These anomalies include vesicoureteral reflux, congenital hydronephrosis, megaloureters, vesical neck contracture, and urethral valves.

REFERENCES

1.   Kunin, C. M. : Prevention and treatment of urinary tract infections, 2nd. Ed. Lea and Febiger, Philadelphia, 1974.

2.   Kunin, C. M. : Epidemiology and natural history of urinary tract infection in school age children. Pediat. Clin. N. A. 18:509-528, 1971.

3. Petersdorf, R. G. , Turk, M. : Some current concepts of uri-
    nary tract infections. Disease-A-Month, December, 1970.

4. Abbott, G. D. : Neonatal bacteriuria: A prospective study in
    1,460 infants. Brit. Med. J. 1:267, 1972.

5. Hanson, L. A. , et al. : Autoantibodies to Tamm-Horsfall Pro-
    tein: A tool for diagnosing the level of urinary tract infection.
    Lancet I:226, 1976.

6. Margileth, A. M. , et al. : Management criteria, documentation,
    and peer review of initial urinary tract infection. Pediatrics
    57:754, 1976.

7. Gillenwater, J. Y. , et al. : Home urine cultures by the dip-strip
    method. Pediatrics 58:508, 1976.

8. Jones, S. R. : Antibody-coated bacteria in urine. NEJM 295:
    1380, 1976.

9. Hallett, R. J. , et al. : Urinary infection in boys. Lancet II:1107,
    1976.

10. Welch, T. R. , et al. : Recurrent urinary tract infection in girls:
    Group with lower tract findings and a benign course. Arch. Dis.
    Child. 51:114, 1976.

11. Drew, J. H. , Action, C. M. : Radiological findings in newborn
    infants with urinary infection. Arch. Dis. Child. 51:628, 1976.

::

CASE 17: FEVER, PAINFUL SWOLLEN JOINTS AND SORE
          THROAT

HISTORY: An 8-year-old boy presented with a one day history of
fever (39°C), associated with painful swelling of the right wrist and
left knee. The patient had a sore throat two weeks prior to the present illness which was treated with salicylates. No cultures were obtained. The past medical history was essentially negative and there
was no history of drug allergy, weight loss, rash, dyspnea, or illness in sibs.

PHYSICAL EXAMINATION: Temperature 39°C, Blood pressure 120/
80 mm Hg, Pulse 110/minute, Respirations 28/minute. The patient
was ill-appearing. He avoided movement of the right wrist and left
knee which were swollen, red, hot and tender. He had a moderately
injected oropharynx without exudate and an enlarged right cervical
lymph node estimated to be 1 x 1 cm. The precordium was active
and a systolic thrill could be felt. Auscultation of the heart revealed
a heart rate of 220/minute, normal heart sounds, and a grade III/VI

holosystolic murmur over the apex not transmitting toward the axilla. The lungs were clear. No rash or hepatosplenomegaly was present and the neurological exam was normal.

LABORATORY DATA: CBC: Hemoglobin = 12 gm%, Hct. 37%, WBC = 16500/cu mm. PMN = 78%, lymphocytes = 18%, monocytes = 2%, eosinophils = 2%. Sedimentation rate = 90 mm/hr. Urinalysis: Normal (no protein or cells). Blood chemistry: Sugar, BUN, electrolytes were normal. Serology: Antistreptolysin O titer = 666 Todd units. C-reactive protein = +2. Chest x-ray: Normal (no cardiomegaly). Throat culture: Negative for group A beta hemolytic streptococci. Blood culture: Negative. Electrocardiogram: Essentially normal except for mild S-T depression and nonspecific T wave changes on V_6. Aspirate left knee: 3 ml of yellow and turbid fluid were aspirated. WBC's/mm^3 = 3000 mainly polymorphonuclear leukocytes. Ratio of (glucose) synovial fluid/blood = 0. 8. Protein = 4 gm/100 ml. Gram stain = negative. Culture = no growth.

QUESTIONS:

1. The most likely diagnosis(es) is (are):
   A. Juvenile rheumatoid arthritis
   B. Septic arthritis
   C. Rheumatic fever
   D. Serum sickness
   E. Sickle cell disease

2. The pathogenic organisms responsible for rheumatic fever are:
   A. Group B beta hemolytic streptococci (Streptococcus agalactiae)
   B. Group C beta hemolytic streptococci
   C. Group A beta hemolytic streptococci (Streptococcus pyogenes)
   D. Staphylococcus aureus
   E. B and C

3. The modified major criteria of Jones for making the diagnosis of rheumatic fever include all the following except:
   A. Carditis and polyarthritis
   B. Chorea
   C. Erythema marginatum
   D. Subcutaneous nodules
   E. Arthralgia

4. Prevention of rheumatic fever recurrence and group A beta hemolytic streptococcal infection is possible by:
   A. Monthly injections of 1. 2 million units of procaine penicillin
   B. Oral sulfonamides (1 gm/day) or oral penicillin V (250 mg. b. i. d.)
   C. Oral tetracycline (250 mg. b. i. d.)
   D. Monthly injections of 1. 2 million units of benzathine penicillin
   E. All of the above except A

5. Treatment of active rheumatic fever includes:
   A. Penicillin and salicylates
   B. Penicillin and glucosteroids
   C. Penicillin and sulfonamides
   D. A and/or B
   E. None of the above

ANSWERS:

1. The most likely diagnosis(es) are (A, C).

Polyarthritis, leukocytosis, elevated sedimentation rate and the presence of C-reactive protein are common findings in rheumatic fever, serum sickness type of hypersensitivity, septic arthritis, rheumatoid arthritis and sickle cell disease. The absence of hepatosplenomegaly, macular rash or small joint involvement helps in differentiating juvenile rheumatoid arthritis (JRA) from rheumatic fever, although JRA can present with fever alone. Moreover, bacteriologic and hematologic findings help to differentiate sepsis and sickle cell disease. The negative history about receiving medications and/or drug allergy helps in ruling out serum sickness. The history and laboratory data presented are compatible with JRA and rheumatic fever. The laboratory findings of the left knee aspirate rules out septic arthritis in which a much higher WBC count, a lower ratio of synovial fluid/blood glucose and positive Gram stain and culture are expected.

2. The pathogenic organisms responsible for rheumatic fever are (C).

Respiratory infection caused by group A beta hemolytic streptococci (Streptococcus pyogenes) of any serotype (as defined by the M protein) that is inadequately treated may result in rheumatic fever. This is reported to occur in approximately 3% of patients or less after a latent period of a few days to 5 weeks. Patients with rheumatic fever have a high antibody response to the soluble streptococcal antigens, namely (streptolysin), hyaluronidase, streptokinase, NADase and DNase B), and to the group A cell wall carbohydrate. The antibody response to the cell wall components of the group A streptococci persist for months to years in patients with valvular heart disease. Moreover, it is thought that cell wall membrane antigens cross react with antigens present in the sarcolemmal sheaths of muscle fibers. Antibodies to these antigens will bind to all muscle tissue (including cardiac tissue) but not to other organs. This antibody also binds to the smooth muscle of blood vessel wall. Heart reactive antibodies are present in the sera of patients with streptococcal infection, connective tissue disease and postpericardiotomy syndrome. However, the levels are strikingly high in patients with acute rheumatic fever as compared to patients with uncomplicated streptococcal infections or streptococcal glomerulonephritis.

3. The modified major manifestations of Jones criteria for the
    diagnosis of rheumatic fever exclude (E).

A diagnosis of acute rheumatic fever based on two major criteria
is stronger than one based on one major and two minor criteria.
Major criteria include carditis, polyarthritis, chorea, erythema
marginatum and subcutaneous nodules. Minor manifestations include
fever, arthralgia, previous rheumatic fever or rheumatic heart disease, positive acute phase reactants and prolonged P-R interval.
Arthralgia or prolonged P-R interval are not valid minor manifestations when polyarthritis or carditis are counted as major manifestations respectively. An antecedent streptococcal infection evidenced
by positive culture for group A streptococci, increased antistreptolysin 0 or other streptococcal antibody or history of scarlet fever
is of prime importance for the diagnosis.

4. Prevention of recurrence of rheumatic fever and group A beta
    hemolytic streptococcal infection is by (B, D).

Recurrence of rheumatic fever may be triggered by another streptococcal infection in as many as 50% of patients who have had previous
rheumatic fever. The rate of recurrence decreases with time after
the initial attack. Monthly injections of 1. 2 million units of benzathin
penicillin is considered as the most effective protection. Oral drugs
such as sulfonamides (1 gram/day) or penicillin V (250 mg. b. i. d.)
if taken regularly are nearly as effective. Five to ten years of chemoprophylaxis is considered sufficient unless the patient has rheumatic
heart disease. In such instances chemoprophylaxis should be continued for life. Patients with rheumatic heart disease undergoing
dental, ear, nose, throat, or genitourinary tract procedures should
receive, in addition to rheumatic fever prophylaxis, prophylaxis for
bacterial endocarditis a day before, the day of, and two days after
the procedure.

5. Treatment of active rheumatic fever includes (D).

Penicillin is thought to be necessary to eliminate any viable streptococci although it has no effect on the severity or duration of acute
rheumatic fever. Moreover, to limit the possibility of irreparable
cardiac injury, suppression of the cardiac inflammatory reaction is
desired. Both salicylates and glucocorticoids suppress the acute
febrile and exudative manifestations of rheumatic fever but neither
has proven effective in diminishing the cardiac damage presumably
because the cardiac inflammatory process was initiated before overt
signs of carditis became apparent. Some authors recommend the use
of glucocorticoids for 2 weeks in patients with rheumatic carditis, to
be followed by salicylates (acetylsalicylic acid 100 mg/kg/24 hrs)
for 4 weeks. Others recommend salicylates only, and reserve glucocorticoids as an additional measure for those in congestive heart
failure and/or pericarditis.

REFERENCES

1. Hoeprich, P. D. (ed.): Infectious Diseases. Chapter 23. Strep-
    tococcosis, p. 255-267. Harper and Row, Hagerstown, Maryland,
    New York, Evanston, and London, 1972.

2. Zabriskie, J. B. : Heart-reactive antibodies. Resident and Staff,
    p. 57-64, April 1976.

3. Kaplan, M. H. and Frengly, J. D. : Autoimmunity to the heart in
    cardiac disease. Current concepts of the relation of autoimmunity
    to rheumatic fever, postcardiotomy and postinfarction syndromes
    and cardiomyopathies. Am. J. Card. 24:459, 1969.

4. Markowitz, M. , Kuffner, A. G. : Rheumatic fever: Diagnosis,
    Management and Prevention. W. B. Saunders, Philadelphia,
    1965.

5. Wannamaker, L. W. , Matesen, J. M. (ed.): Streptococci and
    streptococcal diseases. Academic Press, New York and London,
    1972.

6. Speck, W. T. , et al. : Transient bacteremia in pediatric patients
    after dental extraction. Am. J. Dis. Child. 130:408, 1976.

7. Rosenthal, A. , et al. : Rheumatic fever under 3 years of age:
    A report of 10 cases. Pediatrics 41:612, 1968.

8. Shulman, S. T. , Ayoub, E. M. : The control of rheumatic fever.
    Clin. Pediat. 14:319, 1975.

9. Blackman, N. S. , Kuskin, L. : Prophylaxis in rheumatic and non-
    rheumatic mitral insufficiency. Clin. Pediat. 14:261, 1975.

::

CASE 18: SPASMS IN A 9-DAY- OLD

HISTORY: This was the first hospital admission for a 9-day-old,
6-pound, black female infant. This baby was delivered after an uncomplicated 40 week gestation to a 34-year-old Para 9, Abortus 3,
Gravida 6 mother in a family auto on the way home from a funeral.
The baby breathed and cried spontaneously. She was seen by a local
physician and both patient and mother were then sent home, after
which the baby was considered to be perfectly well for two days. At
the age of 3 or 4 days, jerking movements of the arms and legs were
noted when a loud noise was made in the vicinity. This condition continued but did not increase in severity for the subsequent 5 days when
the mother took 3 siblings of the patient to a physician for evaluation
of a respiratory illness. While in the physician's office, the 9-day-old

baby was observed to have a seizure. She was taken immediately to a local hospital, received oxygen, and intramuscular lincomycin therapy, and fluids were administered subcutaneously by clysis. The patient was then transferred to a referral center.

FAMILY HISTORY: The siblings, ages 15, 13, 8, 5, 4 years were well. Immunization histories of the siblings were not known and the parents had no knowledge of their own immunizations. The family lived in the suburbs of a small city. They used city water and had indoor plumbing. The infant was receiving an evaporated milk formula.

PHYSICAL EXAMINATION: Temperature 38.3°C. Respirations 40-90. Pulse 160-220. Blood pressure 120, systolic palpable in the right arm. Height 40 cm. Weight 2,650 grams, Head circumference 33 cm. A well-developed, small infant whose most remarkable feature was her inability to open her mouth completely. The neck was alternately supple and rigid. The child had intermittent generalized muscular spasms. The chest was clear to auscultation and percussion. The abdomen varied from soft to absolute rigidity of the muscular wall. The umbilicus was observed to be crusted but no purulent material or erythema was present. No organomegaly was noted and the neurological examination showed symmetrically hyperactive reflexes. Every movement of the baby resulted in coarse jerks of the extremities and opisthotonus.

LABORATORY WORK: Hemoglobin, 12.6 grams%; hematocrit, 38%; WBC, 14,900; neutrophils, 34%; lymphocytes, 52%, monocytes, 9%, eosinophils, 5%. Serum chemistires revealed a BUN of 16 mg%; sodium, 145 meq./L; potassium, 5.6 meq./L; chloride, 111 meq. /L; CO_2 content, 23 mm/L; total protein, 7.1 gm%; albumin, 4.0 gm/100 ml; calcium, 10.5 mg/100 ml; phosphorous, 6.1 mg/100 ml; bilirubin, 5.0 mg/100 ml. After initial hydration, the BUN was subsequently recorded as 2-10 mg/ml. The bilirubin declined over one week to 0.4 mg/100 ml. CSF contained 55 rbc, 5 neutrophils, and a glucose was 140 mg./100 ml. No organisms were visible on Gram stain and the culture was subsequently negative. Blood culture was obtained and subsequently reported as sterile. Nasopharynx and stool showed no pathogens. An umbilical swab was obtained and the culture showed S. epidermidis and Proteus morganii.

COURSE IN HOSPITAL: The infant had continuous spasms precipitated by any stimulation. During the first two days of hospitalization 60-80 spasms were recorded and on days 4 and 5 the spasms numbered as many as 120. After a gradual decrease in frequency, no spasms were observed from day 9 through 14. Her appetite increased and she gained weight. She was discharged home on the 21st hospital day.

QUESTIONS:

1. Diagnosis of tetanus neonatorum is apparent in this infant. Immediate therapeutic measures include:
   A. Administration of intravenous glucose
   B. Administration of intravenous calcium gluconate
   C. Maintenance of an adequate airway and prevention of anoxia
   D. Administration of tetanus toxoid

2. Tetanus is caused by Clostridium tetani, a gram-positive, spore forming, anaerobic bacillus. Diagnosis of this infection is made:
   A. Only by isolation of the organism from wound or blood
   B. Primarily by the clinical constellation of symptoms
   C. Retrospectively by demonstration of serological response to the illness

3. Recovery and identification of C. tetani and other anaerobic organisms from clinical materials can be reliably accomplished:
   A. Only when the specimen is collected and immediately placed in anaerobic conditions for transport to the laboratory for subsequent culture under anaerobic conditions
   B. By streaking and plating of the specimen at the bedside onto a blood agar plate, MacConkey's or chocolate agar
   C. By the use of nitrogen filled chamber "glove box", in the bacteriology laboratory after the specimen is routinely obtained

4. Identification of the Clostridum tetani can be accomplished by:
   A. Gas chromatography
   B. Milk digestion
   C. Gram stain of the broth
   D. Growth on blood agar
   E. Toxin production

5. Specific therapy includes:
   A. 4-5 units/kg of tetanus immune globulin, Human (TIG), intramuscularly and by local infiltration
   B. Penicillin
   C. Equine Tetanus antitoxin (TAT), intramuscularly and intravenously
   D. Sedation: chlorpromazine, phenobarbital

6. Active immunization for tetanus is indicated for all infants and children. Indicate whether the following statements are true or false.
   A. Tetanus (the illness)confers immunity to the patient
   B. Infants can receive their first immunization in the first days of life
   C. Tetanus toxoid can be administered with TIG and successfully induce an antibody response

D. Adequate immunization is the receipt of 4 doses of DPT
    administered 3x at 2 monthly intervals, followed by a sub-
    sequent injection approximately 1 year after the third in-
    jection
E. Adults are immunized with the same material (DTP) in a
    similar manner
F. The booster vaccine material Td is administered every 3
    years

7. Tetanus in the U.S.A. is characterized by:
    A. The occurrence in women after abortion or delivery, after
        surgery, including that of G.I. tract, and after amputation
    B. Greatest mortality occurs in neonates and individuals
        > 50 years
    C. A preceding history of puncture wound or laceration in 50%
        cases
    D. Being the sequel of unusual wounds including frost bite, in-
        fected teeth and decubitus ulcers
    E. Occurrence in drug addicts

ANSWERS:

1. (A-C)

After obtaining a single serum specimen for laboratory determinations, rapid therapeutic manuevers would include the intravenous
administration of 50% glucose and calcium gluconate. Since it is
possible that this infant suffers from hypoglycemia, it is important
to give immediate therapy for this possibility. The clinical response of the infant should be instantaneous and the subsequent therapy can be guided appropriately.

The serum phosphate concentration in the neonatal period is frequently higher than in later infancy. Because of the low glomerular
filtration rate, and a relatively high rate of tubular reabsorption of
phosphate, the infant may maintain elevated serum phosphate levels.
This is particularly true if there is a large phosphate load such as
occurs with cows milk feedings. Recurrent convulsions can occur
and diagnosis depends upon the determination of serum calcium and
phosphate levels. Serum phosphorus may be high as 10-12 mg/100
ml. The principal treatment, if the infant is symptomatic is to administer intravenous calcium and subsequently add calcium to the
feedings in such amounts as to reduce the phosphate load. Calcium
phosphate will be precipitated in the intestine and thus the amount
of phosphate absorbed is reduced.

The maintenance of an adequate airway is of primary importance.
This may require endotracheal intubation or tracheostomy. The
amount of sedation will need to be individually adjusted to afford adequate relief from muscular spasms without inducing respiratory

depression. The administration of tetanus toxoid in the setting of
a patient symptomatic with illness has no therapeutic benefit for the
immediate situation.

2. (B)

A clinical constellation of symptoms remains the most reliable
means of diagnosis of this condition. Positive cultures of an infected
wound or umbilicus are useful confirmatory evidence but are frequently negative. This occurs if materials are not properly handled
or if the wound has subsequently healed so that the portal of entry
is no longer apparent. The toxin of C. tetani is extremely potent,
and quantities necessary to produce disease do not produce a significant antibody response in a patient. Therefore, a patient with
tetanus requires subsequent immunization, and serological determinations provide only confirmatory evidence of the absence of antibodies at the onset of illness.

3. (A)

The recovery of anaerobic organisms from clinical material has improved greatly within the last several years. The improvement results primarily from obtaining specimens under strictly anaerobic
conditions. Commercially available carbon dioxide filled tubes can
be carried to the bedside so that the material may be inoculated
directly into them. In addition, the modern bacteriology laboratory
is equipped with a nitrogen filled "glove box" in which all of the subsequent manipulations of the cultures can be formed. These techniques depend upon receiving specimens that have not been exposed
to air in the process of obtaining and transporting them to the laboratory.

4. (A, E)

C. tetani is one of six group IV Clostridia species which have terminal spores and liquify gelatin. Isolation of C. tetani is often difficult. A freshly poured blood agar plate lightly inoculated under an-
erobic conditions will show C. tetani swarming growth in 1-2 days.
The marginal cells are then transferred to broth. The original specimen can be mixed with broth and 0. 1 ml. injected at the base of the
tail of mice. Death or tetanus can sometimes be demonstrated even
though the organism is not detected by culture. Gas chromatography
can identify fermentation products such as acetic and butyric acids
with less proprionic acid, ethyl and butyl alcohols from peptone
yeast extract medium. Milk is only slowly clotted if at all. Lecithin-
ase is not produced but gelatin is liquified.

5.   (A, B, D)

Tetanus immune globulin (human) or TIG should always be used in
preference to equine tetanus antitoxin. The material is supplied as
250 units/vial. The preparations can be administered intramuscularly and infiltrated directly in the area of a defined wound. An op-
timum therapeutic dosage has not been established, although in older
children and adults a dosage of 3,000-6,000 units is recommended.
A retrospective analysis suggests smaller doses are equally effective. Injection of 4-5 units/kg of body weight provides a plasma level
of 0.01 to 0.02 units/ml for four weeks or more. TIG is commercially produced by several manufacturers and should be available in
any hospital setting. If TIG is not available, TAT of equine origin
should be used. It is administered as a single dose of 50,000-100,000
units, with desentization, if necessary, after appropriate testing for
sensitivity. Part of this dose (20,000 units) can be administered intravenously. It is unlikely that newborn infants will be previously
sensitized to equine serum; however, there is a small chance that
they have received transplacental material IgG containing antibodies
to equine serum. Penicillin is appropriate for killing the organisms
and therefore therapy for 10-14 days is usually recommened. Sedation for the newborn baby is individually determined at the time the
illness is being cared for. Chlorpromazine syrup 3 mg. every 6 hrs.,
phenobarbital, 10-20 mg. every 6 hrs.; mephenesin, 130-160 mg.
every 6 hrs.; and diazepam, 0.3 mg/kg. I.V. have been used to control severe spasms.

6.   (A) False. The illness does not confer immunity as the toxin is
a poor antigen, although a potent toxin.

    (B) True. This is impractical, however, because infants in the
first two weeks of life are apparently tolerant to the pertussis component of DPT vaccine. Immunization in the first days of life does
not produce an adequate antibody response to pertussis and these
children appear to be less able to produce antibodies for the subsequent 18 months of life.

    (C) True. If toxoid and antitoxin are administered simultaneous-
ly, they should be administered in separate syringes at different
sites. In adults the standard dose of toxoid (10 Lf/ml) and 250 units
of antitoxin can be given simultaneously.

    (D) True. Tetanus has not been reported in the United States in
individuals with adequate primary immunization. After 4 doses of
tetanus toxoid, antitoxin persists at protective levels for at least 5
years and an ability to react promptly to a booster injection persists
for a longer time.

(E) False. Adults are immunized with tetanus toxoid Td. It contains a smaller dose of diphtheria toxoid and there is no pertussis component. Two injections are given 2 months apart intramuscularly, and a third injection should then be given 6 months to 1 year later. In the U. S., women less than 20 and men older than 50 years are more likely to have antibody titers below the protective threshhold.

(F) False. Booster Doses: Children age 3-6 years receive 1 injection of DPT at the time of school entrance (that would be their 5th injection). Thereafter the recommended dose of Td is administered every 10 years. In management of injuries it is unnecessary to give a booster injection more than every 5 years. Adequate recall of immunity has been demonstrated with a booster injection 25 years past primary immunization. If tetanus immunization is incomplete, that is, less than 2 previous injections of tetanus toxoid, the remainder of the recommended series of injections should be given.

7. (A-E)

The retrospective analysis of reported tetanus [11] in the U. S. documents all of the features cited in this question. Of additional importance is the overall downward trend in morbidity and mortality since 1950. The peak incidence of disease occurs in neonates and those > 50 years, so that the mortality parallels the occurrence of disease.

REFERENCES

1. Garnier, Muller, J., et al. : Tetanus in Haiti. Lancet. pp. 383-386, Feb. 15, 1975.

2. Athavale, V. B. , Pai, P. N. : Tetanus neonatorum - clinical manifestations. J. Pediat. 67:649-657, 1965.

3. Smythe, P. M. , et al. : Treatment of tetanus neonatorum with muscle relaxants and intermittent positive-pressure ventilation. Brit. Med. J. 1:223-226, 1974.

4. McCracken, George H. , Jr. , et al. : Double-blind trial of equine antitoxin and human immune globulin in tetanus neonatorum. Lancet 1:1146-1149, June, 1971.

5. Levine, Leo, et al. : Active-passive tetanus immunization. NEJM 274:186-190, 1966.

6. McComb, James A. , Dwyer, Roderick C. : Passive-active immunization with tetanus immune globulin (Human). NEJM 268: 857-862, 1963.

7. Peebles, Thomas C. , et al. : Tetanus-toxoid emergency boosters. NEJM 280:575-580, 1969.

8.   Edsall, Geoffrey: The current status of tetanus immunization.
     Hosp. Prac. 6 (No. 7): 57-66, July, 1971.

9.   Brooks, Geo. F. , et al. : Tetanus toxoid immunization of adults:
     A continuing need. Ann. Int. Med. 73:603-606, 1970.

10. Blake, Paul A. , et al. : Serologic therapy of tetanus in U. S. ,
     1965-71. JAMA 235:42-44, 1976.

11. LaForce, F. Marc, et al. : Tetanus in the United States. NEJM
     280:569-574, 1969.

:::

CASE 19: HEPATOSPLENOMEGALY AND SKIN RASH IN A NEONATE

HISTORY: The patient was the male product of a full-term gestation
in a 24-year-old para 1, abortion 0, married, black female. Birth
weight was 2820 grams. Pregnancy was uncomplicated with the exception of a history of an erythematous macular rash on the forearms
in the 5th month of pregnancy. Labor and delivery were uncomplicated and initial physical exam was within normal limits except
for scrotal edema. The baby was discharged home on the 3rd hospital day. At 2 weeks of life the patient was seen because of progressive scrotal swelling, noisy breathing, and increase in abdominal
girth.

PHYSICAL EXAMINATION: Temperature 37°C, pulse 100/minute,
respiratory rate 38/minute, weight 2900 grams. An irritable, mini-
mally icteric baby with an erythematous rash over the thorax,
nasal congestion, rapid shallow respirations, and abdominal distention. The child's lungs were clear and heart was regular and
rhythmic. The liver was palpated 4 cms. below the right costal margin and firm. The spleen could be felt 2 cms. below left costal margin. The scrotum was edematous and the remainder of the physical
exam was unremarkable.

LABORATORY DATA: CBC revealed a hemoglobin of 4. 6 gms%,
hematocrit 16%, WBC 44,000 with 68% neutrophils, 24% lymphocytes,
3% stabs, 2% metamyelocytes, 2% myelocytes, 1% myeloblasts. The
platelet count was 182,500 and reticulocyte count was 5.9%. Peripheral
smear showed target cells, marked aniso and poikilocytosis with
microspherocytes, fragmented red blood cells, helmets, and drum
sticks. Sickle prep was negative. Coombs' test was negative.

QUESTION:

1. The differential diagnosis includes:
   A. Leukemia
   B. Congenital syphilis
   C. Congenital herpes simplex infection
   D. Congenital rubella
   E. Congenital cytomegalovirus
   F. Congenital toxoplasmosis
   G. All of the above

Further laboratory studies revealed a positive VDRL test on the baby's serum as well as on the mother's and father's serum. Fluorescent absorption test for syphilis (FTA-ABS) was positive on baby's serum, and the IgM was moderately elevated. Moreover, the patient had elevated liver enzymes and a total protein of 5.7 gms% with an albumin of 2 gms%. Bilirubin was 11.9 mg% total with 4.3 mg% direct. The LP was performed and was normal. X-rays of the long bones revealed a metaphysitis with an adjacent periostitis.

QUESTIONS:

2. Syphilis may be spread by:
   A. Sexual exposure
   B. Kissing
   C. Prenatal infection
   D. Transfusion
   E. Accidental direct inoculations
   F. All of the above

3. Signs of late congenital syphilis include:
   A. Frontal bossing and short maxilla
   B. High arched palate and Hutchinson's teeth
   C. Interstitial keratitis and 8th nerve deafness
   D. Saddle nose and mulberry molars
   E. Rhagades and saber shin
   F. All of the above

4. Non-treponemal serologic tests for syphilis include:
   A. Complement fixation tests (Kolmer and Wassermann)
   B. Flocculation tests (VDRL, Hinton, Kahn, Eagle, etc.)
   C. Treponemal pallidum immobilization (TPI)
   D. Reiter protein complement fixation (RPCF)
   E. Fluorescent treponemal antibody absorption test (FTA-ABS)
   F. Macro and microchemagglutination tests

5. The treatment of neonatal congenital syphilis includes:
   A. Benzathine penicillin-G
   B. Aqueous crystaline penicillin-G
   C. Aqueous procaine penicillin-G
   D. Gentamicin or kanamycin
   E. Tetracycline

6. All patients with early syphilis and congenital syphilis should be encouraged to:
   A. Return for repeat quantitative non-treponemal tests
   B. Undergo neurologic re-evaluation with a repeat CSF examination after 6 months if CNS involvement was initially demonstrated
   C. Have interviews and investigations made with their contacts
   D. Receive accurate information about their veneral disease in order to seek early medical care
   E. All of the above

ANSWERS:

1. The differential diagnosis includes (G).

The TORCH complex (toxoplasmosis, rubella, cytomegalovirus, herpes simplex) and syphilis, when acquired congenitally, as well as congenital leukemia, present with similar clinical signs and symptoms. The clinical signs of early congenital syphilis can be seen at birth but usually manifest themselves 2-4 weeks after delivery. There are 3 syndromes - the flu-like syndrome, the generalized adenopathy, and the rash. The flu-like syndrome in the baby manifests itself as lacrimation (iritis) and "snuffles" with nasal discharge that is thick, tenacious, and possibly hemorrhagic. The nasal mucous membrane has a number of erosions and/or mucous patches as does the oropharynx. The dark field examination of the erosions and discharge will show numerous spirochetes. The baby has a characteristic hoarse cry. The baby may also have an osteochondritis as evidenced by x-ray films. Moreover, a generalized, discrete, non-tender, hard adenopathy may be manifest. Rash in the infant may be maculopapular or papular but in contrast to the rash of acquired secondary syphilis, a bullous eruption may occur. In addition, the infant often has a distended abdomen with hepatosplenomegaly and hemolytic anemia.

2. Syphilis may be spread by (F).

About 95% of all syphilis is transmitted sexually. Kissing a person who has lesions of primary or secondary syphilis on the lips or oral cavity will transmit the disease, since the organisms are most perfuse in mucous membranes. Congenital syphilis occurs prenatally when the mother infects the fetus in utero and may be transmitted at any time in gestation. Inflammatory lesions are rarely, if ever, found

in the fetal tissue prior to 18 weeks of intrauterine life. It has been
recently shown that actual infection of the fetus occurs early in
pregnancy and that the pathogenic changes in the tissues may not
take place until after the 5th month when the fetus becomes immuno-
competent and inflammatory processes associated with plasma cells
can be found. In support of the hypothesis, on the few occasions
when treponemes were found in fetuses before the 5th month there
has been no reaction in fetal tissues. Spirochetes rarely, if ever,
overwhelm the early fetus, causing intrauterine death and expulsion,
and it has been shown repeatedly that syphilis is not a cause of first
trimester losses. Infection from transfusions is rarely seen today
because of the stringent requirement that all blood donors must have
a non-reactive blood test report before their blood can be used.
Moreover, on the conditions of blood bank storage, the spirochetes
of syphilis will die in 24 hours. Finally, accidental direct inoculations are another way of transmitting syphilis.

3.   Signs of late congenital syphilis include (F).

There are at least 14 stigmata that are helpful in the diagnosis of
late congenital syphilis. However, the above mentioned ones are
listed in the order of the frequency of their occurrence. Frontal
bossing of Parrot represent a localized periostitis of the frontal and
parietal bones. This may occur with rickets, and as an isolated lesion is not diagnostic of congenital syphilis. Syphilitic rhinitis,
when extending to the maxilla, prevents this bone from developing
normally, resulting in a concave or shallow-dish configuration in the
middle section of the face and a high arched palate. Short maxilla and
dependent alterations in the palate are not pathognomonic of congenital
syphilis. Saddle nose is the end result of a syphilitic rhinitis that is
usually the first manifestation of early congenital syphilis in the neonatal period. The bones and cartilage of the nasal cavity fail to develop properly, resulting in a repression at the root of the nose -
the so-called saddle nose. Hutchinson's triad of signs which are pathognomonic of late congenital syphilis include diffuse interstitial keratitis, 8th nerve deafness (Labyrinthine disease), and Hutchinson's
teeth. The abnormality in the upper central incisors of the permanent
dentition does not appear until age 6 or older. The teeth are peg-
shaped with the width of the biting surface less than the gingival margin. Interstitial keratitis is rarely present at birth. It is almost always caused by congenital syphilis but occasionally by tuberculosis.
The onset is usually between ages 5 and 25 with symptoms of acute
iritis: pain, tearing and photophobia, followed by clouding of the
cornea and invasion of the surface and stroma by the blood vessels.

The keratitis is not due simply to direct invasion by spirochetes but presumably reflects a local antigen-antibody reaction in a tissue sensitized by transient spirochetal invasion in fetal life. Antitreponemal drugs do not prevent or treat interstitial keratitis, although corticosteroids may suppress it. Eighth nerve deafness is usually not apparent until the second decade of life and is noted in elementary or junior high school students. In many cases the onset of deafness is ushered in by vertigo, followed by loss of hearing for the higher frequencies, and finally for the conversational tones. Rhagades are linear scars seen in the newborn radiating from the angles of the eyes, nose, mouth, chin, anus, and areas of moisture. When rhagades are present there are always other signs of congenital syphilis. Saber shin is an abnormality resulting from periostitis of the anterior and middle portion of the tibia which causes a thickening of the mid portion of the tibia with an anterior bowing of the bone. Saber shins may be seen as a result of rickets, fractures, osteomyelitis, and tumors.

4. Non-treponemal serologic tests for syphilis include (A, B).

The two kinds of antigens used in serologic tests for syphilis are treponemal and non-treponemal. The non-treponemal group includes the complement fixation test such as the Kolmer and Wassermann, and the flocculation tests (VDRL, Hinton, Kahn, Eagle). Treponemal tests include the Treponema pallidum immobilization (TPI) and the Reiter protein complement fixation (RPCF). There are also the immunofluorescent tests, the fluorescent treponemal antibody absorption tests (FTA-ABS), as well as the more recently available macro- and micro hemagglutination tests. Within the non-treponemal group, the flocculation tests are more sensitive, much easier to perform, much more economical, and more widely available than those characterized by complement fixation. Thus, they are generally used to screen for the presence of syphilis, and since they can also be titered, they are useful in monitoring treatment responses in early syphilis. A serum VDRL generally becomes positive 4-6 weeks after infection, usually some 1-3 weeks after the chancre first appears. It may revert to negative 6-24 months after treatment if therapy was effective. Thus it can be used in a general way as a follow-up. Treponemal tests are used to confirm or rule out syphilis when the history and physical exam and flocculation testing defy a definitive onset. Currently, the most common treponemal test is the FTA-ABS, which is the first laboratory index to become positive in early syphilis. It tends to stay positive long after effective treatment. When congenital syphilis is suspected, IgM-FTA-ABS is the test of choice since, if positive, it indicates specific IgM production by the fetus in utero. The newer macro and micro hemagglutination tests compare favorably with the FTA-ABS over all and they are more economical and easier to do. Furthermore, although they are less sensitive in primary syphilis, they are more sensitive in late infections and in previously treated cases. Because neither the treponemal nor the non-treponemal tests are truly specific, false positive reactions can be a problem. Biologic false-positive reactions occur with infections such as malaria, leprosy, viral pneumonia, measles, and infectious mononucleosis; recent smallpox or other vaccinations; and collagen diseases, including systemic lupus erythematosis and polyarteritis nodosa. Basically, any disease that can promote normal or increased immunoglobulins in the bloodstream can also cause a false-positive reaction to one or more of the tests of syphilis. Other treponemal diseases such as yaws, pinta, and bejel yield true positive FTA-ABS results.

5. The treatment of congenital syphilis includes (A, B, C).

In infants with congenital syphilis without CNS involvement, benzathine penicillin-G, 50,00 units/kg IM in a single dose is recommended. However, in infants with congenital syphilis and an abnormal CSF, aqueous crystaline penicillin-G 50,000 units/kg IM or IV daily in 2 divided doses for a minimum of 10 days is recommended; or one can use aqueous procaine penicillin-G, 50,000 units/kg IM daily for a minimum of 10 days. Clinical data on the efficacy of benzathine penicillin in congenital neurosyphilis are lacking, and the procaine or aqueous penicillin regimens are recommended if neurosyphilis cannot be excluded. Since CSF concentration of penicillin achieved after benzathine penicillin are minimal to nonexistant, these revised recommendations seem more conservative and appropriate until clinical data on the efficacy of benzathine penicillin can be accumulated. Other antibiotics are not recommended for neonatal congenital syphilis. After the neonatal period, the dosage of erythromycin and tetracycline for congenital syphilitics who are allergic to penicillin should be individualized, but need not exceed dosages used in adult syphilis of more than 1 year's duration. Tetracycline should not be given to children less than 8 years of age.

6. All patients with early syphilis and congenital syphilis should be encouraged to (E).

Repeating quantitative non-treponemal test 3, 6, and 12 months after treatment is essential. Patients with syphilis of more than 1 year's duration should also have a repeat serologic test 24 months after treatment. All patients with neurosyphilis must be carefully followed with serologic testing for at least 3 years. In addition, follow-up of these patients should include clinical evaluation at 6 month intervals and repeat CSF examinations. Interviewing and investigating the contacts should begin with the infected patient. When the contacts are found, they should be examined and treated. These patients should receive accurate information about their venereal disease.

REFERENCES

1. Holder, W. R. , Knox, J. M.: Syphilis in pregnancy. Med. Clin. N. A. 56:1151, 1972.

2. Silverstein, A. M.: Congenital syphilis and the timing of immuno-genesis in the human fetus. Nature 194:196, 1962.

3. Harter, C. A. , Benirscke, K.: Fetal syphilis in the first trimester. Am. J. Obstet. and Gynecol. 124:705, 1976.

4. Kaplan, J. M. , McCracken, G. H.: Clinical pharmocology of benzathine penicillin-G in neonates with regard to its recommended use in congenital syphilis. J. Pediat. 82:1069, 1973.

5. Jaffe, H. E.: The laboratory diagnosis of syphilis. Ann. Int. Med. 83:846, 1975.

6. Miller, G. N.: Value and limitations of non-treponemal and treponemal tests in the laboratory diagnosis of syphilis. Clin. Obstet. and Gynecol. 18:191, 1975.

7. Treatment of syphilis and gonorrhea. The Medical Letter, Vol. 18, No. 7, March 26, 1976.

8. Center for Disease Control: Syphilis - CDC recommended treatment schedule, 1976. J. Infect. Dis. 134:97, 1976.

::

CASE 20: A NEWBORN WITH STRANGE APPEARANCE AND PETECHIAE

HISTORY: The patient was a 4-pound, 12-ounce baby delivered at the end of 35 weeks gestation to a 16-year-old married Gravida 1, Para O female. Membranes ruptured two days prior to delivery and the only complication of pregnancy was a reported urinary tract infection two months prior to delivery. The delivery was uncomplicated and the Apgar was 9. The infant was noted to have petechiae diffusely distributed over all body surfaces.

CLINICAL EXAMINATION: The child was thought to be irritable with a high-pitched cry and observed to be microcephalic. Pulse 156. Respirations 66. Head circumference 27. 5 cm. Length 43 cm. The anterior fontanelle and sutures were open. Pertinent physical examination included normal cardiac examination, a liver palpable 2 cm. below the right costal margin and a spleen palpable 5 cm. below the left costal margin. By Dubowitz criteria the child was judged to be the product of 35 to 36 weeks gestation.

ACCESSORY LABORATORY INFORMATION: Hemoglobin, 13. 6
grams% with 18 nucleated red blood cells/100 red blood cells. White
blood cells 37, 400/mm^3 with 50% neutrophils, 23% lymphocytes,
12% monocytes, 15% stabs. Platelets 43, 000/mm^3. Urinalysis was
unremarkable. STS negative. The patient was blood Type O and had
a negative Coombs test. Skull films obtained showed periventricular
calcifications. Cerebrospinal fluid showed an icteric spinal fluid
with 5 mononuclear white blood cells, protein 380 mg%, and sugar
45-90 mgm.%. The cultures were sterile for bacteria.

COURSE IN HOSPITAL: The child seemed to stabilize and feed well.
On the 10th day she developed seizures which were documented on
EEG and phenobarbital therapy was initiated.

QUESTIONS:

1. Intrauterine infection is suggested by the following clinical fea-
    tures of this baby's illness: small for gestational age, micro-
    cephaly, hepatosplenomegaly, and petechiae. Differential diag-
    nosis includes:
    A. Rubella virus
    B. Cytomegalovirus
    C. Herpes simplex virus
    D. Coxsackie viruses
    E. Syphilis

2. Evaluation of the baby included "TORCH" titers. The results
    were as follows: Cytomegalovirus CF Abtiter = 1:16, toxoplasmo-
    sis indirect hemagglutination (IHA) antibody titers = 1:64, herpes
    simplex virus Cf antibody titer 1:8, VDRL negative, rubella
    hemagglutinating inhibiting (HAI) antibody titer 1:64. The follow-
    ing statements are true:
    A. These titers indicate infant infection with each of these
        agents except syphilis
    B. Simultaneous determination of maternal antibodies would
        allow differentiation of congenital infection as the titers
        would be higher in the infant
    C. These titers represent evidence of infection (probably mater-
        nal) with each agent except T. pallidum at an undetermined
        time and additional studies are needed

Additional investigation of the possibility of cytomegalovirus infection was instituted. A urine and peripheral white blood cells from
the infant were obtained and found to be positive for cytomegalovirus
by tissue culture isolation of the virus. Complement fixation and indirect hemagglutination antibody titers to CMV were done on the
mother and father and the results are listed below:

	CMV CF	CMV IHA
Mother	1:128	≥ 1:1024
Father	1:64	1:64

Cytomegalovirus was isolated from the mother's urine, the baby's urine, and at a later date from the liver, kidney and spleen of the infant.

QUESTIONS:

3. Indicate which of the following statements are true:
   A. Cytomegalovirus infection as indicated by a CF antibody titer of 1:8 or greater is unusual in adult women
   B. The excretion of cytomegalovirus by the infant in the first several days of life is indicative of intrauterine acquisition of virus
   C. Congenital infection with cytomegalovirus occurs only with primary maternal infection
   D. Cervical and/or urinary excretion of virus by the mother during pregnancy indicates a reason to consider therapeutic interruption of pregnancy because of the frequency of associated infected and affected infants

4. Cytomegalovirus has been isolated from the following materials:
   A. Breast milk
   B. Urine
   C. Cervix
   D. Salvia
   E. Peripheral white blood cells
   F. A variety of tissues of infected infants including liver and lung

5. The following clinical features have been observed in association with congenital cytomegalovirus infection:
   A. Circulating antigen-antibody complexes
   B. Hemolytic anemia
   C. Myeloproliferation prompting a differential diagnosis of congenital leukemia
   D. Biliary atresia
   E. Congenital ascites

6. Auditory difficulties occurring as a result of congenital cytomegalovirus infection may be characterized by:
   A. Complete loss of hearing
   B. A deficit only in high frequencies
   C. Progression of deficit during the first 2-4 years of life
   D. In a few instances isolation of virus from the Reissner's membrane and organ of Corti
   E. Far more frequent occurrence than ocular abnormalities

ANSWERS:

1. (A-E)

The hallmark of intrauterine infection with either rubella or cytomegalovirus is a small for gestational age infant. Either of these
infections may prohibit optimal intrauterine growth. The vast majority of neonatal herpes simplex and Coxsackie virus infections
are acquired during the process of delivery and thus the weight of
infants is usually appropriate for gestational age. Infants with congenital syphilis do not tend to be small for gestational age. Microcephaly is also more characteristic of intrauterine infection with
either rubella or cytomegalovirus. This suggests that brain development has been severely compromised and implies infection of some
duration. The hepatosplenomegaly represents active hepatitis and
splenic involvement as evidenced by the isolation of either of these
agents from tissues of infected infants. The liver is a primary target for infection due to the hematogenous spread of viral (and bacterial) agents occurring via the umbilical vessels. Any of these infections may be associated with thrombocytopenic purpura and these
viruses have been isolated from bone marrow. The hepatitis of
herpes simplex virus infection is usually not present at birth but
again occurs in association with the other symptoms sometime after
the fifth day of life. This feature of HSV related illness often represents the first indication of disseminated intravascular coagulation.
Statistically, cytomegalovirus is by far the most frequent of the
agents listed in the differential diagnosis. Approximately 1% of all
newborn infants may be excreting cytomegalovirus.

2. (C)

IgG antibodies are transported across the placenta and thus the antibody titers in cord serum may represent only maternal experience.
The absence of detectable antibodies may be useful in ruling out an
agent as being of possible etiologic concern. The height of these
antibody titers will not define the presence of infection in the infant.
It is not unusual to observe a quantitatively greater titer of antibody
in fetal serum than in maternal serum at the time of delivery. Additional studies should include a quantitation of the IgM in the infants
serum. It is also possible to obtain specific IgM antibody titers for
toxoplasmosis, syphilis and rubella and sequential determinations
of infant antibody titers may be helpful. Passively transmitted antibodies should decline in the first three to six months of life so that
the baby progressively loses detectable antibodies to the agents
listed.

3. (B)

The prevalence of cytomegalovirus antibodies varies with the population being studied. Approximately 50% of women of lower socioeconomic groups are antibody positive by the age of 13 years and 80%

by age 25 years. Approximately 55% of women of upper socioeconomic groups are positive by the age of 25 years. Thus, cytomegalovirus infection particularly in the lower socioeconomic age groups is common. Evidence is accumulating to indicate that congenital infection with cytomegalovirus may occur in women who are undergoing recurrent cytomegalovirus infection as well as primary infection. Not only have two infected infants been born consecutively to a single mother in at least 3 reported cases, but women who have been documented to excrete cytomegalovirus prior to conception may subsequently have an infected infant. Some evidence would tend to suggest that infants may be more severely affected if infection is transmitted during a primary infection.

Longitudinal evaluation of women during pregnancy has shown that a significant number, from 5-30%, will excrete virus sometime during their pregnancy. Virus tends to be suppressed during the first trimester and excretion is more common in the last trimester. The majority of women who excrete virus do not have a discernible rise in cytomegalovirus antibody titers or have infected infants. Thus, detecting viral excretion during the latter part of pregnancy is of itself not an adequate reason for consideration of therapeutic interruption of the pregnancy.

Infants who have acquired cytomegalovirus during the delivery or in the immediate postpartum months do not excrete virus during the first days of life. Therefore, the excretion of virus in the urine during the first days of life is indicative of intrauterine acquisition of this agent.

4. (A-F)

All of these materials have been shown to contain virus. CMV is most commonly detected in the urine and cervix of pregnant women. The detection of virus in saliva or peripheral white blood cells is less common and may indicate a poorly localized infection. In the immediate postpartum period breast milk may contain virus, and the tissues from infected infants who have been extensively investigated contain virus in virtually all the viscera.

5. (A-E)

Careful studies have shown circulating antigen antibody complexes in congenital CMV infection. There is a tendency for IgM complexes to be more prevalent, and in a very few cases deposition of antibody and complement in the glomeruli of the kidney have been observed at postmortem examination. Hemolytic anemias associated with acquired cytomegalovirus infection are well described. Less frequently a leukemoid response or myeloproliferation has been observed in infants with congenital infection. These cells have enhanced colony forming ability and the significance of these observations is not yet understood. Several infants with congenital biliary atresia with congenital cytomegalovirus infection have been reported. These may constitute one of the insults predisposing to this unfortunate congenital anomaly. Finally, ascites due to obstruction of GU tract or severe hepatic disease in association with congenital cytomegalovirus infection has also been described.

6. (A-E)

The potential magnitude of the sensorineural hearing deficit has only recently been appreciated. A complete loss of hearing as well as a deficit occurring only in high frequencies has been described. Most alarming is the observation that this deficit may progress over the first 2-4 years of life. Virus has been detected in Reissner's membrane and the organ of Corti. The hearing deficit is much more common than any ocular deficits with cytomegalovirus infection. An estimated 5-1000 cases of hearing deficit in infants may be due to CMV each year in the United States. (CMV infection occurs 1/100 deliveries and 10/60 infected babies have had a hearing deficit. Thus, 1 infant/600 deliveries may have a deficit and there are 3×10^6 deliveries in the U. S. per year.)

REFERENCES

1. Reynolds, David, W , et al. : Maternal cytomegalovirus excretion and perinatal infection. NEJM 289:1-5, 1973.

2. Stagno, Sergio, et al. : Cervical cytomegalovirus excretion in pregnant and non-pregnant women: Suppression in early gestation. J. Infect. Dis. 131:522-527, 1975.

3. Reynolds, David W. , et al. : Inapparent congenital cytomegalovirus infection with elevated cord IgM levels. NEJM 290:291-296, 1974.

4. Starr, John G. , et al. : Inapparent congenital cytomegalovirus infection. NEJM 282:1075-1078, 1970.

5. Kumar, Mary L. , et al. : Inapparent congenital cytomegalovirus infection. NEJM 288:1370-1372, 1973.

6. Melish, Marian E. , Hanshaw, James-B. : Congenital Cytomegalovirus Infection. Am. J. Dis. Child. 126:190-194, 1973.

7. Hanshaw, James B. , et al. : School failure and deafness after "silent" congenital cytomegalovirus infection. NEJM 295:468-470, 1976.

8. Embil, J. A. , et al. : Congenital cytomegalovirus infection in
    two siblings from consecutive pregnancies J. Pediat. 77:417-
    421, 1970.

9. Stagno, Sergio, et al. : Pediatrics 52:788-794, 1973.

10. Davis, Larry E. , et al. : Cytomegalovirus mononucleosis in
    a first trimester pregnant female with transmission to the fetus.
    Pediatrics 48:200-206, 1971.

11. Frank, Donald J. , et al. : Fetal ascites and cytomegalic in-
    clusion disease. Am. J. Dis. Child. 112:604-607, 1966.

12. Symonds, Daniel A. , Driscoll, Shirley G. : Massive fetal as-
    cites, urethral atresia, and cytomegalic inclusion disease. Am.
    J. Dis. Child. 127:895-897, 1974.

13. Weinberg, Arthur G. , et al. : Monoclonal macroglobulinemia
    and cytomegalic inclusion disease. Pediatrics 51:518-524,
    1973.

14. Kantor, Gary, L. , et al. : Immunologic abnormalities induced
    by postperfusion cytomegalovirus infection. Ann. Int. Med.
    73:553-558, 1970.

15. Coombs, R. R. H. : Cytomegalic inclusion-body disease asso-
    ciated with acquired autoimmune haemolytic anaemia. Brit.
    Med. J. 2:743-744, 1968.

::

CASE 21: HEPATIC FAILURE IN THE NEWBORN

HISTORY: A 16-day-old, white male infant who was the 1300 gram
product of a 32-week gestation was transferred to a University Medical Center. The infant was born to a 19-year-old Gravida I, Para
0 mother whose pregnancy was complicated by repeated episodes of
vaginal spotting. One month prior to delivery the mother was hospitalized with jaundice and found to have a positive hepatitis B surface antigen test of her serum. The mother subsequently did well
but labor began spontaneously with rupture of membranes four days
prior to delivery of the infant. The child was reported to have good
color and a spontaneous cry. He was considered well until 9 days of
age when icterus was present and phototherapy initiated because of
a bilirubin of 8. 7 mg%. During the subsequent two days, apnea and
bradycardia occurred requiring frequent stimulation. One day prior
to transfer of the infant, rales were heard on physical examination
and chest x-ray revealed right upper lobe infiltration. Penicillin and
kanamycin therapy was initiated and the infant was transferred.

PHYSICAL EXAMINATION: Temperature 36. 8°C. Pulse, 164.
Respirations, 62. Blood pressure, 60/36. Weight, 1145 grams.
Head circumference, $27\frac{1}{2}$ cm. Height, 40 cm. Skin: No observable
rash or cutaneous lesions. Remarkable physical findings included
bilateral coarse breath sounds but no audible rales. The abdomen
had no organomegaly but the liver edge was palpable 1 cm. from
the right costal margin. The infant was alert, demonstrated a good
suck, grasp and Moro reflex.

ACCESSORY LABORATORY DATA: Hemoglobin, 17. 5 grams%,
hematocrit 52%, WBC 12,900, neutrophils, 11%, bands, 50%, lymphocytes, 12%, myelocytes 19%. Platelets 130,000. Bacterial cultures
of the blood, cerebrospinal fluid and urine were sterile. Nose culture grew group B beta hemolytic streptococci. Hepatitis B surface
antigen and antibody was absent from serum.

COURSE IN HOSPITAL: The pneumonia persisted and progressed
after gentamicin and ampicillin therapy were begun. Methicillin
was subsequently initiated 7 days after admission. Pulmonary compromise resulted in progressive changes in support therapy from
nasal CPAP to an increase in the FIO_2 and finally to a respirator.
The infant retained CO_2. He maintained a persistent hyponatremia
with a serum sodium ranging from 119 to 127. His progressive deterioration continued. A second lumbar puncture was performed two
weeks after admission and bacterial cultures were again sterile although the fluid was grossly bloody. During the third week of hospitalization ascites developed with serum SGOT of 134, SGPT of 77,
alkaline phosphatase of 51, and LDH of 496. Paracentesis produced
yellow fluid with characteristics of transudate. Hepatitis surface
antigen was still negative in this serum. During the fourth week of
hospitalization seizures occurred. The semicomatose state of the
infant prompted a serum NH3 determination and a value of 359 was
recorded. Two double exchange transfusions were accomplished but
the NH3 ranged from 206 to 980. During the fourth week of hospitalization, the child became anuric and subsequently expired. The final
serum sample obtained during the three days prior to death of this
infant was hepatitis B surface antigen positive. Viral cultures were
done and the results are listed in Table 21-1.

TABLE 21-1		
DATE	SPECIMEN	
6/28	N/P culture	Herpes Simplex Virus
6/28	Urine, Stool	Herpes Simplex Virus
7/2	Paracentesis site of abdomen	Herpes Simplex Virus

QUESTIONS:

1. Herpes simplex virus infection of the newborn baby is most fre-
quently acquired by:
   A. Transplacental transmission of the virus associated with
      maternal viremia
   B. Acquisition of virus from the infected birth canal
   C. Nosocomial contact within the newborn nursery

2. Infection of herpes simplex virus can produce:
   A. Disseminated disease of the newborn
   B. Congenital anomalies of the newborn
   C. Localized infection of the newborn

3. Infection of the newborn infant is characterized by:
   A. Age at onset of symptoms - birth to 3 weeks, usually about
      6 days
   B. The presence of skin vesicles
   C. Pulmonary infiltrates
   D. Meningitis
   E. Hepatic enlargement

4. Specific laboratory diagnosis of herpes infection of the newborn
   includes:
   A. The presence of intranuclear inclusions/multinuclear giant
      cells in Papanicolaou stained smears of cells from vesicular
      lesions, maternal cervix, conjunctivae, cornea or urine
   B. Isolation of herpes simplex virus from the respiratory tract,
      urine, blood, CSF and other body fluids
   C. Examination of biopsy or autopsy samples of tissue (including
      lung, liver, and spleen) for intranuclear inclusions and iso-
      lation of virus from tissues
   D. Elevation of IgM during the first 2-3 weeks of life
   E. Presence of herpes simplex neutralizing antibodies

5. Attempted therapy of herpes simplex virus infection of the new-
   born should include consideration of:
   A. Halogenated pyrimidines
   B. Immune serum globulin
   C. Purine nucleosides

ANSWERS:

1. (B)

Acquisition of herpes simplex virus by the newborn infant most frequently occurs in association with passage through the birth canal
and contact with infectious virus in this location. There is some evidence to suggest that virus may gain access to the fetus, ascending
from the birth canal, after labor has been in progress for more than

four hours. Although there are a few cases [7,9] indicating that virus
may occasionally be acquired by the transplacental route, these
situations are unusual. There is a single report of apparent nosocomial transmission of herpes simplex virus [3]. For these reasons,
the recommendation has been made that the identification of active
herpes simplex viral infection of the maternal birth canal at the
time of delivery should indicate the need to consider caesarean section. Since the risk of neonatally acquired herpes simplex would appear to be somewhat less if a caesarean section is performed before
labor has progressed for four hours, this recommendation is presently made. Women who have active herpes simplex infection only at
an earlier period of time in their pregnancy should not be subjected
to caesarean section.

2. (A-C)

Several reports have appeared which indicate a small number of
infants with identifiable congenital anomalies are associated with
intrauterine herpes simplex infection [6,11,12,13]. These infants
have congenital malformations of the central nervous system including microcephaly, intracranial calcification, microphthalmus,
retinal dysplasia, and one child has been observed with an associated patent ductus arteriosus and short digits with deformed nails.
These infections are presumed to be a result of transplacental
transmission of virus. Both herpes Type I and herpes Type II have been
implicated as causative of these infections. Disseminated herpes
simplex virus infection of the newborn infant results in visible infection
of the central nervous system, lungs, liver, spleen, skin, and is associated with detectable virus in the nasopharyngeal secretions, urine,
peripheral white cells/ and cerebrospinal fluid. The extent of involvement varies from one infant to another. Infants have been
observed in whom the disease is apparently localized to the central
nervous system, eye, skin, or oral cavity. In general, the outcome
is far better if the disease is localized to the skin, eyes, and/or
oral cavity. Survival is particularly poor in groups with disseminated disease or in disease localized to the central nervous system.

3. (A-E)

The infant usually does well for the first several days of life, during
the incubation period of virus infection. Unfortunately, not all infants
have recognizable vesicular lesions assisting in the recognition of
infection. These visible cutaneous stigmata are present in only 42%
of cases with disseminated herpes and 67% of cases with local central
nervous system involvement. Pulmonary involvement is not unusual
and there is nothing characteristic about the x-ray features suggesting that herpes simplex virus is the causative agent. The pneumonitis
is usually not apparent until the end of the first week of life. The central nervous system involvement may be the dominant clinical feature of the infection. Frank seizures and evidence of increased intracranial pressure may progress rapidly. Herpes virus can usually be

isolated from the cerebrospinal fluid of the neonate whose CSF frequently has a mononuclear pleocytosis with an elevated protein. Of
particular interest is the involvement of the liver and adrenal glands.
This involvement is characterized by focal necrosis with a minimal
amount of inflammation. Although the liver is involved in almost all
fatal cases of neonatal herpes simplex, the infant may not be jaun-
diced during life. Thirty percent of the cases in one series had
neither jaundice or hepatomegaly. The catastrophic nature of the
liver involvement is evidenced by the present case where a rise in
enzymes was minimal and yet the total destruction of the liver was
apparent by the elevation of the serum ammonia, with development
of ascites, and the appearance of disseminated intravascular coagulation.

4. (A-C)

The characteristic features of herpes simplex infection of cells include Cowdry Type A intranuclear eosinophilic inclusion bodies. In
certain tissues, multinucleate giant cells may sometimes be seen as
a result of herpes simplex infection. These pathological features are
not specific for herpes simplex virus and other herpes viruses; for
example, cytomegalovirus and varicella zoster virus can induce
identical changes in infected tissues. Therefore, although the pathology can suggest infection with a herpes agent and the epidemiology
may provide a clinical diagnosis isolation of virus remains the sine
qua non for identifying the etiologic agent as herpes simplex virus.
As indicated in the preceding questions, herpes simplex infection of
the newborn is often disseminated and therefore virus can be isolated
from many sites. It is worth contrasting these findings to those of
infection in an older patient. Herpes encephalitis with localization
in the temporal lobe of the cerebral hemispheres may produce devastating disease. Virus is almost never isolated from the CSF in this
setting, although sporadic reports have indicated that viral antigen
may be detected by immunofluorescence. Herpes simplex virus grows
rapidly in a number of different cell culture systems. It is an easy
agent to isolate and frequently is detectable within 24-48 hours after
obtaining materials from the patient. Virus has also been visualized
by EM examination of vesicular tissue. As in the present case, the
absence of cutaneous vesicular lesions in an extremely ill premature
infant makes it difficult to diagnose this infection unless specific
cultures are obtained. Occasionally it happens that a biopsy of the
liver or other tissues is obtained and the characteristic pathology
then alerts the clinician to the possible presence of herpes simplex
virus. Although the infant may have an elevation of IgM antibodies
during the first several weeks of life, characteristically this is not
detected in cord blood because the infant is acquiring his infection
during parturition. Identification of herpes simplex neutralizing antibodies in the infant's serum does not specify whether the antibodies
are maternal or infant in origin. IgG neutralizing antibodies can
cross the placenta readily and the majority of women of child bearing

age have measurable antibodies. Therefore, the detection of this activity in fetal serum may merely represent maternal experience with the virus. Continued detection of antibody or a rise during the first months of life may offer confirmation of infection if the infant survives.

5. (C)

The extremely high rate of morbidity and mortality with neonatal herpes simplex infection has prompted early attempts to alter the course of this illness. Since many cases of maternal herpetic infection are not recognized clinically, it is often impossible to identify the infant at risk and perform a caesarean section. One halogenated pyrimidine, 5-idoxuridine (IDU) has been tested in a number of clinical situations. Topical application to the conjunctiva appears to alter the course of kerato conjunctivitis caused by herpes virus. The effects of IDU are seen in host cells as well as on viral replication. This phosphorylation of IDU to 5-idoxuridine triphosphate allows its incorporation into DNA. The 5-iodouracil replaces thymine. The 5-iodouracil does not pair with adenine as faithfully as thymine and mismatching occurs during replication and transcription of the substituted DNA. IDU itself also competively inhibits the synthesis of thymidine triphosphate which reduces the overall rate of DNA synthesis. The net result is that there is a reduced amount of DNA synthesized and that it is an altered DNA molecule which functions poorly. The use of this drug is associated with significant toxicity and has not appeared to alter the course of disease in a relatively small number of infants who have been treated. On the other hand, purine nucleosides, particularly adenine arabinoside (Ara-A), has been used for several years in an ongoing controlled clinical trial. The first collected group of cases [4] would appear to indicate that 10-20 mg/kg administered by a continuous 12-hour intravenous infusion for a period of 10-15 days is without significant toxicity to the infant. It is possible that this drug administered early in the course of disease may be efficacious but relatively few infants have been studied to date. The course of HSV infection is not uniform and, therefore, a larger group of infants must be evaluated. This drug is probably the one to be considered if therapy is to be instituted. Immune serum globulin has not been shown to alter the course of neonatal herpes simplex infection and maternal antibody crosses the placenta giving detectable antibody levels to these infants at the time of their illness.

REFERENCES

1. Nahmias, Andre J. , et al. : Herpes simplex virus infection of the fetus and newborn. In Infections of the Fetus and the Newborn Infant. (Saul Krugman and Anne Gershon editors) Vol. 3, pp. 63-77, 1975.

2. Young, Edward J. , et al. : Disseminated Herpesvirus infection.
    JAMA 235:2731-2733, 1976.

3. Francis, Donald P. , et al. : Nosocomial and maternally ac-
    quired herpesvirus hominis infections. Am. J. Dis. Child.
    129:889-893, 1975.

4. Ch'ien, Lawrence T. , et al. : Antiviral chemotherapy and neo-
    natal herpes simplex virus infection: A pilot study - experience
    with adenine arabinoside (Ara-A). Pediatrics 55:678-685, 1975.

5. Nahmias, Andre J. , et al. : Perinatal risk associated with
    maternal genital herpes simplex virus infection. Am. J. Obstet.
    Gynec. 110:825-837, 1971.

6. Sieber, Otto F. , Jr. , et al. : In utero infection of the fetus by
    herpes simplex virus. Pediatrics 69:30-34, 1966.

7. Witzleben, Camillus L. , Driscoll, Shirley G. : Possible trans-
    placental transmission of herpes simplex infection. Pediatrics
    36:192-198, 1965.

8. Hanshaw, James B. : Herpesvirus hominis infections in the
    fetus and the newborn. Am. J. Dis. Child. 126:546-555, 1973.

9. Light, Irwin J. , Linnemann, Calvin C. , Jr. : Neonatal herpes
    simplex infection following delivery by caesarean section.
    Obstet. and Gynec. 44:496-499, 1974.

10. Nehmias, Andrea J. , M. Ousama Tomeh: Herpes simplex
    virus infections. Current Prob. in Ped. IV, No 4, Feb. 1974.

11. Self, Mary Ann, et al. : Congenital malformation of the central
    nervous system associated with congenital type (Type II) herpes
    virus. J. Pediat. 75:13-18, 1969.

12. Florman, Alfred L. , et al. : Intrauterine infection with herpes
    simplex virus, resultant congenital malformations. JAMA
    225:129-132, 1973.

13. Montgomery, John R. et al. : Congenital anamolies and herpes
    virus infection. Am. J. Dis. Child. 126:364-366, 1973.

::

CASE 22: CONGENITAL HEART DISEASE AND MICROCEPHALY

HISTORY: This is the first hospital admission of an 8-day-old baby
girl who was the 2, 211 gram product of a 37 week gestation. Her
mother was 29 years old and para 2-0-1. She worked in a high school
as a clerk in the office. The pregnancy was complicated by an upper

respiratory tract infection at about 4 months, requiring some medications for symptomatic relief. During the 2-3 weeks prior to delivery an elevation in blood pressure and proteinuria was observed.
The mother was hospitalized, received magnesium sulfate, and when
there was no reduction in blood pressure a caesarian section was
performed. A previous child had also been delivered by C section
because of cephalopelvic disproportion. The baby was noted to be
small for gestational age. She was pale with grunting respirations
and required 25% oxygen. The child fed poorly, organomegaly was
noted, and a chest x-ray revealed cardiomegaly with an increase in
pulmonary vasculature. With these findings she was transferred to
a tertiary care center at 8 days of age.

PHYSICAL EXAMINATION: Temperature 37. 2°C. Pulse 180. Respirations 80. Blood pressure 70/44. Weight 2130 grams. Head circumference 31. 5 cm. She was a microcephalic infant without increased transillumination. She had micrognathia and unusually small
eyes. No cataracts were observed. Examination of her chest showed
normal breath sounds. Her heart was large with an active precordium. She had a Grade III/VI systolic murmur heard along the left
sternal border which radiated to the axilla. Abdomen: Liver was
palpable 3 cm. from the right costal margin, the spleen was 4 cm.
from the left costal margin. She was a moderately lethargic infant
with a depressed Moro reflex and poor grasp.

ACCESSORY LABORATORY DATA: Hematocrit 46%. WBC 22, 200
with 53% neutrophils, 3% bands, 35% lymphocytes, 6% monocytes,
2% eosinophils and 1% metamyelocyte. Her bilirubin was 13.0mg%
which gradually decreased over the subsequent 2 weeks in the hospital to less than 1 mg%. Cerebrospinal fluid, blood, and urine were
obtained for bacterial and viral cultures. Throat swab was also submitted for attempted viral isolation and a single serum sample was
obtained for total IgM and antibody determinations. The total IgM
was 40 mg%. VDRL was negative. No intracranial calcifications
were detected. Chromosomes were normal. The cerebrospinal fluid
had a protein of 132 mg%. and a glucose of 124 mg% and there were
no cells.

COURSE IN HOSPITAL: Cardiac catheterization studies demonstrated
and ASD, VSD, and systemic pulmonary artery pressures with a
large left to right shunt. She required digoxin. She developed seizures and phenobarbital therapy was initiated. An EEG showed evidence of multifocal cortical epileptic discharges. She required gavage
feedings because of her inability to suck well. She was discharged
after a prolonged hospitalization which was characterized by poor
weight gain.

QUESTIONS:

1. This small infant with microcephaly, hepatosplenomegaly, and congenital heart disease was suspected of having intrauterine infection. Additional information might be helpful in her evaluation. Indicate which of the following procedures would be appropriate.
   A. Contact with the obstetrician to ascertain what serological tests had been done at the beginning of pregnancy
   B. Attempts to determine if rubella-like illness had been identified in the school or county where she is employed
   C. Serological evaluation of the infant's serum for cytomegalovirus, rubella, and toxoplasma antibodies
   D. Determine the past history of rubella or rubella-like illness in the mother

2. The serological studies on a sample obtained on the 8th day of life revealed a cytomegalovirus CF titer of less than 1:4, rubella hemagglutinating inhibiting antibodies of 1:32, toxoplasmosis titers of less than 1:16 and a negative VDRL. Indicate which of the following statements is true.
   A. The rubella titer of 1:32 indicates congenital infection with rubella virus
   B. The absence of cytomegalovirus CF antibodies rules out the diagnosis of congenital cytomegalovirus infection
   C. Rubella specific IgM hemagglutination inhibiting antibodies would be helpful

3. Attempted definition of intrauterine viral infection by culturing suspected materials should include which of the following?
   A. Culture of peripheral white blood cells
   B. Culture of the urine on human fibroblasts and Vero cells
   C. Culture of the cerebrospinal fluid
   D. Culture of a throat swab

4. Management of this patient includes counseling of the parents with regard to the prognosis for the infant. Indicate which of the following statements is true.
   A. All infants infected with rubella virus have demonstrable congenital anomalies
   B. Infection in the second trimester of pregnancy has no residual effects on the infant
   C. Microcephaly, poor ability to feed and multiple congenital anomalies suggest very strongly that altered developmental retardation will be present
   D. Auditory deficiencies cannot be tested in this age group

5. Rubella immunization was designed to protect the fetus from the teratogenic effects of rubella virus. This is a unique form of immunization since the attenuated virus is administered to children so as to achieve serioimmunity in women by childbearing age. Indicate which of the following statements is true.
   A. The immunization program has not altered the pattern of rubella infection in the United States
   B. Rubella immunization does not prevent reinfection and therefore will not be effective in protection of the fetus
   C. Attenuated virus is not teratogenic and therefore can be administered to adult women
   D. The duration of immunity after rubella immunization is not yet known

ANSWERS:

1. (A-D)

The increasing availability of rubella hemagglutination inhibition tests by state laboratories and other sources provide an accessible means of determining immunity to rubella virus. Consequently, many obstetricians have this antibody test done at the time of an early prenatal visit. In the case under discussion, a negative titer early in pregnancy with a positive titer at the time of delivery would imply recent infection with rubella virus. This would not establish primary infection as it has been demonstrated that an antibody rise can occur with secondary exposure to rubella. In this case no such antibody determination had been performed.

The Department of Human Resources located within the State Health Department receives reports of communicable illnesses which are "reportable". In this case neither rubella virus infection has been reported, nor virus isolated, nor demonstration made of serological conversion in individuals in the county of residence of the patient. It would have been extremely helpful if an outbreak of such disease could have been identified. An infant's serum can be assayed for cytomegalovirus complement fixing antibodies, rubella hemagglutinating inhibiting antibodies and toxoplasmosis antibodies by indirect hemagglutination. If these determinations are negative it mitigates against the possibility of one of these agents being responsible for the infant's condition.

Positive antibody determinations indicate that antibody is present, but it may be maternal IgG globulin which has been placentally transmitted. It is appropriate to ask for a past history of rubella or rubella like infection but the history is notoriously unreliable. In this particular instance, the mother was certain that rubella had been diagnosed twice during her adolescence. The confusion results from exanthema due to other agents such as an enterovirus which is indistinguishable from rubella. In addition, since rubella can occur without a rash the disease may not be recognized. Therefore, the history is not particularly helpful unless perhaps an epidemic of disease is occurring.

2. (C)

As discussed in answer #1, the presence of detectable hemagglutinating inhibiting antibodies to rubella virus indicates that either the mother or the baby has encountered antigen. For that reason, rubella specific IgM hemagglutinating inhibiting antibodies would determine whether the infant was producing the antibodies. Since IgM antibodies do not traverse the placenta such antibodies must be the result of the infants antigenic stimulation. The absence of cytomegalovirus CF antibodies certainly mitigates against this virus as playing a role in the infant's illness, but the complement fixation assay may not be entirely sensitive for IgM antibodies. It is possible that an infant will be transiently antibody negative while excreting virus from the urine or having it detected in peripheral white blood cells. It would be worthwhile to attempt virus isolation from the urine and peripheral white blood cells and to repeat the antibody determination at a later time.

3. (A-D)

Cytomegalovirus has been successfully isolated from saliva or a throat swab, peripheral white blood cells, and urine during the first 48 hours of life in an infant who is congenitally infected. These infants may excrete virus from these sites for years. In addition, rubella virus is isolated from throat swabs, cerebrospinal fluid, and urine. Usually, virus is more easily detectable during the first several months of life and many infants no longer have detectable virus in urine or throat swabs by the age of 6 months. Since cytomegalovirus grows only on human fibroblasts, it is essential to utilize these cells as one culture system. Rubella virus grows on Vero cells; but its detection involves another indicator system with production of cytopathic effect or lack of superimposed infection with a second agent such as an enterovirus, to indicate that rubella virus had interfered with the cytopathic effect of this virus. In this instance, throat swab and urine inoculated into the test systems was able to interfere with cytopathic effect on an enterovirus subsequently inoculated into the cell culture systems. Rubella antiserum neutralized the interference.

4. (C)

The spectrum of disease associated with intrauterine rubella infections includes totally asymptomatic infants without congenital anomalies who have detectable virus excretion. The opposite end of the spectrum includes an undergrown infant with multiple congenital

anomalies as in the present case. Careful longitudinal evaluation of
pregnancies documented to be complicated by rubella virus infection
have shown that infants infected during the second trimester may indeed have detectable abnormalities of development. As the major
organogenesis has already occurred, the deficits involve subtle neurological abnormalities and may not be detected until the child is
several years of age. The visible effects on the central nervous system, observed difficulties feeding and associated congenital heart
disease of this infant suggest very strongly that mental retardation
may be a significant feature of this child's illness. Auditory deficiencies can be tested for in infants of any age, and very reliable
testing is accomplished in the first several months of life. It is important to define this deficiency so that awareness will allow the
parents to optimally correct for this and guide the physician in the
handling of this infant.

5. (D)

Rubella immunization has probably altered the pattern of rubella infection in the United States. Previously, the United States had a epidemiological pattern similar to that of Puerto Rico. Immunization
was not instituted in Puerto Rico where an epidemic of rubella occurred, whereas the United States did not have that outbreak. The
number of reported cases of adult or childhood rubella and congenital rubella has consistently declined since the advent of immunization.
Rubella is recognized less frequently and a national epidemic has not
occurred since 1964. It is correct that rubella immunization does not
prevent reinfection with the virus. Thus far, reinfection of pregnant
women has not been associated with detectable infection of the fetus
or abnormalities. This may represent the very small number of such
pregnancies that have been followed, but in the absence of previous
reports indicating that a mother might have two infected infants it
seems probable that reinfection is much less likely to lead to infection of the fetus. Attenuated virus has been demonstrated to cross
the placenta and to infect the fetus. In the majority of the situations
where this has been studied, the products of conception have been
obtained by therapeutic interruption of the pregnancy. In these instances the period of time after exposure to virus was too short to
allow development of congenital anomalies. The demonstration of
virus in fetal tissues means that under no circumstances should this
attenuated virus vaccine be administered to pregnant women. The
duration of immunity following rubella immunization is not yet known.
It seems likely that the risk of viremia is decreased, although antibody rises following either natural exposure or reimmunization indicate that subclinical infection has occurred. The change in the epidemiology of rubella virus infections in the United States suggests
that immunization has altered the occurrence of congenital infection
and that continued surveillance is mandatory for determining the
future recommendations with this vaccine.

REFERENCES

1. Desmond, Murdina M. , et al. : Congenital rubella encephalitis: Course and early sequellae. J. Pediat. 71:311-331, 1967.

2. Krugman, S. editor: Rubella Symposium, Am. J. Dis. Child. 110:345-476, 1965.

3. Menser, Margaret A. , Forrest, Jill N. : Rubella/high incidence of defects in children considered normal at birth. Med. J. Austr. 1:123-126, 1974.

4. Unsigned Editorial: Rubella Reinfection and the fetus. Lancet May 5, 1973, p. 978.

5. Vesikari, Timo, et al. : Immune response of the neonate and diagnosis by demonstration of specific IgM antibodies. J. Pediat. 75:658-664, 1969.

6. Dudgeon, J. A. : Congenital rubella. J. Pediat. 87:1078-1086, 1975.

7. Lerman, Stephen J. , et al. : Accuracy of rubella history. Ann. Int. Med. 74:97-98, 1971.

8. Krugman, S. : Present status of measles and rubella immunization in the United States: A medical progress report. J. Pediat. 90:1-12, 1977.
::

CASE 23: FEVER, VOMITING, DROWSINESS, NECK STIFFNESS AND HEADACHE

HISTORY: A 5-year-old boy presented with the chief complaint of low grade fever of 2 weeks duration associated with loss of appetite and malaise. Three days prior to admission, he developed a non-throbbing generalized headache, neck stiffness and progressive drowsiness. He became lethargic and had several episodes of vomiting not related to food intake. The past medical history was essentially negative. There was no history of head trauma. The patient lived with his grandmother who gave a history of chronic cough.

PHYSICAL EXAMINATION: Temp. 38. 9°C, pulse 90/minute, B. P. 110/75 mm Hg. , respiratory rate 28/minute, weight 18 kg. Physical examination revealed an ill-appearing, apathetic and drowsy young boy with a stiff neck. Fundi are normal. The patient has positive Kernig's and Brudzenski's signs with increased deep tendon reflexes in both lower extremities. Babinski's sign was negative. There were no localizing neurological deficits. There was no generalized lymphadenopathy. The remainder of the physical examination was within normal limits.

LABORATORY DATA: CBC: Hgb. 12 gm%, Hct. 37%, WBC 12,000/
cu mm, PMN 70%, lymphocytes 28%, monocytes 2%. Urinalysis:
normal. Blood chemistry: normal BUN, sugar, calcium, and electrolytes. Lumbar Puncture: opening pressure 300 mm CSF, CSF
color clear. Cells 70 wbc, 60% lymphocytes. Sugar 28 mg% (blood
sugar 95 mg%), protein 110 mg%. Gram stain - no organism. Culture - no growth. India Ink prep - negative. Chest x-ray: infiltrates
in the right upper lobe. PPD (5 TU) 48 hrs. = 11 mm of induration.

QUESTIONS:

1. The most likely diagnosis is:
    A. Pneumococcal or H. influenzae meningitis
    B. Brain abscess
    C. Viral meningitis
    D. Tuberculous meningitis
    E. Brain tumor

2. The diagnosis of tuberculous meningitis is based mainly on the
    results of:
    A. Intradermal tuberculin test
    B. Chest roentgenogram
    C. History of tuberculous contact
    D. Examination of the CSF
    E. All of the above

3. The recommended therapy of tuberculous meningitis in children
    includes:
    A. Isoniazid, streptomycin and para-aminosalicylic acid
    B. Rifampin, ethionamide and streptomycin
    C. Ethambutol, isoniazid and para-aminosalicylic acid
    D. Rifampin, ethionamide and ethambutol
    E. None of the above

4. The prognosis of tuberculous meningitis depends on:
    A. Early diagnosis
    B. Presenting stage of disease
    C. Appropriate treatment
    D. All of the above
    E. A and C

5. Late sequelae of tuberculous meningitis include:
    A. Mental deficiency
    B. Hydrocephaly
    C. Cranial nerve palsies and/or convulsions
    D. Paresis and/or spasticity
    E. All of the above

ANSWERS:

1. The most likely diagnosis is (D).

Tuberculous meningitis commonly has an insiduous onset with gradual or intermittent increase in symptoms. Fever is almost always
present, often low grade at first and later associated with vomiting.
The most striking symptom is apathy, varying from a general lack
of interest to drowsiness. The first stage of tuberculous meningitis,
in which only general symptoms similar to those of many common
childhood ailments occur, lasts for one to two weeks. The second
stage may start abruptly with signs and symptoms pointing to the
involvement of the central nervous system, which leads over a
period of two to three weeks to stage three. Stage three is characterized by profound disturbance of the central nervous system and
marked changes in sensorium, including coma.

2. The diagnosis of tuberculous meningitis is based mainly on the
   results of (E).

Intradermal tuberculin test, chest roentgenogram, history of tuberculous contact, and examination of the cerebrospinal fluid (CSF) are
all important in the diagnosis of tuberculous meningitis. Positive
tests are most valuable in combination. In critically ill patients,
depression of delayed hypersensitivity to tuberculin varies from
total anergy to reactivity to only an increased dose of tuberculin.
In a series reported by Idriss et al. 93% and 72% of cases of tuberculous meningitis had a positive reaction to the tuberculin skin test
(PPD) and positive pulmonary roentgenographic changes respectively. Cerebrospinal fluid pleocytosis may be absent initially or throughout the course, and a marked polymorphonuclear response may be
observed. In the majority of cases, CSF changes consist of low
glucose, elevated protein and pleocytosis. Hinman, in 1967, found
that the CSF sugar was the first parameter to return to normal after the institution of therapy. This was followed by temperature,
CSF cell count, and lastly CSF protein. Finally, the history of
tuberculous contact is important for both diagnosis and treatment.
A contact infected with a resistant strain should be vigorously
sought since in these instances failure is common if conventional
antimycobacterial agents are used.

3. The recommended therapy of tuberculous meningitis includes
   (A).

Isoniazid (INH), streptomycin, and para-aminosalicylic acid (PAS)
are the three first-line antituberculous drugs recommended for the
therapy of tuberculous meningitis in children. Although alternate
regimens using other antimicrobial agents have gained acceptance
in adult literature for treatment of pulmonary tuberculosis, such
is not the case for tuberculous meningitis in either childhood or

adulthood. Paucity of published experience with second-line antimycobacterial agents in tuberculous meningitis of childhood renders
these drugs inappropriate for use for infections with sensitive Mycobacterium tuberculosis, which comprise approximately 90% of isolates. Patients who harbor or are suspected of harboring isoniazid-
resistant mycobacteria should receive three or four antituberculous
agents, including isoniazid, rifampin and others such as pyrazinamide, streptomycin and ethambutol. Rifampin has many side-effects
which should be taken into consideration. Hepatitis, hemolytic anemia, skin rash and gastrointestinal tract disturbances are the common side-effects. The immunosuppressive effect of rifampin so far
has not been shown to have important clinical significance. However,
other medications such as PAS and barbiturates inhibit the intestinal
absorption of rifampin. CSF concentrations of rifampin are only
slightly above the minimum inhibitory concentration for tubercle
bacilli, though they are somewhat higher in the early stage of meningeal inflammation. Streptomycin and ethambutol only penetrate
well through inflamed meninges and so should be reserved for the
first 6-8 weeks of treatment. Pyrazinamide and ethionamide appear
to penetrate the blood-brain barrier with ease, though both are relatively toxic drugs. Treatment with corticosteroids is indicated in
infants and in patients with advanced disease. Corticosteroids have
been used to decrease the cerebral edema associated with tuberculous meningitis and to attempt to decrease the inflammatory response. [9]

4.   The prognosis of tuberculous meningitis depends on (D).

Appropriate treatment as discussed in the previous answer, early
diagnosis and the presenting stage of disease are extremely important in the prognosis of tuberculous meningitis. The mortality rate
is approximately fifty percent for patients admitted with coma (stage
3), and fifteen to thirty percent for patients admitted with drowsiness
or focal signs in the central nervous system (stage 2). Symptoms
and signs of cerebral involvement which predominate and persist
over those arising from the meninges are early indications of poor
prognosis.

5.   Late sequelae of tuberculous meningitis include (E).

In the series reported by Idriss et al. late sequelae of tuberculous
meningitis affected 53% of the patients and included mental deficiency,
convulsions, cranial nerve palsies, hemiparesis, spasticity, hydro-
cephaly, optic atrophy and diabetes insipidus. Deafness, pituitary
disturbances, hydromyelia due to basal arachnoiditis, and paraplegia
from spinal adhesive arachnoiditis have also been reported.

REFERENCES

1. Idriss, Z. H. , et al. : Tuberculous meningitis in childhood. Am. J. Dis. Child. 130:364-367, 1976.

2. Lehler, H. : The angiographic triad of tuberculous meningitis. Radiology 87:829, 1966.

3. Lincoln, E. M. , Sewell, E. M. : Tuberculosis in children. McGraw-Hill, Inc. , New York, 1963, p. 173.

4. Hinman, A. R. : Tuberculous meningitis at Cleveland General Hospital (1959-1963). Am. Rev. Resp. Dis. 95:670-673, 1967.

5. Steiner, P. , Portugalenza, C. : Tuberculous meningitis in children. Am. Rev. Resp. Dis. 107:22-29, 1973.

6. Editorial: Neurological complications of tuberculosis. Lancet I:1094-1095, 1970.

7. Steiner, M. , et al. : Primary drug-resistant tuberculosis in children: A continuing study of the incidence of disease caused by primarily drug resistant organisms in children observed between the years 1965 and 1968 at the Kings County Medical Center of Brooklyn. Am. Rev. Resp. Dis. 102:75-82, 1970.

8. Visudhiphan, P. , Chiemchanya, S. : Evaluation of rifampicin in the treatment of tuberculous meningitis in children. J. Pediat. 87:983-986, 1975.

9. Escobar, J. A. , et al. : Mortality from tuberculosis meningitis reduced by steroid therapy. Pediatrics 56:1050, 1975.

::

CASE 24: FEVER, HEADACHE AND VOMITING IN A CHILD WITH CHRONIC OTITIS MEDIA AND MASTOIDITIS

HISTORY: An 8-year-old boy with known chronic left otitis media and mastoiditis for the previous 2 years, presented with a history of fever, headache, and projectile vomiting of 5 days duration. One day prior to admission he became drowsy and disoriented. There was no history of drug intake or head trauma.

PHYSICAL EXAMINATION: Temp. 39. 5°C, B. P. 140/90 mm Hg. , Pulse 80/ minute. Patient had purulent discharge from the left ear and a perforated eardrum. Pupils were equal, round, and reactive to light, and examination of fundi revealed bilateral papilledema.

Chest, lungs, heart, and abdomen were within normal limits. On neurological examination the patient was drowsy but responded to painful stimuli. He had generalized weakness but no gross cranial nerve palsy. Deep tendon reflexes were normal and neither clonus or positive Babinski could be elicited. No sensory loss or motor dysfunction.

LABORATORY DATA: CBC: Hgb. 12. 5, Hct. 39%, WBC 10,100/cu mm, PMN's 68%, Lymphocytes 30%, Monocytes 2%. Urinalysis: normal. Blood urea nitrogen and electrolytes were within normal limits. Liver function studies were normal. Lumbar puncture: opening pressure - 280 mm CSF, color - clear, cells - 20 wbc (12 PMN, 8 L), sugar - 60 mg% (serum glucose 100 mg%), protein = 55 mg%, Gram stain - no organism seen, culture - negative. Purulent discharge from left ear revealed gram-positive cocci and gram-negative rods on Gram stain. Proteus sp. and Staphylococcus sp. were cultured from that material. Electroencephalogram: abnormal focus over left posterior quadrant. Left carotid arteriogram: avascular mass in the left temporal region.

QUESTIONS:

1. The most likely diagnosis in this case is:
   A. Brain abscess
   B. Subdural hematoma
   C. Epidural hematoma
   D. Brain tumor
   E. None of the above

2. Cerebrospinal fluid findings in patients with a brain abscess are:
   A. Presence of white blood cells and normal sugar and protein
   B. No cells, low sugar, and normal protein
   C. No cells, normal sugar and normal protein
   D. No cells, normal sugar and high protein
   E. Any of the above

3. The most likely pathogenic organism(s) cultured from a brain abscess would be:
   A. Bacteroides sp. and/or anaerobic or microaerophilic streptococci
   B. Staphylococcus aureus
   C. Proteus sp.
   D. A and/or B

4. The antimicrobial therapy of choice in patients with brain abscess prior to identification of the pathogenic organism is:
   A. Penicillin and cephalothin
   B. Penicillin and gentamicin
   C. Cephalothin and kanamycin
   D. Chloramphenicol and methicillin
   E. Chloramphenicol and penicillin

5. Associated and predisposing conditions in patients with brain abscess are:
   A. Otitis - mastoiditis - sinusitis
   B. Cyanotic congenital heart disease
   C. Bacterial pneumonia
   D. Osteomyelitis
   E. Any of the above

ANSWERS:

1. The most likely diagnosis in this case is (A).

A brain abscess has to be suspected in patients suffering from fever, headache, vomiting and altered state of consciousness. These are the most common presenting signs and symptoms in patients with brain abscess. Moreover, the past history of chronic otitis and mastoiditis should give us a hint since otitis - mastoiditis - sinusitis are the main associated and predisposing conditions to a brain abscess.

2. Cerebrospinal fluid findings in patients with a brain abscess are (E).

There is a wide range of cellular and biochemical changes observed in the CSF of cases with brain abscess. White blood cells could be present with normal sugar and protein in some cases while in others, a low sugar level or an elevated protein might be the only abnormal finding. A normal CSF does not rule out a brain abscess since the focus may not be adjacent to the meninges. Usually, bacteria are neither seen on Gram stain nor isolated on culture of the CSF.

3. The most likely pathogenic organism(s) cultured from a brain abscess is (D).

Adequate techniques for culturing anaerobic organisms have revealed that as many as 90% of all brain abscesses will harbor anaerobic bacteria, most often Bacteroides sp. and anaerobic streptococci. Penicillin resistant staphylococci are also common pathogens and must be considered while choosing the antimicrobial drugs prior to culture results.

4. The antimicrobial therapy of choice in patients with brain abscess prior to identification of the pathogenic organism is (D, E).

Choice of initial antibiotic therapy when the organism is unknown, is determined by the spectrum of likely pathogens and is restricted to drugs which have been shown to penetrate both CSF and brain parenchyma in adequate concentrations. Black et al. found in antibiotic concentration of chloramphenicol, penicillin, and methicillin in brain abscess to be adequate. Similar data were found by Kramer et al. Thus an initial combination of chloramphenicol and methicillin would

give adequate levels and cover for the anaerobic pathogens and
staphylococci that might be resistant to penicillin. If there is no
reason to suspect Staphylococcus aureus, then the combination of
penicillin and chloramphenicol would be adequate.

5. Associated and predisposing conditions in patients with a brain
    abscess are (E).

An infected parameningeal site is the most common predisposing
condition for a brain abscess. Parameningeal foci metastasize
through direct extension or by retrograde thrombophlebitis via
venous channels connecting either the ear structures or sinuses to
the cerebral cortex. In cyanotic heart disease with right to left
shunt, the postulate is that the usual "normal" bacteremia one en-
counters daily, which is in part filtered out by the lungs, will bypass
the lungs and reach peripheral sites, including the brain. Finally,
hematogenous or metastatic spread of infections from distant foci,
such as the lungs (pneumonia), bone (osteomyelitis) or infected
wounds, can cause a brain abscess. Head trauma, cerebrovascular
accident and anoxia have also been included among the predisposing
conditions for the development of a brain abscess.

REFERENCES

1. Samson, D. S. , Clark, K. : A current review of brain abscess.
    Am. J. Med. 54:201-210, 1973.

2. Nager, G. T. : Mastoid and paranasal sinus infection and their
    relationship to the central nervous system. Clin. Neurosurg.
    14:288, 1966.

3. Heineman, H. S. , and Braude, A. I. : Anaerobic infections of the
    brain. Observation on eighteen consecutive cases of brain ab-
    scess. Am. J. Med. 35:682-697, 1963.

4. Kramer, P. W. , et al. : Antibiotic penetration of the brain. J.
    Neurosurg. 31:295-302, 1969.

5. Black, P. , et al. : Penetration of brain abscess by systemically
    administered antibiotics. J. Neurosurg. 38:705-709, 1973.

6. Shaher, R. M. , Denchar, D. C. : Hematogenous brain abscess in
    cyanotic congenital heart disease. Am. J. Med. 52:349-355,
    1972.

7. Gregory, D. H. , et al. : Metastatic brain abscesses. Arch. Int.
    Med. 119:25-31, 1967.

CASE 25: FEVER, VOMITING AND IRRITABILITY IN AN INFANT

HISTORY: A 10-month-old boy was hospitalized because of a 2-day history of fever (102°F), irritability and vomiting. Patient had a mild, upper respiratory tract infection one week prior to the present illness. On admission, he was lethargic and irritable and appeared seriously ill. No history of illness in the family.

PHYSICAL EXAMINATION: Temperature 103°F, respiration 40/minute, pulse 140/minute. The neck was supple and anterior fontanelle was small and flat. The right tympanic membrane was red and bulging and the patient had a mild rhinorrhea. There was no skin rash and the remainder of the physical examination was unremarkable except for slightly hyperactive deep tendon reflexes. There was no clonus or focal neurologic findings.

LABORATORY DATA: CBC: Hemoglobin 12 gms%, hematocrit 38%, WBC 22,000/cu mm with 70% neutrophils, 11% band forms, and 19% lymphocytes. Urinalysis was normal. Blood urea nitrogen and serum electrolytes were within normal limits. Lumbar puncture revealed a cloudy cerebral spinal fluid (CSF) with 8,000 WBC's/cu mm, of which 96% were polymorphonuclear leukocytes. CSF protein was 210 mg%, and CSF glucose was 12 mg% (blood glucose 100 mg%). Gram stain of the CSF revealed many neutrophils and gram-negative diplococci. Aspirate from right middle ear revealed many neutrophils on Gram stain, but no organisms were seen or cultured. Blood culture was negative.

QUESTIONS:

1. The most likely diagnosis of this meningitis is:
   A. Hemophilus influenzae type B
   B. Streptococcus pneumoniae
   C. Staphylococcus aureus
   D. Neisseria meningitidis
   E. Listeria monocytogenes

2. The diseases that are most likely to be confused with Neisseria meningitidis septicemia on the basis of similar skin lesions include:
   A. Rocky Mountain spotted fever
   B. Measles
   C. Rubella
   D. Secondary syphilis
   E. Chicken pox
   F. Varicella

3. Meningococcal disease can manifest itself as:
    A. Acute bacterial pneumonia
    B. Pericarditis
    C. Migratory polyarthritis
    D. Meningitis
    E. Septicemia

4. The recommended antimicrobial regimen for patients with men-
    ingococcemia and/or meningococcal meningitis is:
    A. Ampicillin
    B. Penicillin G
    C. Chloramphenicol in patients with hypersensitivity to penicillin
    D. Tetracycline
    E. Sulfonamide

5. The recommendation of antibiotic chemoprophylaxis for the pre-
    vention of meningococcal disease in household contacts is pre-
    dicted on the following observations:
    A. Attack rate in household contacts is significantly higher
    B. Carrier rate of pathogenic strain in household contacts is
        higher
    C. Close surveillance may be difficult to implement and impos-
        sible to maintain for more than 24 to 48 hours

6. Antibiotics which provide effective chemoprophylaxis for meningo-
    coccal disease are:
    A. Oral ampicillin
    B. Oral penicillin
    C. Oral chloramphenicol
    D. Oral sulfonamide
    E. Oral rifampin and/or minocycline

ANSWERS:

1. The most likely diagnosis is (D).

N. meningitidis has been historically associated with world-wide
epidemic outbreaks of leptomeningeal inflammation for centuries
and has the capacity to produce fulminating illness and death within
a matter of a few hours. The bacterial cells of this gram-negative,
non-motile, non-sporulating organism usually exist as pairs with
their opposing surfaces flattened, giving them the appearance of
"biscuit shaped" diplococci. This organism, which does not require
a selective growth media when isolation from blood or CSF is sought,
also grows on chocolate agar, Mueller-Hinton medium, and the selective culture medium of Thayer and Martin which contains polymixin
and other antimicrobial agents. Selective culture media inhibit growth
of saprophytic Neisseriaceae and other organisms of the genitourinary and upper respiratory tract. Identification of the family Neisseriaceae usually depends on biochemical and serologic (immunologic)

tests. N. meningitides ferments glucose and maltose, whereas N. gonorrhoeae ferments only glucose. Both are oxidase and catalase positive. Most strains of N. meningitidis that cause clinical disease elaborate antigenic capsular polysaccharides, and encapsulated N. meningitides give a quelling reaction or form specific precipitates when mixed with appropriate antisera. The different serotypes of N. meningitidis are groups A, B, C, D, X, Y, and Z. In the past, group-A strains have been responsible for world-wide epidemic outbreaks of illness. Sporadic occurrence of disease due to group B and C organisms is responsible for the majority of meningococcal disease in the U. S. A. Group A epidemics in Scandinavia, Africa and Brazil have been enormous.

2. The diseases that are most likely to be confused with Neisseria meningitidis septicemia on the basis of similar skin lesions include (A-D).

The cutaneous lesions of meningococcal septicemia characteristically are petechial or purpuric in nature. These lesions generally have a peripheral distribution and can occur initially over the volar surfaces of the wrists and forearms, on the palms or over lower legs or ankles, and over the soles. Furthermore, they may not have the hemorrhagic component in their early evolution, in which case they may be indistinguishable from typical macules or papules. Therefore, lesions of meningococcemia that appear in atypical locations and lack any petechial or purpuric appearance may be confused with the cutaneous lesions or exanthems of a number of other diseases such as Rocky Mountain spotted fever, measles, rubella, and in the adult, secondary syphilis. It is always advisable to aspirate a representative lesion under aseptic conditions, and Gram stain and culture the tissue fluid. The presence of segmented neutrophils and gram-negative cocci or diplococci within these phagocytic cells or lying free in the tissue fluid is highly suggestive of Neisseria meningitidis infection. Studies by light, electron, and immunofluorescent microscopy of biopsied specimens of the skin from patients with acute meningococcemia who exhibited mainly maculopurpuric lesions, revealed endothelial necrosis, thrombosis, and necrosis of other elements of the vascular wall such as muscle cells. Immunoglobulins and complement were also found in the vascular wall in most cases.

3. The manifestations of meningococcal disease include (A-E).

Although the name of this organism denotes its importance as a cause of leptomeningeal inflammation, other forms of disease such as acute meningococcal septicemia, primary acute bacterial pneumonia, and inflammation involving serous membranes causing pericarditis and migratory polyarthritis may be caused by this organism. Meningococcemia may progress to septic shock (Waterhouse-Friderichsen Syndrome) with adrenal hemorrhage, intravascular coagulopathy, irreversible circulatory failure, and a characteristic high mortality rate. Resistance to clinical meningococcal disease is correlated with the presence of serum antibodies as measured by radioimmunoassay, which appear to prevent invasive disease. Cell mediated immune functions as well as the complement system also contribute to some extent, particularly with respect to the degree and durability of the immune state.

4. The recommended therapeutic regimen for the patients with meningococcemia or meningitis are (A-C).

Because of the emergence of sulfonamide resistant strains of groups C, B, and A meningococci, and since so far no strain of Neisseria meningitidis has been shown to carry a plasmid or exhibit resistance to penicillin class drugs, large doses of intravenous crystalline penicillin are recommended as therapeutic regimens for patients with meningococcemia or meningitis. For individuals in whom hypersensitivity to penicillin precludes the use of this class of antimicrobial drug, chloramphenicol therapy is a good alternative. In 1973, sulfonamide resistance was found in 75% of group C isolates, 57% of group A, 20% of B, and 4% of Y isolates. Thus, sulfonamides are no longer considered effective therapeutic agents except when the target organism is demonstrably and reliably known to be sulfonamide sensitive.

5. The recommendation of antibiotic chemoprophylaxis for the prevention of meningococcal disease in household contacts is predicated on (A-C).

Studies have shown that the carrier rate of meningococcal disease in household contacts of a case is significantly higher than the carrier rate in the general population in endemic and epidemic disease. The carrier rate of the pathogenic strain in household contacts of cases is 4-5 times that observed in the general population. Meningococcal carriers are probably at least risk of contracting systemic illness from homologous strains of meningococci, since meningococcal carriage produces an antibody response. The high carriage rate in household contacts, however, leaves those contacts who are not carriers with an increased risk of acquiring infection and illness. This chemoprophylaxis during the first 24 to 48 hours after diagnosing the index case is very important since many secondary cases occur within 3 days. Difficulties in surveillance are especially prominent in developing countries with scarce medical resources where socioeconomic factors, coupled with scarcity or unavailability of medical care, may preclude effective surveillance. In areas of adequate access to medical care, however, surveillance is often chosen over chemoprophylaxis for control of contacts of sporadic civilian cases.

6. Antibiotics which may provide effective chemoprophylaxis are (D-E).

Although penicillin and ampicillin are highly effective in treating the illness, they are not sufficiently effective in eradicating the carriage state to warrant their use of chemoprophylaxis. Studies from several laboratories suggest that any effective antimicrobial drug must be present in all secretions of the upper respiratory drugs in a concentration exceeding that required to inhibit the growth of Neisseria meningitidis. Sulfonamide derivatives are readily secreted by the parotid and accessary saliva glands, where as the penicillin and virtually all other antimicrobial drugs are not. Oral rifampin is an exception and resembles the sulfonamide in that it is found in high concentration in oral secretions and tears. Minocycline is another drug that produces greater than minimum inhibitory concentrations for meningococci in the saliva. Thus, rifampin and minocycline would be expected to prevent acquisition of meningococci as well as to eradicate strains that may be carried. It seems neither of these regimens is without major problems, however. Treatment with rifampin for more than several days results in emergence of rifampin resistant strains of N. meningitidis in a significant proportion of patients. No minocycline resistant strains have been isolated from carriers undergoing treatment, but the occurrence of significant and frequent drug reactions after the administration of even a single dose of minocycline poses a severe limitation on its use in asymptomatic household contacts of cases. The development of groups A and C meningococcal polysaccharide vaccines during the past several years has produced an important and powerful tool for the control of meningococcal epidemics. Moreover, some advocate use of these vaccines with chemoprophylaxis for household and other intimate contacts of cases under endemic or epidemic circumstances. Group B capsular polysaccharide is relatively non-immunogenic, and injection of reasonably good preparations of group B polysaccharide elicited little or no antibody response.

REFERENCES

1. Artenstein, M. S. , et al. : Prevention of meningococcal disease by group C polysaccharide vaccine. N. Engl. J. Med. 282:417, 1970.

2. Artenstein, M. S. : Prophylaxis for meningococcal disease. JAMA 231:1035, 1975.

3. Goldschneider, I. , et al. : Human immunity to the meningococcus. I. The role of humoral antibodies. J. Exp. Med. 129:1307, 1969.

4. Goldschneider, I. , et al. : Human immunity to the meningococcus. II. Development of natural immunity. J. Exp. Med. 129:1327, 1969.

5. Gotschlich, E. C. , et al. : Human immunity to the meningococcus. III. Immunogenicity of Group A and Group C meningococcal polysaccharides in human volunteers. J. Exp. Med. 129:1367, 1969.

6. Beam, W. E. , et al. : The effect of rifampin on the nasopharyngeal carriage of Neisseria meningitidis in a military population. Infect. Dis. 124:39, 1971.

7. Munford, R. S. , et al. : Eradication of carriage of Neisseria
    meningitidis in families: A study in Brazil. J. Infect. Dis.
    129:644, 1974.

8. Sotto, Mirian N. , et al. : Pathogenesis of cutaneous lesions in
    acute meningococcemia in humans: Light, immunofluorescent,
    and electron microscopic studies of skin biopsy specimens. J.
    Infect. Dis. 133:506, 1976.

9. Guttler, R. B. , et al. : Effect of rifampin and minocycline on
    meningococcal carrier rates. J. Infect. Dis. 124:199, 1971.

10. Drew, T. M. , et al. : Minocycline for prophylaxis of infection
    with Neisseria meningitidis: High rate of side effects in recip-
    ients. J. Infect. Dis. 133:194, 1976.

11. McCormick, J. B. , Bennett, J. V. : Public health considerations
    in the management of meningococcal disease. Ann. Int. Med.
    83:883, 1975.

12. Lepow, M. L. , and Gold, R. : Current status of vaccines
    against the meningococcus. Prev. Med. 3:449, 1974.

::

CASE 26: THREE-YEAR-OLD BOY WITH A 4-DAY HISTORY OF
          STIFF NECK AND LOW-GRADE FEVER

HISTORY: This 3-year-old Caucasian boy presented with a four-day
history of stiff neck and low grade temperature. He had been in excellent health until one week prior to admission when he became
less active, refused his meals, and seemed mildly feverish. His
parents thought he was developing "the flu" and they treated him
with aspirin and a proprietary "cold pill".

Four days prior to his admission the youngster awoke complaining
of a stiff neck. His parents assumed initially that this was positional
and represented a "muscular stiffness". These symptoms persisted
in conjunction with increasing irritability and periodic lethargy. He
vomited once, and thereafter a pediatrician was consulted. The
presence of fever and nuchal rigidity was confirmed.

All members of the immediate family and all playmates were well,
and there was no known exposure to communicable diseases. Past
history was unremarkable and the review of systems revealed nothing beyond the presenting complaints. Immunizations were up to
date and complete for DPT, poliomyelitis and measles.

Family pets included a dog, 2 cats, tropical fish, and a small painted
turtle, as well as a red herring recently purchased in a local store.

PHYSICAL EXAMINATION: Temp - 38. 5°C. , R - 25, Pulse 90 regular, BP 95/60. This well-developed youngster was not in acute distress. He was alert but quite irritable. There was no rash other than a few fine petechiae on the upper extremities. There was marked nuchal rigidity. No parotid or submaxillary swelling was seen. Eye grounds were normal, as were the tympanic membranes. The throat was not inflamed. The lungs were clear to percussion and auscultation and the heart size, rate and rhythm were normal, without murmurs or thrills. The abdomen was soft and without organ enlargement or localized tenderness. Cranial nerves, reflexes, and modalities of sensation were normal.

LABORATORY DATA AND TESTS: White blood count total = 12, 500 per cu. mm. Differential: neutrophils 68%, bands 7%, lymphocytes 25%. Chest x-ray negative.

Urinalysis: trace of protein and acetone, negative for sugar. Sediment revealed an occasional leukocyte and epithelial cell and a rare erythrocyte and hyaline cast.

Lumbar Puncture: Opening pressure was normal. The opalescent fluid contained 2000 white blood cells per cu. mm., predominantly polymorphonuclear in morphology. Sugar 20 mg% (corresponding blood sugar 90 mg%) Protein 40 mg%. Gram Stain: revealed a few gram-negative bacteria described as "coccobacillary" and occasionally grouped in pairs.

Electrolytes were unremarkable. Liver function tests were normal as was the pancreatic amylase. Blood cultures were drawn. An intravenous drip was begun and antibiotics administered: Ampicillin (400 mg/kg/24 hours), Chloramphenicol (100 mg/kg/24 hours).

A provisional diagnosis was made of meningococcal meningitis. The following day all aerobic cultures of the CSF were growing bacteria, which were described as gram-negative coccal or diplococcal forms when smeared from the small colonies appearing on solid media. In contrast the bacteria in the liquid culture medium looked like short stubby bi-polar staining rods (also gram-negative).

QUESTIONS:

1. The most likely cause of this infection is which one or more of the following?
    A. Neisseria meningitidis
    B. Neisseria gonorrhoeae
    C. Hemophilus influenzae type B
    D. Acinetobacter (Mima polymorpha)
    E. Dual infection with Neisseria meningitidis and Hemophilus influenzae type B
    F. None of the above

2. Bacteria were identified as Acinetobacter. These bacteria are
    easily recovered from man and are common saprophytes.
    A. True
    B. False

3. Since these bacteria are sometimes resistant to ampicillin,
    chloramphenicol must be continued in the present case at least
    until the sensitivity patterns have been determined.
    A. True
    B. False

4. The recovery of Acinetobacter from the CSF in this case suggests:
    A. The cultures were contaminated with skin organisms
    B. That this child may be suffering from an immunodeficiency
        condition, previously unrecognized
    C. The need for a careful re-examination of the child to search
        for possible dermal sinuses
    D. That these bacteria may acquire virulence through transfer
        of R factors

When the skull was carefully examined, a tiny crusted lesion was found
in the midline of the occiput (Fig. 26.1). Skull x-rays were obtained,
and an associated underlying bony defect was noted (Fig. 26.2).

QUESTION:

5. The most likely cause of the appearance of this occipital skin
    lesion and associated skull defect is:
    A. The result of child abuse or a forgotten and neglected injury
    B. A dermoid sinus and cyst
    C. Invasive midline granuloma
    D. Cat scratch disease with secondary invasion of the granu-
        lomatous lesion by saprophytes

ANSWERS:

1. (C, but A, B, D, E are also possible)

The commonest gram-negative coccobacillary organism causing
meningitis in a healthy 3-year-old child is H. influenzae B. Unfortunately, the microscopic appearance can be deceptive, and
other organisms such as Acinetobacter (Mima polymorpha) are
not distinguishable. Mima polymorpha are gram-negative cocco -
bacillary organisms which are morphologically variable as their
name implies and are often mistaken for N. meningitidis. They
have been called Mima polymorpha, Herellea, Bacterium anitratum,
BSW, Diplococcus mucosus and Neisseria Winosgradkyi. In the
recent classification of Bergey's Manual, these organisms are now
in Genus IV of the Neisseriaceae family and are referred to as
Acinetobacter. These organisms are catalase-positive, oxidase-
negative, and therefore are distinguished from oxidase-positive
genera; i.e. Moraxella, Branhamella, and Neisseria.

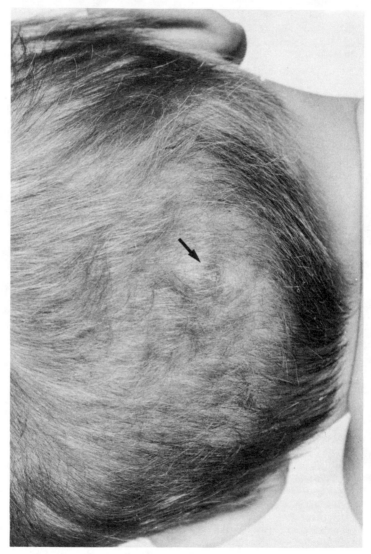

FIG. 26.1: View of the occiput showing small crusted lesion of skin near midline.

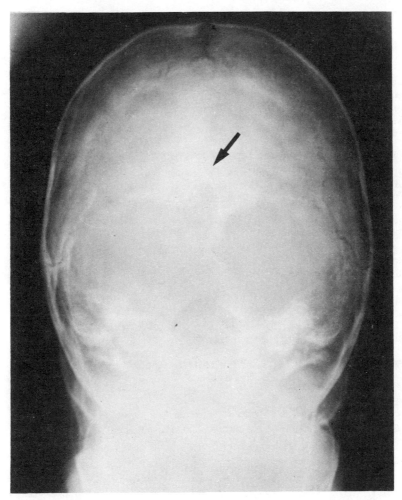

FIG. 26. 2: Skull x-ray showing underlying bony defect.

2. (A)

These bacteria are commonly found on healthy skin (especially that of the scalp) and have been recovered from the male and female urogenital tracts, as well as from conjunctivae.

3. (A)

It is of practical importance to await identification of these organisms as Acinetobacter by their oxidase reaction because of possible penicillin (ampicillin) resistance. Since H.influenzae B is the commonest organism causing meningitis in this age group, chloramphenicol therapy is initiated. Final identification and sensitivity testing may allow adjustment of therapy to ampicillin.

4. (C)

Although serious Mima polymorpha disease has occurred in healthy patients [1,6], one should always be suspicious of a structural or functional disorder of host defense mechanisms in the presence of these infections.

In the present case, skin contaminants are virtually ruled out as a source of the positive cultures because of the appearance of consistent bacterial forms in the original CSF smear and the abundance of the growth of Mimeae on all media.

The history and the initial physical examination eliminates the existence of all but the most subtle immune deficiency states.

Saprophytic bacteria do not "acquire virulence" or become invasive in nature through genetic transfer.

A careful re-examination of the child is mandatory, in particular to search for evidence of a skin defect.

5. (B)

The midline punctum of the skin of the occiput and the associated skull defect are characteristics of a dermoid cyst and sinus [5].

The epithelial and neuro-ectodermal layers separate during the fourth week of embryonic life. Any failure of the separation to occur completely will result in a defect involving the skin and central nervous system. Since the process of separation occurs along the mid-dorsal aspect of the embryo, these persistent connections and defects are usually found along the midline of the skull and back. The defects may be superficial or deep ranging from the epidermis (epidermoids) to the dermis, and involving any layer and level of the central nervous system into and including the spinal canal or ventricles. Dermoids are defined by the inclusion of nests of deeper

skin derivatives such as sebaceous glands and hair. The external
opening of a dermoid sinus may contain hairs, and in some cases
may be surrounded by skin exhibiting increased pigmentation or a
hemangioma. Cysts may occur along or at the inner end of the sinus
in connection with or within the central nervous system. If the
cyst is not free to drain through the sinus, it can present as a mass-
lesion [2].

When the connection of the central nervous system and skin is complete with an open sinus - as it was in the present case - there is a
continual and recurrent risk of infection by organisms resident on
the skin [3].

FINAL NOTE: In the present case the Acinetobacter was ampicillin-
sensitive and the meningitis resolved uneventfully. Subsequently
neurosurgical exploration demonstrated the dermoid sinus and cyst
which were successfully removed. The cyst was within the posterior
fossa displacing the cerebellum. The patient recovered without
significant sequelae.

REFERENCES

1. Hermann, G. III, Melnick, T.: Mima polymorpha meningitis in
    the very young. Am. J. Dis. Child. 110:315-318, 1965.

2. Matson, D. D., Ingraham, F. D.: Intracranial complications of
    congenital dermal sinuses. Pediatrics 8:463-474, 1951.

3. Mount, L. A.: Congenital dermal sinuses as a cause of menin-
    gitis, intraspinal abscess and intracranial abscess. JAMA 139:
    1263-1268, 1951.

4. Reynolds, R. C., Cluff, L. E.: Infection of man with Mimea.
    Ann. Int. Med. 58:759-767, 1963.

5. Shanks, S. C., Kerley, P. (Eds).: A textbook of X-ray Diagnosis.
    Vol. 1. H. K. Lewis & Co., Ltd., London, 1969, p. 131-133.

6. Waite, Comdr. C. L., Kline, Lt. A. H.: Mima polymorpha men-
    ingitis. Am. J. Dis. Child. 98:379-384, 1959.

:::

CASE 27: CHRONIC PROGRESSIVE NEUROLOGICAL DISORDER
        IN AN ELEVEN-YEAR-OLD BOY

HISTORY: An eleven-year-old boy, the second of a family of four
children and healthy, unrelated Caucasian parents, was noted by
his parents to be absent-minded and forgetful since his return to
school from summer camp 12 weeks previously. Inquiry from his

school teachers indicated that for several months his work had become untidy and less accurate, and that he was less outgoing in his
relationships with his classmates. The family physician was consulted and no abnormality was found on physical examination. There
appeared to be no predisposing emotional factors. The boy was sent
to the school guidance counselor and was urged to increase his dili-
gence and attentiveness. Pediatric consultation was prompted by
further progression of the episodes of forgetfulness and apparent
intellectual deterioration.

There was no history of head injuries. Neither he nor any other
member of the family had been receiving drugs or medications.
There was no family history of neurological disease. There were
no household pets. Specific inquiry elicited that 10 months ago he
had become an enthusiastic fisherman and had made some of his
own fishing tackle, including lead weights.

Past medical history was unremarkable other than the appearance
of "shingles" 2 years previously. Immunizations were complete
for diphtheria, pertussis and tetanus as well as for poliomyelitis,
but he had not received measles vaccine. There was a history of
measles (uncomplicated) at 18 months of age and varicella at age
3. There was no history of allergic disease in the patient or the
family.

PHYSICAL EXAMINATION: This was a drowsy and withdrawn afebrile youngster with normal vital signs (including blood pressure).
There was no nuchal rigidity. He was occasionally disoriented in
place and time and found it difficult to concentrate during the examination. Upon one occasion he appeared to be slow in recognizing
his father. The physical examination was otherwise entirely unremarkable except for slight difficulty with finger-to-nose and heel-
to-shin tests, and subtle, inconstant, very brief uncontrolled movements of some fingers and the right wrist.

LABORATORY DATA: Urine analysis, blood counts, serum chemistries (including fasting blood sugar), serum copper, ceruloplasmin
and lead, as well as x-rays of the skull, chest, wrist, and abdomen
were all normal. The intradermal intermediate strength PPD test
was negative. The VDRL and Mono spot tests were negative. Computerized axial tomography was normal.

Lumbar puncture: normal pressure. Fluid was clear and colorless
without cells and was negative for culture (bacteria including anaerobes, mycobacteria, and fungi). CSF sugar 80 mg, with corresponding blood sugar of 95 mg%. Protein 50 mg%. There was a first zone
colloidal gold curve.

EEG (Fig. 27.1) revealed severe abnormalities with recurring irregular generalized complexes containing slow waves at $1\frac{1}{2}$ - 3 per second with irregular (approximately one second in duration) bursts of
high voltage at intervals of about 10 seconds.

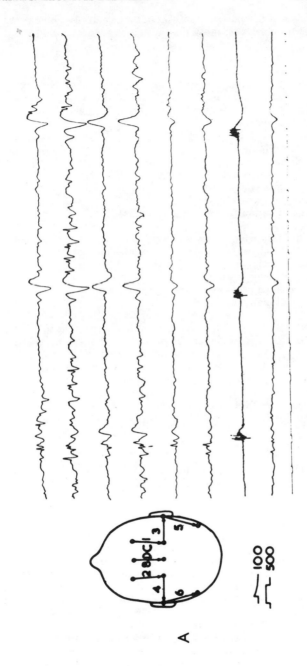

FIG. 27. 1: EEG (6 channels) top and Polymyograph (2 recordings) bottom illustrating recurring irregular generalized complexes (EEG) and associated bursts of muscle action potentials.

Polyelectromyogram: showed some myoclonic activity coinciding
with the periodic bursts on the EEG.

QUESTIONS:

1. The following is a list of conditions of infectious or possible in-
    fectious etiology which may be relevant to this case. Which one(s)
    on this list can probably be ruled out at this point?
    A. Cerebral abscess
    B. Chronic meningitis
    C. Late complications of congenital or acquired syphilis
    D. Chronic herpes simplex encephalitis
    E. Subacute sclerosing panencephalitis (SSPE)
    F. Creutzfeldt-Jakob disease
    G. Multiple sclerosis
    H. Progressive multifocal leukoencephalopathy

2. Which of the following procedures or tests would you request at
    this time?
    A. Muscle biopsy
    B. Virus antibody tests on serum
    C. Virus antibody tests on cerebrospinal fluid
    D. Virus cultures on the CSF

FURTHER INVESTIGATIONS: Serum samples were sent to the state
laboratory for serology and were reported as showing no evidence
of recent infection with: influenza A and B, herpesvirus hominis
(H. simplex), varicella zoster, adenovirus, arbovirus, mycoplasma,
Epstein-Barr virus, cytomegalovirus, rubella.

The measles CF and HI antibody on serum and cerebrospinal fluid
(CSF) are listed below:

	SERUM	CSF
Measles CF	2048	256
Measles HI	256	4

QUESTIONS:

3. The most likely diagnosis was therefore SSPE and a brain biopsy
    was carried out for absolute confirmation. Which one or more
    of the following tests of the biopsy specimen may be useful?
    A. Light microscopy
    B. Electron microscopy
    C. Virus culture employing co-cultivation techniques
    D. Immunofluorescent staining
    E. Intracerebral inoculation of steroid-treated mice

4. The diagnosis is confirmed and it can now be stated that the
   expectation for this youngster is:
   A. Complete recovery with or without sequelae following a
      course of steroid therapy
   B. Complete or at least partial recovery after a course of
      therapy with systemic idoxuridine
   C. Progression to coma and death
   D. Possible prolonged survival with permanent brain damage

ANSWERS:

1. At this point the history and findings are so characteristic of
   SSPE that any of the alternative diagnostic choices appear con-
   siderably less likely. The best answer to the question is E;
   (A - D) and (F - H) can all probably be ruled out.

Brain abscess or tumor may present in a very obscure manner, but
the absence of localizing or lateralizing findings on the EEG, the
CAT scan and the physical examination reduce the likelihood of an
intracerebral abscess or tumor.

Chronic meningitis is eliminated by definition since the examination
of the CSF has failed to reveal direct evidence of meningeal inflammation (lack of cells).

The late complications of congenital lues might be accompanied by
a first zone colloidal gold curve. The findings of nonreactive VDRL
has not ruled out this possibility, since only approximately 75% of
persons with neurosyphilis have a reactive VDRL. An FTA-ABS
should now be done on sera, and a VDRL on CSF in order to rule
out neurosyphilis.

Herpesvirus hominis encephalitis usually presents as an acute and
rapidly progressive disorder and is often characterized (particularly
with the passage of time) by the development of focal signs often
referable to one or the other temporal lobe. Herpesvirus infections
of the central nervous system are relatively common (probably the
most frequent cause of severe encephalitis) and may present in a
very obscure manner often unassociated with recognizable diagnostic features. However, the progress of herpesvirus hominis encephalitis is rarely chronic, and the destructive lesions in the brain associated with H. simplex cytopathic effects often lead to the presence
of erythrocytes in the cerebrospinal fluid [5].

Creutzfeldt-Jakob disease is a transmissable presenile dementia
caused by an as yet undefined "slow virus", and is not reported at
this early age [6]. Subacute multifocal leukoencephalopathy is a rare
degenerative condition of the central nervous system associated with
the presence of a Papova virus. It is a condition which has always
been associated with malignant lymphoproliferative disease and/or

diminished host immune capacity [7, 8]. Multiple sclerosis is a condition frequently exhibiting a remitting pattern often beginning with an attack of optic neuritis. In the present case, the course and the EEG findings are inconsistent with this diagnosis.

In the present case, the progress, EEG findings, myoclonus, and CSF colloidal gold pattern were entirely consistent and characteristic of the disease SSPE. Virtually all patients with this condition have a history of prior measles or measles immunization [9]. Frequently, as was true in the present case, the episode of measles has occurred at a relatively early age.

It has been suggested that SSPE patients manifest subtly aberrant (depressed) immunologic function, though it is uncertain whether these immunologic changes predate and underlie the neurologic condition, or reflect an earlier impact of the basic pathogenesis of the disorder [10]. In this regard, it is noteworthy that the present patient had experienced a reactivation of varicella-zoster virus (shingles) two years prior to the recognition of neurologic symptoms.

2. (B, C)

The most useful diagnostic tests at this point would be those for virus antibody levels in serum and CSF, particularly antibody (HI, neutralizing or CF) to measles virus. Virus cultures would be entirely negative in these circumstances and there are no diagnostic changes in muscle pathology associated with SSPE. Serum CF antibody to measles is markedly elevated in SSPE and measurable CF antibody is usually found in CSF as well. These findings probably reflect the chronic presence in SSPE brains of measles virus antigens (Fig. 27. 2), though in the absence of any active replication of this or a related virus.

3. (A - D)

Light microscopy may show the typical intranuclear inclusions associated with this condition. EM can be employed to demonstrate the presence of packed arrays of intranuclear nucleocapsids which resemble the tubular structures of measles and related myxoviruses and paramyxoviruses. Virus cultures employing co-cultivation of explants of brain from affected individuals with sensitive feeder layers has in some instances actually yielded measles-like virus[12, 13]. Finally, immunofluorescence may be used to demonstrate the presence in affected cells of measles antigens, or at least antigens which cross-react with measles.

The intracerebral inoculation of steroid-treated mice has no place in this diagnostic workup.

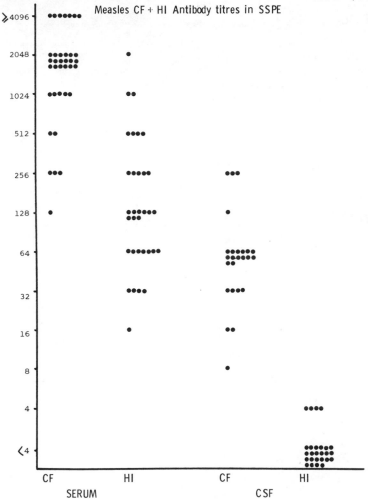

FIG. 27. 2: Comparison of titers of measles CF and HI antibody in serum and cerebrospinal fluid in a series of cases in SSPE (Dr. W. C. Marshall, Great Ormond St. Hospital For Sick Children, London). These titers demonstrate the high serum HI and CF titers. In the cerebrospinal fluid measles antibody is always detectable. Several studies suggest that CSF CF antibody titers may be the single most practical serological method for identification of the patient with SSPE. Neutralizing antibody titers are even more consistent but less readily available. Measles HI titers in CSF are also elevated, although the study cited demonstrates patients with low or undetectable titers.

4. (C, D)

The majority of patients with SSPE progress to a state of decerebrate rigidity, coma and death, and although it can be stated that
complete recovery does not occur, there are some cases in which
there appears to be an arrest in the progression of the disease.
There is as yet no evidence that any form of therapy will ameliorate,
arrest, or reverse the course of SSPE, although some claims have
been made for the efficacy of Transfer Factor [14]. The occurrence
of occasional spontaneous arrest of the disease progress underlines
the hazards which attend interpretation of uncontrolled treatment
trials of this relatively rare condition.

REFERENCES

GENERAL:

1. Bell, W. E. and McCormick, W. F. : Neurologic infections in
   children. Major Problems in Clinical Pediatrics Vol. 12. W. B.
   Saunders, Philadelphia, 1975, (Chap. 17: Chronic viral infections of the central nervous system).

2. Gajdusek, D. C. : Slow virus disease of the central nervous system. Am. J. Clin. Path. 56:320-330, 1971.

3. Jabbour, J. T. , et al. : Epidemiology of subacute sclerosing
   panencephalitis. JAMA 220:959-962, 1972.

4. Metz, H. , et al. : Subacute sclerosing panencephalitis. Arch.
   Dis. Child. 29:554-557, 1964.

SPECIFIC:

5. Symposium: clinical spectrum of herpes simplex virus infections.
   Postgrad. Med. J. 49:375-439, 1973.

6. Roos, R. , et al. : The clinical characteristics of Creutzfeldt-
   Jakob disease. Brain 96:1-20, 1973.

7. Richardson, E. P. , Jr. : Our evolving understanding of progressive multifocal leukoencephalopathy. Ann. N. Y. Acad.
   Sci. 230:358-364, 1974.

8. Zu Rhein, G. M. , Chou, S. M. : Particles resembling papova
   viruses in human cerebral demyelinating disease. Science
   148:1477-1479, 1965.

9. Brody, J. A. , Detels, R. : Subacute sclerosing panencephalitis:
   a zoonosis following aberrant measles. Lancet II: 500-501,
   1970.

10. Gerson, K. L., Haslam, R. H. A: Subtle immunologic abnormalities in four boys with subacute sclerosing panencephalitis. NEJM 285:78-82, 1971.

11. Sever, J. L., Zeman, W.: Serological studies of measles and subacute sclerosing panencephalitis. Neurology 18:95-97, 1968.

12. Barbosa, L., et al.: Isolation of measles virus from brain cell cultures of two patients with subacute sclerosing panencephalitis. Proc. Soc. Exper. Biol. Med. 132:272-277, 1969.

13. Payne, F. E., et al.: Isolation of measles virus from cell cultures of brain from a patient with subacute sclerosing panencephalitis. NEJM 281:585-589, 1969.

14. Lawrence, H. S.: Transfer factor and cellular immunity to virus infections. Perspectives in Virology IX, Academic Press, 1975, p. 135-151.

15. Sever, John L., et al.: Diagnosis of subacute panencephalitis: the value and availability of measles and antibody determinations. JAMA 228:604-606, 1974.

::

CASE 28: FEVER, LETHARGY IN AN ELEVEN-MONTH-OLD GIRL

HISTORY: This eleven-month-old Caucasian girl presented with symptoms of fever and lethargy. She had been in excellent health prior to the present illness. The neonatal and developmental history was unremarkable and all immunizations were complete and up-to-date. The family was in general excellent health and there was one female sibling, aged three years. There was no history of drug allergies or sensitivities and no known exposure to serious communicable disease, including tuberculosis.

All members of the family, including the patient, had recently experienced a mild respiratory illness characterized by a low-grade fever. The last remnants of this "cold" had faded within the few days prior to the present illness.

On the day of presentation the patient seemed well upon awakening, ate a good breakfast, and played quietly all morning. By noon she appeared slightly flushed and "cranky" and was not interested in eating. She was irritable, felt warm, and was found to have a rectal temperature of 40°C. She was seen at a local clinic, sent home with reassurance to mother that this was a "virus infection," and that fever should be controlled with aspirin. Upon arrival at home the temperature had risen to almost 41°C, and the infant appeared "gray and limp". She vomited once, was sponged with tepid water and taken to a local hospital emergency room. Physical examination was said to reveal no specific abnormalities other than a persistently elevated temperature and lethargy. Chest x-ray was negative. White blood cell count was 7300 with a normal differential. Lumbar puncture revealed clear fluid with no cells and no bacteria seen on Gram stain. Blood, CSF and nose and throat cultures were obtained, and because of the child's floppy appearance and high fever she was referred to a medical center for further evaluation.

PHYSICAL EXAMINATION: Temperature 40°C; Pulse 110; Resp: 50. The patient was well-developed, well-nourished, and slightly restless. She had normal body measurements for age. The skin was pale, dry and very warm. The fontanelle was not distended. Nuchal rigidity was difficult to evaluate. The remainder of the examination was entirely unremarkable.

LABORATORY DATA: (four hours after earlier evaluation in community hospital): White blood count, 11,500. Differential - neutrophils 80%; stabs 4%; lymphs 16%; platelets and erythrocyte morphology normal. Chest x-ray - normal. Lumbar puncture - normal pressure. Clear fluid - 2 lymphocytes, 1 neutrophil, negative Gram stain. CSF was sent for protein, sugar and culture. Blood was sent for culture, electrolytes and sugar. Urine: negative other than a trace of protein.

QUESTIONS:

1. The family history of a recent prior "cold", now resolved, may have played which of the following roles in the pathogenesis of this child's disease?
   A. The present illness is a recrudescence of the same virus infection, a typical biphasic pattern
   B. The present illness reflects a new virus infection - probably Roseola infantum
   C. The present illness represents a secondary systemic bacterial infection
   D. The present illness is a postinfectious allergic complication of the resolving illness

2. Additional diagnostic assistance may be provided by:
   A. Countercurrent immunoelectrophoresis (CIE) run on samples of blood and CSF against antiserum to the "K" antigen of E. coli
   B. CIE on blood, urine and CSF against polysaccharide antigens of Hemophilus influenzae type B, Streptococcus pneumoniae (pneumococcus), and Neisseria meningitidis (meningococcus)
   C. Performance of a limulus endotoxin test

3. Faced with this clinical situation you should:
   A. Admit the child to hospital, start an intravenous drip and administer ampicillin (400 mg/kg/day) pending culture reports

B. Reassure and send the child home, with instructions for the parents to return or call as needed

C. Admit the child to hospital overnight for observation, but without specific therapy until cultures are reported

D. Admit the child to hospital, start an intravenous drip, and administer ampicillin (400 mg/kg/day) as well as chloramphenicol (100 mg/kg/day) pending the culture reports

E. Administer steroids immediately because this illness represents a serious allergic reaction

The following morning both sets of blood and CSF cultures were positive, and smears of the culture fluid revealed pleomorphic gramnegative rods.

QUESTIONS:

4. These bacteria will probably be identified as:
   A. Bordetella pertussis
   B. Escherichia coli
   C. Hemophilus influenzae (type B)
   D. Pseudomonas aeruginosa
   E. Staphylococcus aureus
   F. Listeria monocytogenes

5. At this point one should:
   A. Administer IV fluids at maintenance level (urine output plus insensible water loss) and continue the therapy as defined in the answer to question #3
   B. Continue to administer the antimicrobial therapy but speed up the IV to deliver at least 3 - 4 liters per meter^2 per day to provide adequate renal flow
   C. Start IV steroids and/or mannitol to prevent intracerebral edema

6. All other family members should now be treated in the following manner:
   A. Culture nose and throat and treat specific pathogens if any are recovered
   B. Treat all family members with sulfamethoxasole for 2 days
   C. Treat all family members with ampicillin for 2 days
   D. None of the above

7. After the culture is reported, which of the following should be done?
   A. Complete and send in a report form to the state PHS laboratory
   B. Notify and treat prophylactically all close contacts
   C. Display an announcement in your office warning of the occurrence of meningitis in the community
   D. Nothing further should or need be done

ANSWERS:

1. (C)

Bacterial pneumonia, meningitis, or other significant septic conditions frequently follow the occurrence and recent resolution of a
nonspecific illness (possible viral infection). The history in this
case is characteristic of such a progression of events and suggests
that a high level of suspicion must be maintained under these circumstances, particularly with the suggestive shift to the left in normal leukocyte count and the apparently unremarkable spinal fluid
findings. Babies in the pre-eruptive phase of roseola infantum may
have obscure high fever but are almost always found playing happily
and acting reasonably well.

2. (A, B)

Considerable assistance may be provided by CIE determinations to
detect in body fluids the presence of bacterial antigens. The "K_1"
antigen is shared by several bacteria, but the usefulness of this
test is presently limited to the newborn period because the E. coli
found to be invasive in this age group are predominantly of K_1 serotype. Antisera also are available to surface polysaccharide of Hemophilus influenzae type B(polyribose phosphate), Streptococcus
pneumoniae and Neisseriae meningitidis. The CIE procedure may
be performed upon serum, urine, CSF, or other body fluids, and
the result can be derived in a matter of just a few hours. A positive
test is usually diagnostic of recent or active infection by the indicated pathogen, but cross reactions with other antigens and nonspecific reactions are not rare. A negative test does not rule out a
specific infection caused by these bacteria and cannot exclude infections caused by other pathogens which do not share these antigens
(for example, staphylococci and beta-hemolytic streptococci). [3,4,5]
Although the polysaccharides of H. flu B and pneumococci persist
in body fluids, the K_1 antigen does not.

3. (D)

Cultures of blood and CSF having been obtained, an IV drip and antimicrobial therapy should be started. The antibiotics of choice for
this child are ampicillin and chloramphenicol. There is no solid
clinical evidence to suggest that this combination of antibiotics is
antagonistic in clinical application. These medications provide adequate coverage for infections caused by most bacterial pathogens
common to this age group. Although ampicillin alone provides adequate antimicrobial coverage in many H. influenzae B infections, the
increasing recognition of systemic infection with ampicillin-resistant
forms necessitates the use of chloramphenicol when H. influenzae B
is a potential pathogen. Ampicillin is employed concurrently because
of potential gram (+) pathogens. After the antimicrobial sensitivities
have been determined, the therapy may be modified. [6,7]

One cannot admit and treat every baby with fever, but in this case considerable reliance was placed upon what must be called clinical judgement. The shift in the leukocyte count and differential over four hours must be viewed with suspicion. If CSF is examined very early in overwhelming bacterial meningitis and sepsis, there may be no detectable pleocytosis. All such specimens, however, must be examined with Gram's stain and cultured.

4. (C)

The bacteria in the culture are almost certainly H. influenzae type B. Specific rapid identification is facilitated by the performance of a quellung test or slide agglutination employing specific capsular anti-serum. [2]

5. (A)

Fluids should be restricted to minimize intracerebral edema. However, in the absence of acute signs of increased intracranial pressure, steroids and mannitol should not be administered. [1]

6. (D)

No specific measures need be taken with respect to the family unless there is the appearance of additional illness apparently infective in origin. In the latter case, thorough examination must be performed and appropriate cultures taken. [1]

7. (A)

One of the most important but often neglected responsibilities of physicians is to report cases such as these to the Public Health Authorities so that appropriate measures may be taken and data of epidemiologic significance may be assembled and made available to health workers and to the community at large. Reportable illnesses in the individual states may vary and in North Carolina H. influenzae B meningitis is reportable. Meningococcal disease is nationally reportable.

REFERENCES

GENERAL:

1. Feigin, R. D. , Dodge, P. R. : Bacterial meningitis: newer concepts of pathophysiology and neurologic sequelae. Pediat. Clin. N. A. 23:541-556, 1976.

2. Editorial (Marshall, W. C.): Hemophilus influenzae infections. Brit. Med. J. 1:462, 1974.

3. Robbins, J. B.: Hemophilus influenzae type B: disease and immunity in humans. Ann. Int. Med. 78:259-269, 1973.

SPECIFIC:

4. Ingram, D. L., et al.: Countercurrent immunoelectrophoresis in the diagnosis of systemic diseases caused by Hemophilus influenzae type B. J. Pediat. 81:1159, 1972.

5. Robbins, J. B., et al.: Escherischia coli K-1 capsular polysaccharide associated with neonatal meningitis. NEJM 290:1216-1220, 1974.

6. Nelson, J. D.: Should ampicillin be abandoned for treatment of Hemophilus influenzae disease? JAMA 229:322-324, 1974.

7. Jacobson, J. A., et al.: Epidemiologic characteristics of infections caused by ampicillin-resistant Hemophilus influenzae. Pediatrics 58:388-391, 1976.

::

CASE 29: RECURRENT HIGH FEVER IN A 21-MONTH-OLD GIRL
          WITH ACUTE LYMPHOBLASTIC LEUKEMIA IN
          REMISSION

HISTORY: Acute lymphoblastic leukemia was diagnosed in this 21-month-old girl in Pakistan three months previously. She had been given one transfusion of fresh whole blood. Thereafter prompt remission of her malignancy had been achieved by combination drug therapy. Her parents then brought her to the United States for further management. At the time of the present referral there were no hematologic abnormalities referable to her malignancy and hospitalization and infectious disease consultation were sought because of the occurrence of three episodes of high fever (temperature over 39°C), each lasting 24 hours, six and four days prior to the referral and again on the day of admission. In between these episodes of fever she appeared remarkably well.

Although malaria was common in the general area of Pakistan from which the child was sent, the parents were unaware of any cases among family members or in the immediate vicinity of their home.

PHYSICAL EXAMINATION: Other than fever accompanied by shaking chills, the physical examination was entirely unremarkable.

LABORATORY DATA: Hb. 10 gms.%; WBC 3000; Differential 55% neutrophils, 45% normal-appearing lymphocytes; platelets 150,000.

QUESTIONS:

1. Which of the following would you NOT investigate with urgency
    in this case?
    A. Malaria
    B. Tuberculosis
    C. Bacterial sepsis
    D. Virus infection
    E. Recurrence of leukemia

2. What investigations would you carry out?
    A. Blood count and marrow aspiration
    B. Urinalysis
    C. Skin tests
    D. Blood, stool, nose and throat, CSF, and marrow cultures
        for bacteria, mycobacteria and fungi
    E. Thick and thin smears of blood for parasites
    F. Chest x-ray
    G. All of the above

These tests were done and it was immediately noted that the thick
smear revealed malarial parasites. Examination of the thin smears
revealed that the parasites were present in enlarged erythrocytes.
Fine basophilic stippling was seen in the parasitized red blood cells
(Schuffner's dots) and the parasites were morphologically characteristic of Plasmodium vivax.

At this early stage it was not felt to be unusual that splenomegaly
and hepatomegaly were absent. It should be recalled that a history
had been obtained of a single transfusion of fresh whole blood in the
initial therapy of her leukemia in Pakistan.

QUESTIONS:

3. This child's malarial infection may have resulted from:
    A. Transmission from an infected mosquito
    B. Transmission from infected blood
    C. Either A or B, or both

4. Which drugs would you use for treatment?
    A. Quinine
    B. Chloroquine phosphate
    C. Trimethoprim-Sulfisoxazole
    D. Atabrine

5. Is any additional form of therapy required after acute, non-
    falciparum, mosquito-induced malarial disease is brought under
    control?
    A. Yes
    B. No

Is any additional form of therapy required after acute, trans-
fusion-induced malaria is brought under control?
C. Yes
D. No

6. If the answer to question #5 includes A, which of the following
drugs would you administer in the case of vivax malaria?
A. Primaquine
B. Quinine
C. Proguanil
D. Atabrine

7. Drug resistance has been reported in the case of which of the
following malarial parasites?
A. P. vivax
B. P. falciparum
C. P. malariae
D. P. ovale
E. All of these

ANSWERS:

1. (D)

The fever pattern in the present case is very unlikely to result from
any known virus infection. As a matter of fact, the fever pattern is
really only characteristic of malaria among the generic disease
types listed. However, in a child with altered host defenses (underlying disease and/or therapy) it is essential to investigate each of
the other possibilities listed.

2. (G)

Having answered question #1, it is apparent that all of the tests
listed will be required in order to effectively investigate these
possibilities.

3. (C)

Although the most likely cause of malarial transmission remains
the bite of an infected mosquito, blood from a carrier-donor may
also carry and transmit parasites and, in this case, could have been
the source of the infection.

4. (B)

Chloroquine phosphate administered for three days is the drug of
choice for treatment of non-falciparum malarial infection.

5. (A, D)

P. falciparum is not accompanied by an exo-erythrocytic phase and requires only acute therapy. All other forms of malaria usually require the eradication of tissue forms after the treatment of the acute erythrocytic disease. However, since erythrocytic parasites of blood-induced infections do not re-enter the liver in human malaria, primaquine therapy is not required in any form of transfusion induced malaria.

6. (A)

There is no satisfactory alternative to primaquine treatment for malarial exo-erythrocytic eradication, although other anti-malarials can be useful in the treatment of an acute attack. In the present case, due to the uncertainty of the means of acquisition, a course of primaquine is indicated.

7. (B)

Chloroquine resistance has been reported in falciparum malaria. In the case of chloroquine resistance, or in an instance where there exists uncertainty concerning drug sensitivity patterns, quinine is the drug of choice and may be lifesaving.

FINAL NOTE: Although little malaria is seen in the USA today, it is well to remember when treating individuals coming from elsewhere that the prevalence and incidence of malaria remain largely unchanged (or even increased) in much of the world. Protozoan parasites more commonly found in the United States, such as Toxoplasma gondii and Pneumocystis carinii, can and do cause significant disease among children with disseminated malignancies.

REFERENCES

1. Bruce-Chwatt, L. J. , et al. : Malaria; epidemiology, laboratory diagnosis, chemoprophylaxis and chemotherapy. Brit. Med. J. 2:91-98, 1971.

2. Feigin, R. D. , Shearer, W. T. : Opportunistic infection in children. I & II, The compromised host. J. Pediat. 87:507-514, 677-694, 1975.

3. Hughes, W. T. , et al. : Infectious disease in children with cancer. Pediat. Clin. N. A. 21:583-615, 1974.

4. Miller, L. H. : Transfusion Malaria. In: Transmissible Disease and Blood Transfusion. Greenwalt, T. J. , Jamieson, G. A. (Eds.) Grune and Stratton, New York, 1974, pages 241-266.

CASE 30: PULMONARY INFECTION AND ACUTE HEMIPLEGIA
IN A 2-9/12-YEAR-OLD BOY WITH ACUTE LYMPHO-
BLASTIC LEUKEMIA

HISTORY: The patient was entirely well until five months ago when
he developed pallor, cervical adenopathy and purpura. Acute lymphoblastic leukemia was diagnosed and anti-leukemic therapy instituted. Remission was achieved and he continued on maintenance
anti-leukemic treatment. Two months ago he developed cough,
breathlessness and signs of a right upper lobe consolidation. Chest
x-ray revealed a right upper lobe pneumonia which was treated with
multiple antibiotics. Resolution was slow and subsequent films
showed persistence of the opacity in the right lung field (Fig. 30. 1).
As no further resolution was occurring and persistent fever and
weight loss continued, a thoracotomy was done and a large abscess
was found and drained. The aspirated contents of the abscess were
odorless. A chest tube was left in place on suction. The pus was
examined microscopically and was cultured. Gram stain revealed
some gram-positive cocci, a few gram-negative bacilli, and many
gram-positive branching narrow bacilli, some of which showed
occasional acid-fast segments.

QUESTION:

1. What form of antimicrobial therapy would you initiate post-
    operatively while the culture studies were in progress?
    A. Anti-tuberculous therapy with two drugs
    B. Anti-fungal therapy with amphotericin B
    C. Antibacterial therapy to cover a broad range of gram-posi-
        tive and negative organisms
    D. No specific therapy pending cultures
    E. Penicillin therapy as appropriate for mixed flora, perhaps
        including Actinomyces or Nocardia, recognizing the latter
        organism will require sulfonamide therapy

The postoperative orders had initiated therapy with ampicillin and cloxa-
cillin and the patient seemed to improve. Subsequently the cultures were
interpreted as showing a predominant growth of Nocardia asteroides.

QUESTION:

2. In the light of this laboratory finding, would you make any changes
    in the therapy, and if so, what would your choice be?
    A. Do not make a change until sensitivites are determined
    B. Stop present drugs and begin high dosage penicillin and linco-
        mycin
    C. Stop present therapy and begin tetracycline
    D. Stop present therapy and start erythromycin
    E. Stop present therapy and start chloramphenicol
    F. Stop present therapy and initiate treatment with sulfonamides
        (includes TMP-SMX)

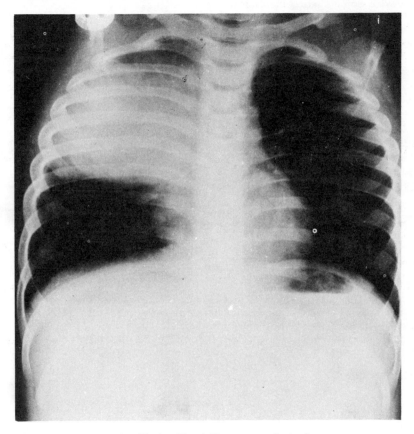

FIG. 30.1: Chest X-ray on admission.

In the present case, the therapy was changed on the basis of the sensitivities and the patient continued to improve. He remained in hematologic remission with no evidence of bleeding. Shortly after a readjustment of his chest drainage tube 12 days postoperatively, he became febrile, had a generalized seizure, and upon recovery remained drowsy and manifested a left hemiplegia. Fundoscopy revealed some engorgement of his retinal veins.

QUESTIONS:

3. What is likely to have happened?
   A. He has had a febrile convulsion
   B. He has dislodged an embolus resulting in cerebral vessel thrombosis, infarction, and cerebral infection with possible formation of an abscess
   C. He had developed acute bacterial meningitis
   D. He has CNS leukemia
   E. This is a not uncommon toxic manifestation of vincristine, which he was receiving for his malignant disease

4. Which of the following investigations would you perform to clarify this situation?
   A. Skull X-ray
   B. EEG
   C. Lumbar puncture
   D. Computerized axial tomography (CAT scan)
   E. Cultures of blood and CSF
   F. All of these

All these studies were done and revealed: CSF and skull X-ray - normal. EEG - a definite abnormality over the posterior left hemisphere. CAT scan - two small areas of altered density (one right frontal and the other left occipital) consistent with the presence of small abscesses (Fig. 30. 2). Cultures - all negative.

QUESTIONS:

5. Should antibiotic therapy be altered in light of these findings?
   A. Yes
   B. No

6. The following are several True-False statements concerning some characteristics of Nocardia asteroides:
   A. Grows only anaerobically
   B. Produces infectious granulomata which may discharge pigmented granules
   C. Belongs to the group of actinomycetes which can cause a form of "Madura foot" or mycetoma
   D. Is commonly found in nature and is highly communicable

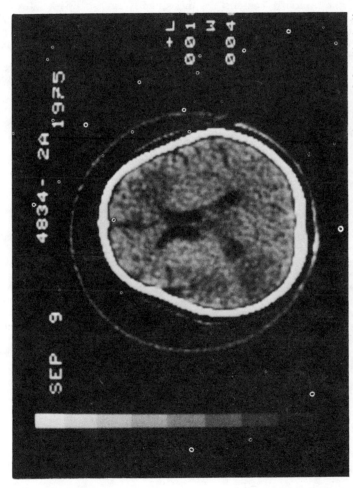

FIG. 30. 2: Computerized Axial Tomography (CAT) Scan showing areas of altered density in the right frontal and left posterior brain.

ANSWERS:

1. (E)

Initiate a course of antibacterial therapy directed against the mixed flora visualized on Gram stain. If the child was extremely toxic, sulfonamides could be used simultaneously as therapy for possible Nocardia. Aminoglycosides are infrequently necessary as enteric gram-negative organisms are an infrequent occurrence in solitary pulmonary abscesses. The predominant organism identified in culture was <u>Nocardia asteroides</u>, a recognized pathogen, particularly in individuals with compromised immune function. [2,4,5]

2. (F or A)

The drainage procedure has been responsible for the significant improvement in his status. Although Nocardia species show variable sensitivity to several antibiotics, the therapy of choice continues to be sulfonamide. A presumptive change to sulfonamide can be made initially or after sensitivity testing. In the present case, the recovered Nocardia proved highly sensitive to trimethoprim-sulfisoxazole and that was the therapy chosen.

3. (B, E)

It is likely that during the tube manipulation an embolus - potentially infected - was dislodged. This fragment(s) would be expected to travel via the pulmonic veins to the left heart and thence via the systemic outflow tract to the brain and/or the rest of the body via the aorta and general circulation. The likelihood of a cerebral abscess must therefore be considered. Nocardia asteroides has a propensity for the induction of pulmonary abscesses, empyemas, and secondary brain abscesses. Vincristine toxicity could also present in this manner, but in view of the preceding history, cerebral embolization and abscess becomes the first possibility to explore.

4. (F)

All of the procedures listed are potentially useful in clarifying the nature of this sudden occurrence. If a CAT scan[3] were not available, similar though probably less exact data could be derived from arteriography. In view of the retinal venous engorgement, the lumbar puncture should be performed with appropriate caution.

5. (B)

The occurrence and recognition of these small infarcts and presumed abscesses does not warrant a change in the antimicrobial therapy.

6.   (A) False. Nocardia asteroides grows aerobically on simple media such as beef-heart infusion blood agar plates.

(B) True. Nocardia may produce pigmented granules very similar to the "sulfur granules" found in infection with actinomycosis. Preparations of these granules are useful for identifying the presence of branching filamentous forms, though by this means distinction of these organisms is not possible.

(C) True. Classic "Madura foot" or mycetoma is a chronic suppurative granuloma of tissue and bone, often involving the extremities. The infection, which may be caused by streptomyces or by Nocardia species of actinomycetes, leads to gradual deformity, though unassociated with significant systemic symptoms.

(D) False. Nocardia are common in nature and are not considered highly communicable. Perhaps it would be more correct to say that they are ordinarily not invasive, though probably very easily and frequently transmitted in nature.

FINAL NOTE: The symptoms referable to the central nervous system gradually resolved and no neurosurgical approach was deemed warranted because of the small size of the lesions, the evidence for more than one focus, and the continued improvement. The lung abscess resolved and the patient was discharged to continue his antileukemic therapy.

Serious infections occur frequently in immunologically abnormal hosts. We are not surprised when such an occurrence overtakes a patient with a generalized malignancy in relapse. This child experienced an invasive infection while in hematologic remission. This illustrates that these patients, even when in marrow remission, are probably not normal with respect to certain basic defense mechanisms. With the development of more aggressive anti-leukemia treatment and the prolongation of remissions and survival, the risk of infectious complications will increase. [6] The relative roles in these complications of treatment and the underlying disease state may be difficult to identify.

REFERENCES

1.   Conant, N. F.: Manual of Clinical Mycology, 3rd edition. W. B. Saunders, Philadelphia, 1971.

2.   Feigin, R. D., Shearer, W. T.: Opportunistic infection in children. I & II, The Compromised Host. J. Pediat. 87:507-514, 677-694, 1975.

3. Gomez, M.R. , Reese, D. F. : Computerized tomography of the head in infants and children. Pediat. Clin. N. A. 23:473-498, 1976.

4. Hart, P. D. , et al. : The compromised host and infection. 2. Deep fungal infection. J. Infect. Dis. 120:169-191, 1969.

5. Hughes, W. T. , et al. : Infectious Disease in children with cancer. Pediat. Clin. N. A. 21:583-615, 1974.

6. Simone, J. V. , et al. : Fatalities during remission of childhood leukemia. Blood 39:759-770, 1972.

7. Ziad, H. Idriss, et al. : Nocardiosis in children. Report of 3 cases and review of the literature. Pediatrics 55:479-484, 1975.

8. Orfanakis, M. G. , et al. : In vitro studies of the combined effect of ampicillin and sulfonamides on N. asteroides and results of therapy in 4 patients. Antimic. Agts. & Chemother. 1:215, 1972.

9. Finland, M. , et al. : Synergistic action of ampicillin and erythromycin against Nocardia asteroides: Effect of time of incubation. Antimic. Agts. & Chemother. 5:344, 1974.

10. Baikie, A. G. , et al. : Systemic nocardiosis treated with trimethoprim and sulfamethoxazole. Lancet II:261, 1970.

11. Bach, M. C. , et al. : Pulmonary nocardiosis therapy with minocycline and erythromycin plus ampicillin. JAMA 224-1378, 1973.

::

CASE 31: RESPIRATORY STRIDOR, FEVER, SORE THROAT, AND PAIN ON SWALLOWING IN A YOUNG CHILD

HISTORY: A $3\frac{1}{2}$-year-old female presented with inspiratory respiratory stridor of 6 hours duration. Two days prior to admission she developed fever (38. 5°C) and sore throat. Over the ensuing 36 hours she was observed to have increasing pain, an inability to swallow secretions, and progressive shortness of breath. The patient's past medical history and family history was unremarkable. Her immunizations were up-to-date.

PHYSICAL EXAMINATION: Temperature 39°C, B. P. 110/78 mm Hg, Pulse 110/min. , Respiratory rate 30/min. The patient was anxious, maintained a rigid upright position with her neck hyperextended and mouth open, drooling saliva. The neck was stiff, apparently tender and attempts at flexion were resisted. A careful and gentle examination of the oropharynx revealed multiple petechiae on the soft palate,

inflamed tonsils without visible foreign body. The tonsillar pillars
were symmetrical and no exudate or membrane were noted over the
tonsils or pharynx. Cervical lymph nodes were slightly enlarged and
the remainder of the physical examination was within normal limits.

LABORATORY DATA: CBC: Hgb = 12gm%, Hct = 38%. WBC = 25,000/
cu mm, PMN = 84%, lymphocytes = 16%. Urinalysis: Normal. Serum
BUN, sugar and electrolytes were normal. X-ray of the lateral
neck revealed swelling of the epiglottis. Cultures of both nasopharynx
and blood yielded type B H. Influenzae.

QUESTIONS:

1. The most likely diagnosis in this case is:
   A. Foreign body aspiration
   B. Asthmatic bronchitis
   C. Laryngotracheobronchitis (croup)
   D. Acute bacterial epiglottitis

2. The agent almost exclusively implicated in this disease is:
   A. Adenovirus
   B. Streptococcus pneumoniae
   C. Influenza B
   D. Hemophilus influenzae (type B)

3. Successful management of this condition is by:
   A. Antimicrobial agents
   B. Tracheostomy
   C. Antimicrobial agents and prompt relief of airway obstruction
      by nasotracheal intubation or tracheostomy
   D. Steroids

4. The antimicrobial agent of choice is:
   A. Penicillin
   B. Tetracycline
   C. Cephalothin
   D. Ampicillin or chloramphenicol

ANSWERS:

1. The most likely diagnosis is (D).

Signs and symptoms common to foreign body aspiration, croup and
bacterial epiglottitis are irritability, restlessness, stridor, hoars-
ness, croupy cough, and at times cyanosis. However, when a patient presents with marked toxicity, high fever and a characteristic
posture with hyperextension of the neck, protrusion of the tongue
and saliva drooling from the mouth, then the diagnosis of acute bacterial epiglottitis should be suspected. There is usually an associated leukocytosis frequently with a left shift. Although a lateral x-ray

of the neck may be of interest, the patient should not be sent to x-ray during the initial evaluation unless accompanied by physicians and means of alleviating airway obstruction are available. He should instead receive prompt supportive therapy and always be in a position allowing prompt recognition and treatment of respiratory compromise.

2. The agent almost exclusively implicated in this disease is (D).

Encapsulated (Pittman type B) H. influenzae is the causative organism which may be isolated from blood; pharynx of patients with edematous epiglottitis contains numerous submucosal microabscesses and blood cultures in 50% of the cases, which supports the septicemic nature of this disease. Other organisms e. g. , pneumococci, staphylococci or streptococci, have been implicated rarely and only on the basis of nasopharyngeal or throat culture results. Diphtheritic croup, although rare in the U. S. must be kept in mind since in Mexico, South America and parts of the Middle East as well as in southern areas of the U. S. there still occur episodic outbreaks. The syndromes of acute laryngitis or laryngotracheobronchitis due to agents such as parainfluenzae, influenzae, or adenovirus are clinically and etiologically distinct from H. influenzae epiglottitis.

3. Successful management of this condition is by (C).

Appropriate antimicrobial agents and prompt relief of airway obstruction go hand-in-hand for successful management of acute bacterial epiglottitis. From 1940 through the late 1960's, tracheostomy was employed only when indicated as an emergency measure. Mortality in the early series varied from 8 to 40%, and patients were at significant risk of sustaining neurologic sequelae secondary to hypoxia. Margolis et al. recommended the use of immediate tracheostomy for all patients with this disease to eliminate mortality due to acute airway obstruction. Removal of the tracheostomy tube is usually possible within a couple of weeks. An alternative to prophylactic tracheostomy was described by Traff and Tos who employed routine nasotracheal intubation for 48 hours. Adjunctive therapy with corticosteroids has been employed in an attempt to decrease epiglottal edema but the results of therapy with steroids are inconsistent. These drugs should not be substituted for antibiotics or for relief of airway obstruction in patients with severe respiratory distress.

4. The antimicrobial agent of choice is (D).

Because H. influenzae type B is the predominant pathogen in this disease, the antibiotic of choice is presently chloramphenicol. Recently, strains of H. influenzae resistant to ampicillin have been reported in cases of epiglottitis and meningitis. Thus, adequate sensitivity testing of H. influenzae type B to ampicillin is important. If the organism is proven to be ampicillin sensitive, one may elect to shift from chloramphenicol to ampicillin. Parenteral therapy is essential in the first 48-72 hours, regardless of the antibiotic chosen, because oral administration may be impossible in the toxic child with severe sore throat and adequate inhibitory levels of the antimicrobial agent are assured with parenteral administration. When septicemia is present, the total course of antimicrobial therapy needed is usually 10 days without occurrence of additional complications.

REFERENCES

1. Berenberg, W. , Kevy, Sh. : Acute epiglottitis in childhood (A serious emergency, readily recognized at the bed side - review of 42 cases). NEJM 258:870, 1958.

2. Addy, M. G. , et al. : Hemophilus epiglottitis: Nine recent cases in Oxford. Brit. Med. J. 1:40, 1972.

3. Norden, C. W. , Michaels, R. : Immunologic response in patient with epiglottitis caused by Hemophilus influenzae type B. J. Infect. Dis. 128:777, 1973.

4. Poole, C. A. , Altman, D. H. : Acute epiglottitis in children. Radiology 80:798, 1963.

5. Robbin, J. B. : Hemophilus influenzae type B: Disease and immunity in humans. Ann. Int. Med. 78:259, 1973.

6. Milko, D. A. , et al. : Nasotracheal intubation in the treatment of acute epiglottitis. Pediatrics 53:674, 1974.

7. Margolis, C. Z. , et al. : Routine tracheotomy in Hemophilus influenzae type B epiglottitis. J. Pediat. 81:1150, 1972.

8. Ampicillin - resistant Hemophilus influenzae. Center for Disease Control, Morbidity and Mortality Weekly Report 23:99, 1974.

9. Andrew, J. D. , et al. : Acute epiglottitis: Challenge of a rarely recognized emergency. Brit. Med. J. 2:524, 1968.

::

CASE 32: APLASTIC ANEMIA AND FEVER

HISTORY: A 10-year-old boy who had aplastic anemia diagnosed 3 months prior to admission has presented with ecchymoses, epistaxis and petechiae. His hematologic evaluation revealed a hemoglobin of 10.2 gm%, a reticulocyte count of 2.2%, a WBC of 2,400 with 1% neutrophils and 99% lymphocytes, and a platelet count of $15,000/mm^3$. Bone marrow performed at that time was extremely hypocellular and the patient was receiving daily oxymetholone, prednisone alternate days and occasional transfusions of fresh whole blood. During a three-day period prior to admission the patient developed a fever of 40°C, a sore throat, malaise, pin pointed petechial rash over the trunk and extremities and decreased activity.

PHYSICAL EXAMINATION: Temperature 38. 4°C, pulse 104/minute, respirations 28/minute, blood pressure 120/60 mm Hg. The general appearance was that of an acutely ill, cushingoid white male. HEENT revealed extensive bilateral conjunctival hemorrhages, tiny petechiae present on the mucous membranes of the oral cavity, and large erythematous tonsils. There were numerous petechiae present over all extremities with an ecchymotic tender area, about 3 cm. in diameter, present on the back of the right calf muscle. The lungs were clear, the heart regular and rhythmic, the liver and spleen were not enlarged and there were no focal neurologic signs.

LABORATORY DATA: Hemoglobin 8. 1 gms%, hematocrit 27%, WBC 1,000/mm^3 with 3% neutrophils and 97% lymphocytes. Platelet count 1,500/mm^3. Urinalysis was within normal limits as were the serum electrolytes and BUN.

COURSE IN THE HOSPITAL: After drawing blood for culture and taking a throat culture, the patient was begun on intravenous gentamicin, carbenicillin, and keflin. He also received platelets and fresh whole blood transfusions. Over the course of the next week, the blood culture grew Enterobacter sp and Klebsiella sp. The patient's subcutaneous bleeding and conjunctival hemorrhages resolved somewhat as an apparent response to therapy. Subsequent blood cultures were negative. Two weeks after admission, the patient was noted to have extensive oral thrush and he was begun on oral mycostatin.

QUESTIONS:

1. Factors contributing to severity of infection in patients with aplastic anemia are:
   A. Virulence of organisms
   B. Number of organisms
   C. Overgrowth of resistant organisms selected by antibiotics
   D. Absolute neutrophil counts

2. The causative agents of serious infections in patients with altered neutrophil function tend to be:
   A. Gram-negative bacteria
   B. Gram-positive bacteria
   C. Fungi
   D. Actinomycetes
   E. Viruses
   F. Protozoa (Pneumocystis carinii)
   G. Others (Mycoplasma)

3. Nonspecific enhancers of resistance in man may include:
    A. Viral interference
    B. Interferon
    C. Interferon inducers
    D. Bacterial interference
    E. Bacterial products such as endotoxins
    F. Transfer factor
    G. Well-defined chemicals (dinitrochlobenzene, levamisole,
        and vitamin C)

4. The nature and type of infections in patients with altered immun-
    ity include:
    A. Otitis, sinusitis, pharyngitis, gingivitis, and esophagitis
    B. Meningitis and/or pneumonia
    C. Intra-abdominal infections
    D. Urinary tract infections
    E. Sepsis and skin infections

5. Appropriate antibiotic regimens for fever of unknown origin in
    immunocompromised patients before cultures and sensitivities
    have returned may include:
    A. Oxacillin, carbenicillin, and gentamicin
    B. Oxacillin, gentamicin, and clindamycin
    C. Penicillin, carbenicillin and gentamicin
    D. Clindamycin or chloramphenicol may be added to any of
        these regimens if a Bacteroides species is suspected

ANSWERS:

1. Factors contributing to severity of infection in patients with
    aplastic anemia and/or cancer are (B-D).

Unlike patients with normal host defenses, patients with aplastic
anemia acquire infections which are both severe and frequent. There
is a wide range in the virulence of infecting organisms, some of
which do not ordinarily infect healthy persons. Treatment with one
or more antibiotics may result in suppression of normal flora of the
gastrointestinal tract, and allow increased numbers of such organisms
as Pseudomonas aeruginosa, Klebsiella - Enterobacter - Serratia,
and Proteus species. Life threatening infections can occur when
large numbers of these organisms are aerosolized into the bronchi.
Streptococci and staphylococci which usually respond promptly to
appropriate antibiotics may cause severe infections in patients with
absent or decreased polymorphonuclear cell function. A lack of
opsonins may contribute to increased risk from these infections so
that primary infection with an organism may be more severe than
reinfection with an organism to which the host has antibodies. The
function of the neutrophils, not only their total count, is critical;
myelocytes and metamyelocytes can phagocytize and kill bacteria,
but with far less efficacy than mature neutrophils. Altered lymphocyte or mononuclear cell function can result from chemotherapy of

the aplastic anemia. In patients with aplastic anemia and low platelets, there is a higher frequency of breakdown of skin and mucous
membranes. Sepsis with normal bowel flora may follow undetected
ulcers in the gastrointestinal tract. Infections often occur, too frequently, because of indwelling intravascular or urinary bladder
catheters, bone marrow aspiration, or biopsies. Even giving ene-
mas or inserting rectal thermometers may result in sufficient trauma
to the anal tissue, paving the way for subsequent life-threatening
infections.

2. The causative agents of serious infections in patients with al-
    tered neutrophil function tend to be (A-C).

Pseudomonas aeruginosa, Escherichia coli, Proteus, Klebsiella,
Serratia marcescens, and Bacteroides species are gram-negative
bacteria responsible for serious infections. The extent to which a
particular strain can establish an infection will depend on the degree
of compromise of the host. Pseudomonas aeruginosa is a well-es-
tablished contaminent of the hospital environment, especially in
moist areas such as sinks, toilets, and respiratory equipments.
Pseudomonas causes vasculitis of small vessels. This gives the
characteristic lesion (ecthyma gangrenosa) which begins as an erythematous maculopapule that becomes vesicular. The vesicle is sometimes hemorrhagic and when it ruptures, a well demarcated gangrenous ulcer appears. A bluish-black escar forms over the ulcer.
Serratia marcescens previously considered non-pathogenic, appears
to be an increasing threat to the altered host. Diphtheroids are frequent contaminants of clinical cultures and are a part of the normal
intestinal, skin, and mucous membrane flora, and they too are capable of producing serious infection in the compromised host. Multiple organism septicemia, with more than 1 species of bacteria, may
also occur in these patients.

Viruses of the herpes virus group which include varicella-zoster
virus, herpes simplex virus, and cytomegalovirus, are double-
stranded DNA viruses which cause life-threatening infection in children with altered cell mediated immunity. Varicella is a highly contagious primary infection and is a serious and potentially fatal infection in children with cancer. Thus, prevention is the primary
objective for control of this disease. At present, passive immunization with zoster immune globulin is effective in the modification
of varicella if administered within 72 hours of exposure. Herpes
simplex virus, which causes localized surface lesions, can also
disseminate to cause pneumonitis, encephalitis, hepatitis and/or
generalized cutaneous lesions. Cytomegalovirus frequently causes
symptomatic infection in immunosuppressed patients which probably represents activation of endogenous infection. Protozoal infection (Toxoplasma gondii, Pneumocystis carinii), opportunistic
mycotic infections (Candida albicans, Aspergillus fumigatus, and
Cryptococcus neoformans), and actinomycetes have all been documented etiologic agents in patients with altered cellular and/or
humoral immune functions.

3. Nonspecific enhancers of resistance in man include (A-G).

Nonspecific enhancers are those whose effects are not limited to a single receptor system. They do not need to be effective against a universe of pathogens but may function alone or as adjuvants with specific antigens to increase an immune response. In part, they probably work because they increase the number of performing cells or increase their rate of performance. They might work by increasing a local inflammatory action, by stimulating chemotaxis, by activating the complement or properidin systems, by increasing the rate of phagocytosis, by activating intracellular lysozymes, by inducing interferon, or by modifying cell membranes of B or T lymphocytes so that they may be more responsive and so yield larger amounts of immunoglobulins or lymphokines. (However, in most instances it is not known how this is accomplished.) A demonstration of viral interference is the observation that small pox vaccination is blocked in infants between 11 and 36 months of age when vaccinia virus was inoculated 9 to 15 days after they had been given an attenuated live measles virus vaccine. Interferons are proteins whose synthesis is induced in a wide variety of cells by viral infection. They do not act directly on viruses but on host cells wherein they reduce the ability of the virus to replicate. Interferons induced by cells of 1 species do not generally protect cells of another species against infection. Bacterial population of the respiratory or gastrointestinal tract may act to inhibit the growth of pathogenic microorganisms as long as this flora is not altered by antibiotic treatment. A lysate of Staphylococcus aureus has recently been reported to have a nonspecific enhancing effect on cell mediated immunity. Similarly, an attenuated strain of Mycobacterium bovis (Bacille-Calmette-Guerin, or BCG) is now receiving most attention as an enhancer of nonspecific resistance especially for certain tumors. Unfortunately, since this is a live vaccine, generalized infections sometimes occur in individuals who were severely immunosuppressed. Finally, transfer factor which is present in lysates of human peripheral blood leukocytes has the capacity to transfer specific immunologic memories for cutaneous delayed hypersensitivity from sensitive donors to nonsensitive recipients. Chemicals such as dinitrochlorobenzene, levamisole, and vitamin C are other nonspecific enhancers of resistance which could be important for individuals of great risk when there is not a prior knowledge of what needs to be resisted.

4. The nature and types of infection in patients with altered immunity include (A-E).

Generally, fever is more apt to be associated with infection when cancer and/or immunosuppression is severe or of long duration. Head and neck infections, meningitis, pneumonia, intra-abdominal infections, urinary tract infections, and skin infections are common in immunosuppressed patients and every effort should be made to obtain a specific microbial diagnosis since superinfection with more antibiotic-resistant bacteria is not an uncommon occurrence in these patients.

5. Antibiotic regimen for life-threatening infections until cultures
    and sensitivities return include (A-D).

The treatment on infections in patients with immunosuppression, as
in any other patient, is aimed at the specific microorganism causing the infection. However, although the diagnosis of a specific
organism is always attempted, empirical therapy is mandatory when
a patient appears to have a life-threatening infection without an evident source. Therefore, one tries to use broad spectrum antibiotics
to cover most gram-positive and gram-negative organisms including
Staphylococcus aureus and Pseudomonas. Once a specific microbial
diagnosis is made, one or more of the antibiotics could be discontinued. The length of therapy varies with the type of infection, the
organism involved, and the host defenses. Finally, preventive measures remain of primary importance since although the majority of
infections are probably endogenous, large numbers of potential
pathogens may be passed from one patient to another on unwashed
hands. Tuberculosis prophylaxis is frequently overlooked and is
particularly important in patients with immunosuppression and a
positive tuberculin skin test.

REFERENCES

1. Armstrong, D. , et al. : Infectious complications of neoplastic
    disease. Med. Clin. N. A. 55:729-754, 1971.

2. Hughes, W. T. , et al. : Infectious disease in children with can-
    cer. Pediat. Clin. N. A. 21:583-615, 1974.

3. Feigin, R. D. , et al. : Opportunistic infection in children (3 parts)
    J. Pediat. 87:507-514, 677-694, 852-866, 1975.

4. Florman, A. L. et al. : Non-specific enhancers of resistance in
    man. J. Pediat. 87:1094-1102, 1975.

5. Gold, E. : Infections associated with immunologic deficiency dis-
    ease. Med. Clin. N. A. 58:649-659, 1974.

6. Young, R. C. , et al. : Management of infections in patients with
    leukemia and lymphoma. Sem. Hema. 9:141, 1972.

7. Pole, J. G. , et al. : Granulocyte transfusion in treatment of
    infected neutropenic children. Arch. Dis. Child. 51:521-527,
    1976.

CASE 33: VOMITING AND IRRITABILITY IN A NEWBORN INFANT

HISTORY: A 30-year-old gravida 1, para 1, abortion 0, young lady
gave birth to a 3,500 gram, male infant at term after an uneventful
labor and delivery. Physical examinations at birth and at 8 hours
of age were essentially normal. At 18 hours of age the newborn began vomiting and refusing to feed and a few hours later he was noted
to be irritable. At 30 hours of age the baby was lethargic, seizure
activity was noted and a lumbar puncture was performed.

PHYSICAL EXAMINATION: Temperature 37. 8°C, B. P. 90/70 mm
Hg, pulse 110/minute, respiration rate 36/minute. Head circumference was 37. 5 cm. and anterior fontanelle was bulging. HENT
was within normal limits. Neck supple. Lungs clear no rales. Heart
regular rhythmic. Liver and spleen were not enlarged, and the remainder of the physical examination was essentially negative.

LABORATORY DATA: Hemoglobin concentration = 14. 5 gm%, WBC
was 13,500/mm^3 (60% neutrophils, 29% lymphocytes, 4% monocytes,
and 7% band forms). Urinalysis normal. Serum BUN, sugar and
electrolytes were normal. Chest x-ray was negative. Lumbar puncture revealed cloudy spinal fluid with 2,800 WBC's/mm^3 containing
98% neutrophils; the glucose was 30 mg% (blood glucose 90 mg%),
and the total protein was 150 mg/100 ml. Gram stain of the CSF revealed many WBC's with gram-positive cocci in chains. Both CSF
and blood were sent for culture.

QUESTIONS:

1. The most likely diagnosis is:
   A. Sepsis
   B. Viral meningitis
   C. Bacterial meningitis
   D. A and/or C
   E. None of the above

2. The agent(s) most commonly implicated in this disease is (are):
   A. Staphylococcus aureus
   B. Streptococcus pyogenes
   C. Group B beta hemolytic streptococcus (Streptococcus agalac-
      tiae)
   D. Listeria monocytogenes
   E. E. coli

3. The antimicrobial agent of choice is:
   A. Penicillin
   B. Ampicillin
   C. Tetracycline
   D. Penicillin/ampicillin and gentamicin
   E. Chloramphenicol
   F. Cephalothin

4. Factors involved in the immune response to group B beta hemolytic streptococci are:
   A. Specific IgG and nonspecific opsonins
   B. Type specific IgM agglutinins
   C. Both

ANSWERS:

1. The most likely diagnosis in this case is (D).

The most frequent signs and symptoms associated with neonatal septicemia and/or meningitis are jaundice, poor feeding, gastrointestinal symptoms, respiratory symptoms, lethargy, fever, seizures, and hepatomegaly, in that order. The presence of a cluster of signs should be highly suggestive of sepsis and/or meningitis and an evaluation for infection, including a lumbar puncture, is indicated. Approximately half of children with neonatal meningitis have WBC's within the range of 10,000 to 25,000/mm^3. Differential leukocyte counts were variable but a rise in unsegmented neutrophils is a valuable clue to presence of infection. The WBC and differential counts do not distinguish between the gram-positive and gram-negative infections. The presence of leukocytes [3,5] and bacteria in gastric aspirate or external ear aspirate have been thought to indicate amnionitis and to represent an infant who has an increased risk of developing infection. Although prematurity, prolonged rupture of membranes and obstetrical complications are major risk factors, the presence of these findings does not establish the diagnosis of sepsis.

2. The agents most commonly implicated in this disease are (C, E).

Group B beta hemolytic streptococci (Streptococcus agalactiae) have become, in recent years, a frequent cause of septicemia and/or meningitis in neonates and young infants. This organism was recovered from both the blood and CSF of the patient presented above. The incidence of this disease has been increasing significantly every year and of all bacterial meningitis in the newborn its incidence rose from 33% in 1970, to 50% in 1971, to 65% in 1972, and to 70% in 1974 as reported from Houston. In many instances, meningitis due to group B streptococci equals or has surpassed in frequency that due to E. coli. The spectrum of illness of this disease varies from asymptomatic colonization of serious and fatal disease. The incidence of this disease is approximately one to two per one hundred colonized newborn according to several series, and 3 per 1000 of all live born infants. Major sites of involvement include septicemia, meningitis, arthritis, pneumonia, empyema, osteomyelitis, ethmoiditis, cellulitis, and conjunctivitis. There are two distinct age-related syndromes. The first is early onset disease which occurs during the first week of life and is frequently associated with maternal obstetrical complications such as prolonged rupture of membranes. It is associated with severe multisystem involvement. Apnea and shock occur within the first 24 hours of life. The mortality rate is as high as 75%. The late onset disease occurs after the first week of life, it involves the meninges most commonly, and the mortality rate is 25%. Group B streptococci are of 5 main serotypes (Ia, Ib, Ic, II and III). Types I and III organisms are common types in early onset disease. Type III organisms predominate from patients with involvement of the central nervous system in both early and late onset disease.

Attempts have been made to differentiate early onset disease of group B streptococcal pneumonia from hyaline membrane disease. Features more common for streptococcal disease were rupture of amniotic membranes for more than 12 hours after delivery, the presence of gram-positive cocci in gastric aspirate, and/or external auditory canal, apnea and shock in the first 24 hours, and the need for lower peak inspiratory pressures on a volume cycle respirator. However, x-ray features are usually indistinguishable from hyaline membrane disease, and on pathologic evaluation, most newborns with streptococcal pneumonia have no histologic evidence of hyaline membrane disease co-existing with their bacterial pneumonia unless they had hyaline membrane disease earlier.

3.   The antimicrobial agent of choice is (D).

Tube dilution sensitivity studies of group B streptococci have shown a median minimal inhibitory concentration (MIC) range of 0. 03 - 0. 06 micrograms/ml. However, when the minimal bactericidal concentration (MBC) was studied, the median range was at least 8 times the MIC. This differed from group A streptococci in which the MIC and MBC do not differ by more than 2 dilutions with penicillin or ampicillin. Moreover, a few strains of group B streptococci demonstrated a synergistic effect between penicillin/ampicillin and gentamicin in half of the strains. In the remaining strains, either an additive or a no effect was observed with this combination of antibiotics. Finally, kinetic studies (timed killing assays) demonstrated enhanced killing of group B streptococci by the addition of an aminoglycoside to penicillin or ampicillin.

4.   Factors involved in the immune response to Group B streptococcal challenge are (C).

Nonspecific opsonins, specific IgG and specific agglutinins (IgM), as well as the phagocytic ability of the polymorphonuclear leukocytes and the cellular immune response, are all essential in host defense against groupB streptococcal disease. Maternal antibodies to the capsular polysaccharide of groupB streptococci probably have a role in protecting the newborn from group B streptococcal disease. Studies have shown that invasive disease occurred frequently in neonates who were born to mothers colonized by Type III organisms if neither the infant nor mother had anticapsular antibody. In contrast, of the mothers who were vaginal carriers and had antibody to Type III capsule, none of the babies developed disease. The studies suggested that transplacental transfer of maternal antibody protects infants from invasive group B streptococcal disease, and that the infants of mothers deficient of these antibodies and also colonized are at risk of invasive disease.

In some studies, the colonization rates of the mothers vary from 25%-30%, as do those of their newborns, with an attack rate of 3/1,000 of all newly born infants or 1:100 of colonized newborn. These findings emphasize the extent of the problem presented by this emerging epidemic disease.

REFERENCES

1. Alojipan, L. C. , Andrews, B. F. : Neonatal sepsis. Clin. Pediat. 14:181-185, 1975.

2. Yow, M. D. : Epidemiology of Group B Streptococcal Infections, 1975. Progress in Clinical and Biological Research, Vol. 3, Infections of the Fetus and Newborn Infant, p. 159, Ed. by Krugman and Gershon, 1975.

3. Feigin, R. : The perinatal group B streptococcal problem: More questions than answers. NEJM 294:106, 1976.

4. Howard, J. B. , McCracken, G. H. : The spectrum of Group B streptococcal infections in infancy. Am. J. Dis. Child. 128:815, 1974.

5. Baker, C. J. , Kasper, D. L. : Correlation of maternal antibody deficiency with susceptibility to neonatal Group B streptococcal infection. NEJM 294:753-756, 1976.

6. Ablow, R. C. , et al. : A comparison of early-onset Group B streptococcal neonatal infection and respiratory-distress syndrome of the newborn. NEJM 294:65-70, 1976.

7. Baker, C. J. , Barrett, F. F. : Transmission of Group B streptococci among parturient women and their neonates. J. Pediat. 83:919-925, 1973.

8. Barton, L. L. , et al. : Group B beta hemolytic streptococcal
    meningitis in infants. J. Pediat. 82:719-723, 1973.

9. Dorand, R. D. , Adams, G. : Relapse during penicillin treatment
    of Group B streptococcal meningitis. J. Pediat. 89:188-190,
    1973.

10. Schauf, V. , et al. : Antibiotic-killing kinetics of Group B strep-
    tococci. J. Pediat. 89:194-198, 1976.

11. Akenzua, G. , et al. : Neutrophil and band counts in the diagnosis
    of neonatal infections. Pediatrics 54:38-42, 1974.

:::

CASE 34: POLYARTHRITIS IN AN 18-DAY-OLD INFANT

HISTORY: The mother was a 22-year-old Indian who was Para 2,
gravida 2, Type A, Rh positive and STS negative. She had received
obstetrical care for 6 months prior to delivery. Her pregnancy was
uncomplicated until 5 days prior to admission, when she developed
"false labor". Shortly thereafter she complained of severe joint pains
and a rash manifest by papules on her palms and soles. One day
prior to delivery the mother developed a fever of unknown etiology.
Labor began spontaneously, lasted 13 hours, and the 3,147 gram
male infant was delivered without difficulty at a gestational age of
40 weeks. The infant was kept in isolation for 24 hours after delivery because of the maternal fever and rash. The mother received
antimicrobial agents of an unknown type for the three days of hospitalization. The infant had received silver nitrate ophthalmic drops.
He had an elevated bilirubin and was observed for 4 days in the hospital before discharge home with his mother.

At 10 days of age the infant was observed to be irritable and cried
during diaper changes. At 14 days of age swelling of his left hand
was observed. There was pain with movement of the fingers. In the
next four days his feet and right elbow also became painful, visibly
swollen and red. The patient was then seen by his pediatrician at 18
days of age and referred to a tertiary care center.

PHYSICAL EXAMINATION: Heart rate 170. Respirations 60. Temperature 37. 5°C. Weight 3, 350 grams. Length 51. 2 cm. Head circumference 34 cm. He was a well-developed, well-nourished male
infant who was irritable when moved. His skin was notable for a
pustular rash in the right inguinal area. No conjunctivitis was present. Pertinent physical findings included a liver which was 5 cm.
below the right costal margin. No splenomegaly was observed. The
right elbow and ankle were swollen, warm, tender and red with a
limited range of motion. External rotation and other movement of
the hip joints elicited crying and it was obvious that movement of
these joints was painful for the infant.

LABORATORY INFORMATION: Hemoglobin, 15.2 grams. WBC.
19,950 with 60% neutrophils, 35% lymphocytes, 5% monocytes.
Urinalysis was within normal limits. X-ray examination showed
soft tissue swelling around the right elbow joint without any visible
changes of bone. The soft tissue swelling of the right ankle and foot
were also apparent. Aspiration of the right ankle joint produced fluid
with several hundred polymorphonuclear white blood cells and gram-
negative cocci were visible within cells. The rash in the right groin
was cultured and Gram stain revealed neutrophils but no visible
bacteria.

QUESTIONS:

1. Polyarticular arthritis in a newborn infant should evoke a con-
   sideration of the following pathogenic bacteria:
   A. Streptococcus agalactiae
   B. Staphylococcus aureus
   C. Neisseria gonorrhoeae
   D. Treponema pallidum
   E. E. coli
   F. Hemophilus influenzae type B

2. Neisseriaceae are fastidious organisms and the following condi-
   tions would improve the recovery of the organism in the bac-
   teriology laboratory:
   A. 5-10% CO_2
   B. Moisture during incubation
   C. Chocolate agar
   D. Thayer-Martin medium
   E. Anaerobic atmosphere
   F. Provision of X and V factors
   G. Direct plating of the synovial fluid and prompt transport to
      the laboratory

3. Differentiation of species of the Neisseriaceae genus are made in
   the laboratory on the basis of the following tests:
   A. Catalase
   B. Oxidase
   C. Sugar fermentations
   D. Morphological characteristics of the colonies and appearance
      of the Gram stained organisms

4. Acquisition of this N. gonorrhoeae by the infant could have occurred:
   A. From the mother in the process of delivery
   B. From fomites in the nursery
   C. From the mother in the postpartum period
   D. From the baby sitter

5. Portals of entry of Neisseriaceae in the newborn include:
   A. Conjunctivae
   B. Mucous membranes of the respiratory tract
   C. Mucous membranes of the gastrointestinal tract
   D. Skin abrasions
   E. Needle inoculation

6. Further evaluation of the infant should include:
   A. VDRL
   B. FTA-ABS-IgM
   C. ASO titer
   D. Blood culture
   E. Nasogastric aspirate for microscopic examination and cul-
      ture

7. Complete care of the infant should also dictate the necessity for
   an evaluation of other members of the family. Indicate which of
   the following statements is (are) correct:
   A. The father may be excluded as he is asymptomatic
   B. The mother has been treated but requires additional evalua-
      tion
   C. The local health department is notified of the diagnosis of
      N. gonorrhoeae infection to allow them to pursue the investi-
      gation
   D. Notification of social service and legal authorities of the
      presence of gonorrheal infection is important to investigate
      possible molestation of the infant

8. Ideal antimicrobial therapy of this infant would be:
   A. Oral penicillin for 10 days in a dosage of 100,000 units/kg/
      24 hours
   B. Intramuscular benzathine penicillin in a dosage of 500,000
      units
   C. Parenteral administered aqueous penicillin (100,000 units/
      kg/24 hr. x 10 days)
   D. Gonococci are increasingly resistant to penicillin and am-
      picillin therapy should be employed

ANSWERS:

1. (A-F)

The presence of polyarthritis first manifest at 10 days of age must
be considered as infection and rapid definition of the etiological agent
is essential to optimally treat this baby. The mother's history is
helpful since the presence of fever and skin lesions around the time
of delivery is typical of N. gonorrhoeae infection. Women are more
likely to become symptomatic at the time of their menses and during
the last trimester of pregnancy. It should be emphasized, however,
that asymptomatic women can also infect their infants. Neither the
mother nor infant were severely toxic and this is probably more

characteristic of infection with N. gonorrhoeae than with S. aureus.
Syphilis can result in limitation of motion of the extremities or
pseudoparalysis in an infant but objective joint findings (that is,
effusion and erythema) are usually absent. [1] Aspiration of the joint(s)
provides the opportunity of direct visualization of the responsible
pathogen. In particular, if his involvement is suspected, aspiration
and possibly drainage will be essential to prevent necrosis of the
femoral head. Fortunately, N. gonorrhoeae is not invasive or destructive to articulating cartilage or bone when treated with appropriate
antimicrobial therapy. Therapeutic open drainage is usually not essential in therapy of N. gonorrhoeae pyogenic arthritis at any age if
it is correctly treated. This infant was normal to physical examination at the time of discharge and remains so for 5 years of followup.
In contrast, E. coli and S. agalactiae may be rapidly invasive and
destructive, and drainage is often necessary. H. influenzae is being
rarely identified as cause of sepsis/meningitis in newborn infants
and should be remembered as an unusual pathogen. The absence of
epiphyseal cartilage in infants allows osteomyelitis to extend from
the metaphysis to the epiphysis and into the joint space in infants
who are less than 1 year of age. Thus, the bony destruction is frequently apparent on roentgenologic examination when pyarthrosis is
present. X-rays of an infant with symptomatic congenital syphilis
may reveal characteristic periosteal elevation and diffuse involvement of many bones. These evaluations can proceed after the initial
work-up and institution of therapy.

2.   (A-D, G)

All of these conditions will improve the rate of recovery of N. gonorrhoeae. These organisms will grow equally well on chocolate agar
and Thayer-Martin (T-M) medium. The latter consists of chocolate
agar with antimicrobial agents (vancomycin, colistimethate, nystat-
in) added to inhibit the growth of common saphyrophytic organisms
inhabiting such sites as the vagina or pharynx. Synovial fluid and
other normally sterile sites (CSF) can be cultured even more effectively on chocolate agar because of presence of some inhibitors in
T-M medium. Neither anaerobic conditions nor X and V factors
enhance growth of Neisseria sp.. X and V factors are needed for
Hemophilus sp.

3.   (C, D)

All species of the Neisseria genus are gram-negative diplococci,
but N. sicca tends to have wrinkled appearing colonies contrasting
to smooth colonies of N. gonorrhoeae, N. meningitidis, N. lactim-
ica, N. subflava, N. mucosa and N. flavescens. All members of
the genus are catalase and oxidase positive. N. gonorrhoeae ferments
only glucose whereas N. meningitidis ferments glucose and maltose.
N. lactamica ferments lactose in addition to glucose and maltose.
N. flavescens does not ferment any of the sugars, whereas N. sicca,

N. mucosa and N. subflava all ferment glucose, maltose, and with variability sucrose and fructose. They do not ferment lactose.

4. (A-D)

Infection with T. pallidum occurs throughout pregnancy as the hematogenous route of infection is most commonly the pathway by which a baby is infected. Only rare instances of acquisition during delivery are recorded and presumably result from contact with a primary lesion in the maternal GU tract. Similarly, European literature documents diffuse listeriosis of the newborn which results from hematogenous dissemination of infection during pregnancy. With these two exceptions the intrauterine conceptus is generally protected from bacterial infections including the bacterial flora of the maternal GU tract. It is most frequently after membranes have ruptured that bacteria gain access to the amniotic fluid and subsequently to the infant. N. gonorrhoeae has been cultured from the external auditory canal and the gastric aspirate of the newborn, indicating that amniotic fluid probably contained these organisms[7, 9] N. gonorrhoeae infection of conjunctivae has also been observed in occasional infants delivered by cesarean section[6] showing that such infection can be acquired without passage through the birth canal. One epidemic of gonococcal disease in a newborn nursery was apparently related to fomite contamination with these organisms. [9] It is also possible for an infected adult (the mother or other responsible care taker) to transmit infection to the baby via contaminated secretions and inadequate personal hygiene. This mother's illness suggests symptomatic gonorrhea and too little information is available to assess her antimicrobial therapy. She may or may not have been effectively treated. The 10 day incubation period is perhaps a little longer than anticipated with infection transmitted during delivery but is still within the acceptable time period for this mode of transmission.

5. (A-D)

In theory, organisms might be introduced by any of the portals listed. Needle inoculation is presently not substantiated in the newborn. Organisms have been cultured from conjunctivae, nasopharynx, rectum, and amniotic fluid in selected circumstances. [6, 8, 12] Skin abrasions are cited although neither local lesions nor positive cultures are reported in recent literature.

6. (A, D)

The mother's VDRL is reported to be negative, but it could have been obtained prior to delivery during the months of prenatal care. All infants should have a VDRL done at birth. Since there is one documented venereally transmitted illness, N. gonorrhoeae in this infant, the chances are increased that a second may also be present.

If the VDRL is positive, quantitation and assessment of IgM antibodies (FTA-ABS-IgM) will assist in defining the presence of infection in the infant. A blood culture should be done at the time of admission to attempt recovery of bacterial pathogens. A naso-gastric
aspirate at 18 days of age will not be helpful.

7. (B, C)

Certainly, the physician discusses the infection with the parents
when accurate identification of the organism is made. This should
obligate the parents to have appropriate examinations and bacterial
cultures. Males may also be asymptomatic carriers of the organism
and therefore the male sexual partner(s) need to be investigated.
Notification of the local Public Health authorities enlists the aid of
those skilled in case findings and knowledgeable in management of
gonococcal infections. Infections of a newborn does not usually en-
voke concern for possible molestation of a child. In older infants
and children, fomite transmission or sexual molestation may be
responsible for transmission of this infection.

8. (C)

Parenteral administration of crystalline penicillin G achieves adequate serum, CSF, and tissue levels of antibiotics. No gonorrhea
infections are readily treatable with parenteral aqueous penicillin.
The organisms causing bacteremia with arthritis in adults are unusual in their uniform susceptibility to very small amounts of penicillin. [13,14] This is noteworthy in the face of demonstrated increases
in the amount of penicillin (often achieved by simultaneous administration of Benemid) necessary to kill many GU strains of N. gonorrhoeae. Benzathine penicillin will produce constant low levels of
penicillin which are likely to be inadequate for therapy in systemic
infection with N. gonorrhoeae. At the present time, the erratic absorption of penicillin from the gastrointestinal tract and absence
of information to substantiate its efficacy in therapy of systemic infection prohibit this mode of therapy.

REFERENCES

1. Rothner, David A. , Klein, Norma: Parrot's pseudoparalysis,
    Revisited. Pediatrics 56:604-605, 1975.

2. Fink, Chester W. : Gonococcal arthritis in children. JAMA
    194:123-124, 1965.

3. Kohan, Daniel P. : Neonatal gonococcal arthritis: Three cases
    and review of the literature. Pediatrics 53:436-440, 1974.

4. Glaser, Stephen, et al. : Gonococcal arthritis in the newborn:
    Report of a case and review of the literature. Am. J. Dis. Child.
    112:185-188, 1966.

5. Kleiman, Martin B. , Lamb, George A. : Gonococcal arthritis
    in a newborn infant. Pediatrics 52:285-287, 1973.

6. Nickerson, C. W. : Gonorrhea amnionitis. Obstet. Gynec. 42:
    815-17, 1973.

7. Scanlon, J. W. : Diagnosis of gonorrhea infection by culture of
    the external ear canal in the newborn. Clin. Pediat. 10:528-
    529, 1971.

8. Handfield, Hunter H. , et al. : Neonatal gonococcal infection.
    I. Orogastric contamination with Neisseria gonorrhoeae. JAMA
    225:697-701, 1973.

9. Cooperman, Morris B. : Gonococcus arthritis in infancy: A
    clinical study of 44 cases. Am. J. Dis. Child. 33:932-948,
    1927.

10. Thompson, T. R. , et al. : Gonococcal ophthalmia neonatorum:
    Relationship of time of infection to relevant control measures.
    JAMA 228:186-188, 1974.

11. Frazer, A. D. , Morton, J. : Gonococcal stomatitis. Brit. Med.
    J. 1:1020-1022, 1931.

12. Armstrong, John H. , et al. : Ophthalmia neonatorum: A chart
    review. Pediatrics 57:884-892, 1976.

13. Weisner, Paul J. , et al. : Low antibiotic resistance of gonococci
    causing disseminated infection. NEJM 288:1221-1222, 1973.

::

CASE 35: DIFFUSE ABDOMINAL TENDERNESS

HISTORY: This is the first hospital admission for a 14-month-old,
black male with a chief complaint of bowel problems for one week.
The patient was considered normal and in perfect health until one
month prior to admission when he developed a pyarthrosis for which
he received intravenous medication for 5 days in a hospital near his
home. No positive blood culture, attempted aspiration of the knee
or further diagnostic studies were obtained to define the etiology of
this infection. The symptoms subsided, and he was again completely
well, receiving no medications for the two weeks preceding the present admission.

Six days prior to admission, the patient began to have 3 watery
stools per day for the next 3 days. The diarrhea then subsided and
on the night before admission he developed grunting respirations,
fever of 101° F and was his usual self. He was seen in a hospital
emergency room where Tylenol was prescribed. Examination within

the following 12 hours revealed diffuse abdominal distension and mild dehydration leading to hospital admission for therapy with intravenous fluids and subsequent transfer to a tertiary care center.

PHYSICAL EXAMINATION: Pulse 172. Respirations 72. Blood Pressure 190/60. Weight 11. 6 kg. He was a grunting, tachypneic, obtunded, black male child. Edema of the extremities was noted. The abdomen was massively distended and tense. No bowel sounds were audible. There was no detectable organomegaly or masses. No herniae were present and rectal examination was negative.

LABORATORY DATA: Hematocrit 43%, WBC. 15, 200 with 6% bands, 54% neutrophils, 38% lymphocytes. BUN 27. Sodium, 128 meq./L. Potassium, 7. 0 meq. /L. , and CO_2 13 meq. /L. Admission x-rays revealed a normal chest film. Flat and upright views of the abdomen showed no free gas and no extraluminal gas. The loops of bowel were not widely separated and the appendix was visualized when a barium enema was accomplished. The interpretation of the x-ray findings was a non-obstructive ileus. Urinalysis is normal.

QUESTIONS:

1. The clinical presentation of this infant focuses attention on the abdomen. Differential diagnosis should include:
    A. Gastroenteritis
    B. Pneumonia
    C. Appendicitis
    D. Peritonitis
    E. Diabetes mellitus

2. Additional laboratory and diagnostic procedures which would help to define the status of the child would be as follows:
    A. Lumbar puncture
    B. Abdominal paracentesis
    C. Blood cultures
    D. Examination of the urine
    E. Liver scan

Several drops of abdominal fluid obtained by paracentesis showed a large amount of protein with polymorphonuclear cells and no organisms visible on Gram stain.

QUESTION:

3. Antimicrobial therapy was initiated and a reasonable choice of agents would be:
    A. Penicillin
    B. Streptocmycin
    C. Keflin
    D. Kanamycin
    E. Clindamycin

The patient continued to deteriorate with a major motor seizure occurring within 24 hours after admission. His hematocrit fell to 24% and his WBC diminished to 2, 500. Serum albumin fell to 1. 7 grams. The admission blood culture was reported to be growing group A beta hemolytic streptococci. X-rays of the abdomen on the 7th hospital day revealed a large dilated loop of small bowel. A second abdominal paracentesis produced yellow fluid with 4, 000 WBC and visible gram-positive cocci. The fluid had no red blood cells and did not have a foul odor.

QUESTION:

4. The deteriorating status of the patient and presence of peritonitis demand further decisions concerning his therapy. An appropriate plan would be to:
    A. Take the patient immediately to the operating room
    B. Antimicrobial therapy should be changed to include coverage for fungal infection and gram-negative rods
    C. This illness is consistent with primary peritonitis and no alteration of therapy is necessary
    D. Consideration of arterial occlusion and vascular compromise of the intestine with necrosis prompts surgical intervention

Surgery was performed and massive mesenteric adenopathy was observed. The bowel was intact from the duodenum to the sigmoid colon. The liver and spleen were normal in appearance. The patient expired 24 hours after surgery.

QUESTION:

5. Postmortem examination revealed:
    A. Suppurative lymphadenitis involving the mesenteric and retro-peritoneal lymph nodes
    B. Chains of gram-positive cocci were seen in the peritoneal tissue but did not grow on culture
    C. Acute vasculitis and hemorrhagic infarcts of the right and left lungs
    D. Acute tubular necrosis of the right and left kidney

ANSWERS:

1. (A-E)

The examination of the infant will establish priorities and the severity of his illness places gastroenteritis far down on the differential diagnosis list unless the complication of perforation of the G. I. tract has occurred. Pneumonia in children may cause severe abdominal pain, presumably due to diaphragmatic irritation, but physical findings suggestive of pneumonitis should be apparent. Diabetes mellitus can present in children with severe abdominal pain and a rigid abdomen. The illness can often be diagnosed before acidosis intervenes, but in children of the age of this infant the progression of acidosis may be extremely rapid. Urinalysis, serum ketone and glucose determinations will establish the diagnosis. Appendicitis is a possibility and is to be considered as the possible antecedent event leading to intestinal perforation and peritonitis. Clinically peritonitis is present and demands instant attention. Definition of underlying disease such as the nephrotic syndrome or perforated viscus depends upon additional diagnostic procedures.

2. (B-E)

Abdominal paracentesis is a simple procedure which can be safely performed and will yield invaluable information. The gross characteristics of the fluid will give a clue to the circumstances. A perforated viscus usually produces malodorous, purulent fluid with exudative characteristics and a mixture of gram-positive and gram-negative organisms on Gram stain. This material ultimately grows enteric bacteria and a mixture of anaerobic bacteria. Vascular compromise may produce bloody fluid, and sequentially with perforation of the viscus typical fecal peritonitis will be present, as described above. Primary peritonitis, defined as peritonitis occurring as the result of hematogeneous dissemination without a perforated viscus, produces an exudative fluid. This fluid is usually serous in appearance with a homogenous population of organisms which may be visible on Gram stain of sediment from centrifuged specimen. S. pneumoniae and S. pyogenes are frequently the organisms or primary peritonitis in children. In children with underlying nephrosis a variety of organisms can be causative in primary peritonitis, but only one organism will be responsible in each patient. Thus, the visualization of a uniform population of bacteria which is characteristic of primary peritonitis may help to prevent an unnecessary laparotomy in a critically ill patient. Total cell count (RBC and WBC), differential WBC count, and chemistries (amylase, protein, sugar) should be performed on fluid and recorded. Culture of fluid on blood agar plate, MacConkey or EMB plate, broth for anaerobic and aerobic organisms (eg. chopped meat or thioglycolate) and anaerobic blood agar plate, should be meticulously performed.

3. (D, E)

Clindamycin is effective therapy against S. pneumonia, S. pyogenes, and S. aureus and the majority of anaerobic organisms in the gastrointestinal tract. Kanamycin (gentamicin) is an effective agent against the majority of the Enterobacteriaceae and would be a logical drug to employ until culture results are available. If perforation of a viscus can be ruled out initially and gram-positive organisms are seen on Gram stain, then penicillin might be selected as the initial form of therapy. It is tempting to relate antecedent pyarthrosis to the present illness. Positive identification of the pathogen by culture supportive tests such as ASO titer, or antigen detection in blood or synovial fluid could have influenced choice of drugs in initial therapy.

4. (C)

This decision is a difficult one. At the time he is considered for surgery the severity of his condition and the presence of one dilated
loop of bowel was thought to represent necrotic intestine. This influenced responsible physicians to perform surgery. Retrospectively,
the S. pyogenes, non-feculent nature of the fluid obtained by paracentesis, and the normal gastrointestinal x-rays present on admission when peritonitis existed should have presented a compelling
picture of primary peritonitis.

5. (A-D)

These features are all consistent with primary peritonitis. The gas-
rointestinal tract was totally intact. The mesenteric lymph nodes
are greatly enlarged. The chains of gram-positive cocci visible in
he retroperitoneal tissues further validate the role of group A beta
hemolytic streptococci in this illness. No other bacteria were iden-
ifiable in antemortem cultures, tissue pathology or postmortem
bacteriology. Primary streptococcal peritonitis was seen in the preantibiotic area and the mortality approached 100%. One of the strik-
ng features of the illness in this toddler was the first several days
of fever and rather vague upper respiratory tract and G. I. complaints. The streptococcus is an organism producing a number of
extracellular substances. The role of these streptolysins, hyaluron-
dase and DNase B in the pathogenesis of disease is uncertain. The
human host does make antibodies to these proteins as well as to the
polysaccharide of the bacterial cell wall. The organism remains
exquisitely sensitive to penicillin and is readily killed by achievable
serum levels of drug. Decreased vascularity will reduce the access-
bility of the organism to the drug. In the presence of significant
necrosis, debridement becomes an important part of therapy of soft
issue infections with this organism.

REFERENCES

1. Litshutz, B. , Lowenburg, H. : Pneumococcic and streptococcic
   peritonitis. Report of 23 cases in infancy and childhood. JAMA
   86: Part I, 99-104, 1926.

2. Pollock, Leo H. : Primary streptococcic peritonitis. Arch. Surg.
   33:714, 1936.

3. Keefer, Chester S. , et al. : Significance of hemolytic streptococcic bacteremia. A study of 246 patients. Arch. Int. Med. 60:
   1084-97, 1937.

4. Leopold, Jerome S. , Kaufman, Robert E. : Acute "Primary"
   streptococcus peritonitis. J. Pediat. 10:45-61, 1937.

5. Newell, Edward, T. , Jr. : Primary streptococcus and pneumococcus peritonitis in children. A study of 61 cases with the report of two interesting recoveries. J. Surg. Gynec. and Obstet.
   68:760, 1939.

6. McDougal, W. Scott, et al. : Primary peritonitis in infancy and
   childhood. Ann. Surg. 181:310-313, 1975.

7. Wilfert, Catherine M. , Katz, Samuel L. : Etiology of bacterial
   sepsis in nephrotic children. 1963-67. Pediatrics 42:841-43,
   1968.

8. Burech, Dennis L. , Kouranyi, Katlin I. , Haynes, Ralph E. :
   Serious Group A streptococcal disease in children. J. Ped.
   88:972-4, 1976.

9. Smith, Edward W. P. , et al. : Varicella gangrenosa due to Group
   A Beta hemolytic streptococcus. Pediatrics 57:306-310, 1976.

::

CASE 36: RECURRENT TACHYCARDIA

HISTORY: The patient is an $11\frac{1}{2}$-year-old girl with a rapid heart
beat who was considered to be in excellent health until she developed
shortness of breath, pallor, and was observed to have a heart rate
of greater than 200 beats/ min. She was hospitalized at a local hospital and the arrhythmia documented to be paroxysmal atrial tachycardia. She was treated unsuccessfully with varying combinations
of digoxin, propranolol, Procainamide, Dilantin, and Lidocaine. Her
electrocardiogram did not reveal Wolff-Parkinson-White Syndrome,
and the patient was discharged on digoxin, 0. 125 mg. every day,
plus Inderal, 5 mg. four times daily. She continued to feel weak and
have an intermittent rapid pulse. She required emergency room consultation and administration of "an unknown drug" two weeks after
her hospital discharge. A second hospitalization 6 weeks later for
persistent tachycardia resulted in the transfer of her care to a tertiary care center. She had no history of fever, rash, arthritis, arthralgia, or chest trauma, and no known history of rheumatic fever.
She had received 4 DPT immunizations during childhood. No other
member of the family was known to be ill.

PHYSICAL EXAMINATION: Pulse 180. Respirations 30. Temperature 37. Blood pressure 100/60. The patient was a well-developed,
well-nourished, white girl who appeared anxious and frightened. The
remainder of the physical examination was within normal limits with
the exception of the regular tachycardia. No hepatosplenomegaly was
present.

LABORATORY DATA: Hemoglobin 13. 8 grams. Hematocrit 40.7%;
WBC 6,800 with 28% polys, 65% lymphs, 4% monos, 1% eosinophil
and 2% atypical lymphocytes. There was an adequate number of
platelets and normal red cell morphology. BUN, glucose, and electrolytes were within normal limits. SGOT=50, CPK=130. Latex fixation LE cell preparation, and antinuclear factor were negative. The
ASO titer was less than 100 and the antihyaluronidase was 132. EKG
showed a rate of 180 with a left bundle branch block pattern. Chest
x-ray was within normal limits.

Viral antibody titers to Coxsackie B viruses were obtained on 2 occasions over a 1-month period of time (Sera 1 & 2 in Table 36-1).
The child needed hospitalization at two 6-month intervals during the
next year. Each time, arrhythmias were uncontrolled and a Lidocaine
intravenous infusion as well as quinidine was required. A fourth hospital admission was necessitated 14 months after initial referral and
a pacemaker was implanted. At the time of the 4th admission 2 sera
were obtained during a one week period (Sera 3 & 4 in Table 36-1).

TABLE 36-1						
COXSACKIE B NEUTRALIZING ANTIBODY TITERS						
	B1	B2	B3	B4	B5	B6
0 Serum 1	<1:10	<1:10	<1:10	<1:10	1:40	
1 mo Serum 2	<1:10	<1:10	<1:10	<1:10	1:80	
14 mo Serum 3	<1:10	1:20	<1:10	<1:10	<1:10	<1:10
14½ mo Serum 4	<1:10	1:640	<1:10	<1:10	1:160	<1:10

QUESTIONS:

1. The diagnosis of myocarditis has been made because of the ar-
    rhythmias and the electrocardiographic changes. The possible
    etiologies would include:
    A. Diphtheria
    B. Acute rheumatic fever
    C. Juvenile rheumatoid arthritis
    D. Lupus erythematosus
    E. Viral myocarditis
    F. Sarcoidosis

2. An ASO titer of less than 100 units excludes the diagnosis of
    acute rheumatic fever.
    A. True
    B. False

3. Viruses associated with myocarditis include:
   A. Coxsackie B viruses
   B. Influenza viruses
   C. Varicella viruses
   D. Polio viruses
   E. Mumps virus
   F. Adenoviruses
   G. Echoviruses

4. Attempts to substantiate a viral etiology of myocarditis should include:
   A. Nasopharyngeal and stool cultures
   B. Blood culture
   C. Acute and convalescent sera for antibody titers
   D. Cultures of available pericardial fluid
   E. Cultures of close family members

5. "Antibody screening" for enterovirus antibodies as performed by the majority of available diagnostic facilities can reliably exclude enteroviruses as etiologic agents.
   A. True
   B. False

6. Antibody titers as cited in Table 36-1 reveal the following:
   A. The first two sera establish the diagnosis of Coxsackie B5 myocarditis
   B. The first two sera demonstrate the patient has encountered Coxsackie B5 at an unknown time
   C. Sera 3 and 4 show infection with both Coxsackie B2 and B5 occurring during the sampling interval
   D. Sera 3 and 4 demonstrate infection with Coxsackie B2 which is temporally related to these two specimens
   E. The Coxsackie B5 antibody rise in sera 3 and 4 may recall of previous experience

7. Pathogenesis of viral myocarditis remains to be established. Indicate which of the following statements are true:
   A. Recovery of infectious virus from the myocardium indicates that viral replication is the cause of observed damage
   B. Recovery of virus at the time of myocarditis is infrequent after the first two weeks of illness
   C. The pathology of acute myocarditis is diagnostic of enterovirus infection
   D. Experimental evidence would indicate that sensitized lymphocytes may be responsible for myocardial damage

8. Prognosis of children with viral myocarditis is:
   A. Always benign
   B. May be fatal
   C. Complete recovery occurs without apparent sequelae
   D. Longitudinal evaluation of children with proven viral myocarditis is not presently available

ANSWERS:

1. (A-F)

Diphtheria is known to produce cardiac arrhythmias including partial
or complete heart block, bundle branch block or extra systoles clas-
sically occurring during the second and third weeks of illness. It
would be exceedingly unusual for the primary illness to pass unrec-
ognized in this apparently healthy child. In addition, her immunization
history includes at least 4 injections of DPT vaccine which should
ensure her immunity against diphtheria toxin. Although acute rheumatic fever must be considered and carditis is the most serious manifestation of this disorder it would seem unlikely in this child. In most
cases acute carditis is associated with a fever and leukocytosis. The
degree of illness is frequently striking. Cardiac enlargement and
auscultatory findings of a murmur are often identified. The commonest arrhythmias would appear to be prolongation of the conduction
time with arrhythmias as the result of the dropped beats or less often
complete heart block. This child lacks the other manifestations of
acute rheumatic fever. Carditis is reported in approximately 10%
of cases of rheumatoid arthritis but is usually associated with other
findings of the illness. Although rheumatoid arthritis can present in
a variety of ways in this child there are no findings of fever and no
suggestion of joint disease. The carditis may be associated with a
prolongation of the QT and PR segments as well as distortion of the
ST segment of the EKG. Although sarcoidosis and lupus erythematosus can cause carditis, in the absence of skin rash, fever, arthralgia,
hepatosplenomegaly, lymphadenopathy or pulmonary disease with
normal renal function, these diagnoses seem unlikely but further laboratory tests will be considered. Viral myocarditis is frequently a
diagnosis of exclusion. The degree of illness varies considerably and
there are no specific hallmarks of disease of viral etiology unless
pathognomonic features of illness such as mumps and varicella are
present. This diagnosis remains a difficult one to confirm.

2. (B)

Evidence of preceding group A beta hemolytic streptococcal infection
is one of the minor criteria used to help establish the diagnosis of
rheumatic fever. The ASO titer is only one of several laboratory
tests which may define preceding streptococcal infection. These
tests include a throat culture for the presence of organisms, anti-
DNase antibodies and antihyaluronidase antibodies.

3. (A-G)

Case reports establishing the temporal relationship of infection with
a variety of viruses have infrequently associated such agents as influenza, varicella, mumps, adenoviruses, and echoviruses with myocarditis. The illnesses of varicella and mumps have identifiable clinical characteristics allowing their identification with some certainty

on the basis of the clinical illness. These occurrences are indeed
unusual and probably the most consistent observations relate to
viruses of the picornavirus group. Although the literature documents
the occurrence of myocarditis in poliovirus infection, it was not a
prominent cause of severe morbidity or mortality. Postmortem
pathology documented typical inflammatory changes but virus was
never isolated from the myocardium. Infrequently, arrhythmias or
congestive heart failure contribute to problems of patients with polio.
Postmortem pathology documented typical inflammatory changes,
but Coxsackie B viruses have been isolated from the myocardium,
and animal models for Coxsackie virus induced myocarditis exist.

4. (A-D)

The enteroviruses are transmitted through the gastrointestinal tract
and are excreted for significant periods of time in the secretions of
the pharynx and in the stool. Fecal excretion of virus tends to be of
greater duration and as with polio, for example, can last for several
months in a normal individual. Therefore, examination of materials
from the gastrointestinal tract may allow identification of an enterovirus in this location. Failure to demonstrate virus does not rule
out this etiology. This does not establish the etiologic relationship of
the virus to the myocarditis. A blood sample can be cultured as patients have been shown to be viremic with a number of the enteroviruses. Usually, viremia precedes the clinical evidence of visceral
involvement with these agents and therefore virus is not detectable at
the time clinical illness is apparent. The yield of positive results is
extremely small but certainly viremia would be significant in such a
patient. Acute and convalescent sera should be obtained in an attempt
to document a change in antibody titer to a responsible agent. It should
be noted that unless an enterovirus is isolated from the patient, antibody screening techniques are inadequate to rule out the possibility
of such infection (see answer #5). All available body fluids (e.g. pleural fluid or pericardial fluid) should be cultured as a positive culture
is of great significance to the patient, and viruses have been isolated
from these materials. Close family members can certainly be sur-
veyed for the presence of virus and this may be helpful in view of the
epidemiology of these infections. This will not establish a causative
role in the patient but may allow serological testing of the patient and
documentation of infection with the same virus.

5. (B)

The 6 Coxsackie B viruses are available in many diagnostic laboratories so that sera specimens can be tested for the presence of neutralizing antibodies to these six viruses. The problem is multiplied
many folds when it is realized that 25 Coxsackie A viruses and 33
echoviruses are known to exist. No laboratory has the ability to perform individual neutralization tests to identify serological changes
in serum specimens to these viruses. At the present time, complement fixation assays do not provide an alternative means of antibody

assay as the antigens are not purified and are not sufficiently cross
reactive to accurately demonstrate antibodies to the majority of enteroviruses. Complement fixation assays have been employed with a
single antigen and although an antibody change to the antigen employed
may occasionally be observed, its absence does not rule out the possibility of enterovirus infection.

6. (B, D, E)

Sera 1 and 2 show titers of 1:40 and 1:80 against Coxsackie B5. This
two-fold change in antibody titer is within the range of variability of
the assay procedure. The presence of this antibody documents the
experience of this child with Coxsackie B5 antigen, but at an unde-
termined point in time. Sera 3 and 4 demonstrate a significant rise
in both antibodies to Coxsackie B2 and to Coxsackie B5. Since Coxsackie B5 antibodies were known to be present for the preceding
year, and a fall in titer occurred during this interval, it is most
likely that the serological rise observed 14 months later represents
recall of previous experience. This type of recall of a different serotype of Coxsackie virus has been documented previously in many individuals. The striking rise of antibodies to Coxsackie B2 would appear to represent recent infection with this agent. It does not establish the role of the viral infection in the exacerbation of her cardiac
arrhythmia but certainly provides evidence of temporally related
Coxsackie B2 virus infection.

7. (A, B, D)

Infectious virus has been recovered from the myocardium in unusual
instances and it is difficult to discount the role of replicating virus
in this situation. On the other hand, examination of material after 9
to 10 days of illness usually fails to demonstrate the presence of
virus. This occurs at a time when the inflammatory response is continuing and the patient may succumb. This would seem to indicate
progression of illness. The pathology of acute myocarditis attributed
to enterovirus infection is entirely nonspecific. Enteroviruses do not
cause the intranuclear inclusions or multinucleate giant cells which
are characteristic hallmarks of other types of viral infections and
are easily recognizable as virus related. The lack of specificity of
enterovirus infections is true of any tissue examined including the
meninges, liver, or lungs. Therefore, mononuclear cell infiltration
and an apparent perivascular cuffing does not assist the pathologist
in his attempt to assign an etiologic agent to the disease process.
Cultures must be obtained. Several experimental models utilizing
Coxsackie viruses would indicate that lymphocytes play an important
part in the pathogenesis of myocardial damage. [16] Infected mice can
terminate virus infection independently of T-lymphocyte function.
Early antibody synthesis occurs normally in T cell deficient mice.
Either T cell depletion or administration of antilymphocyte globulin
decreased inflammation of heart and increased survival of the mice.
These provocative animal data remain to be extended to human disease.

8. (B-D)

Infants with acute Coxsackie myocarditis in the neonatal period have
succumbed with their illness during the first month of life. This
rapidly fatal illness is one which has been studied, and the overwhelming nature of the viral invasion is apparent as the central nervous system and other viscera are also involved. The acquisition of
viral myocarditis later in childhood is more difficult to study. There
is some evidence to suggest that infection with the Coxsackie viruses
may be more common than previously expected. The documentation
of viral myocarditis is usually accomplished by serological means
as in the present case. Published reports of sequential evaluations
of patients with documented serological conversion to a specific virus
are not available in the pediatric literature. Several adult studies
would tend to indicate that such illness leaves a broad spectrum of
pathology. Some persons have no detectable heart disease and others
may have a chronic progressive course of myocardial degeneration
with death due to congestive heart failure.

REFERENCES

1. Galpine, J. F. , Mac Wilson, W. C.: Occurrence of myocarditis
    in paralytic poliomyelitis. Brit. Med. J. 2:1379-81, Dec. 1959.

2. Jungeblut, Claus W.: Newer knowledge of the pathogenesis of
    poliomyelitis. J. Pediat. 37:109-128, 1950.

3. Van Reken, David, et al.: Infectious pericarditis in children.
    J. Pediat. 85:165-169, 1974.

4. Lerner, Martin A. , Wilson, Francis M.: Virus myocardiopathy.
    Prog. Med. Virol. 15:63-91, 1973.

5. Gear, James, Measroch, Veronica: Coxsackie virus infections
    of the newborn. Prog. Med. Virol. 15:42-62, 1973.

6. Kilbourne, Edwin, et al.: The induction of gross myocardial le-
    sions by a Coxsackie (pleurodynia) virus and cortisone. J. Clin.
    Invest. 35:362-70, 1956.

7. Kibrick, Sidney, Benirschke, Kurt: Acute aseptic myocarditis and
    meningoencephalitis in the newborn child infected with Coxsackie
    virus group B, type III. NEJM 255:883-889, 1956.

8. Whitehead, J. E. M.: Silent infections and the epidemiology of
    viral carditis. Am. Heart J. 85:711-13, 1973.

9. Schmidt, Natalie, J. , et al.: Association of group B Coxsackie
    viruses with cases of pericarditis, myocarditis or pleurodynia
    by demonstration of immunoglobulin M antibody. Inf. and Imm.
    8:341-8, 1973.

10. Haas, Joel E. , Yunis, Eduardo J. : Viral crystalline arrays in human coxsackie myocarditis. Lab. Invest. 23:442-6, 1970.

11. Cherry, James D. , et al. : Paroxysmal atrial tachycardia associated with echo 9 virus infection. Am. Heart J. 73:681-6, 1967.

12. Nathanson, Gerald, et al. : Benign neonatal arrhythmias and Coxsackie B virus infection. J. Pediat. 86:152-153, 1975.

13. Rodriguez, Torres Ramon, et al. : A sensitive electrocardiographic sign in myocarditis associated with viral infection. Pediatrics 43:846-852, 1969.

14. Berkovich, Sumner, et al. : Virologic studies in children with acute myocarditis. Am. J. Dis. Child. 115:207-212, 1968.

15. Kibrick, Sidney, Benirschke, Kurt: Severe generalized disease (encephalohepatomyocarditis) occurring in the newborn due to infection with Coxsackie virus group B. Evidence of intrauterine infection with this agent. Pediatrics 22:857-875, 1958.

16. Woodruff, Jack F. , Woodruff, Judith J. : Involvement of T-lymphocytes in the pathogenesis of Coxsackie virus B3 heart disease. J. Imm. 113:1726-1734, 1974.

:::

CASE 37: A NINE-MONTH INFANT BOY WITH FAILURE TO
          THRIVE AND RECURRENT DIARRHEA PRESENTING
          WITH SEVERE DYSPNEA, CYANOSIS AND COUGH

HISTORY: This 9-month-old male infant, the first child of healthy unrelated parents, was slow to gain weight and suffered from recurrent bouts of loose stools since age three months. Two weeks ago he developed a dry nonproductive cough and shortness of breath. His family physician had prescribed and he had received Ampicillin for one week. Nevertheless his respiratory symptoms were worsening.

PHYSICAL EXAMINATION: BP normal; Pulse 90 and regular; Temperature 98. 6; Resp. 80/min. This was a thin, wasted, pale, white, male infant with a prominent troublesome dry, nonproductive cough. He was tachypneic and mildly cyanotic. There was evidence of oral "thrush" (white placques were visible on his tongue, palate, and buccal mucosa). There were no palpable lymph nodes. Examination of the chest revealed rapid shallow respirations and harsh vesicular breathing without adventitious sounds. No cardiac murmurs were heard.

LABORATORY DATA: Hemoglobin 9. 6 gm%, WBC 1600 total (1300 neutrophils, no bands, 300 lymphocytes). Platelets normal, erythrocytes slightly hypochromic. Electrolytes unremarkable. Blood gases, pH 7. 42; pCO_2 33. 4; Bicarbonate 20. 8; PO_2 48 (breathing 38% inspired O_2). Chest x-ray: Lung fields revealed a diffuse hazy "ground glass" appearance without evidence of hilar enlargement or cardiomegaly (Fig. 37. 1). An immunodeficiency was suspected on the basis of the reduced appearance of lymphoid tissue, the evidence of pulmonary infection, and the failure to thrive accompanied by chronic diarrhea. These suspicions were confirmed in further immunological studies. Immunoglobulin analysis revealed:

    IgM < 4 IU/ml (34 micro grams per ml)
    IgA < 3 IU/ml (43 micro grams per ml)
    IgG   15 IU/ml (120 micro grams per ml)

He had an absolute lymphopenia and lymphocytes could not be induced to transform with exposure to phytohemagglutinin, concanavallin A, and pokeweed mitogens.

QUESTIONS:

1. This child has a diffuse lung infection; which of the following generic groups is least likely to be etiologic?
    A. Bacteria
    B. Viruses
    C. Mycoplasma
    D. Protozoa

2. What one or more additional investigations would you carry out (in what order) to define the etiology of the infection?
    A. None, since if the infection is not bacterial it can only be treated with nonspecific measures
    B. Direct examination of a sample of lung tissue or aspirate (open biopsy or needle aspirate) for culture (bacteria, fungi, mycoplasma and viruses) and pathologic study
    C. Nose and throat swab and tracheal aspirate samples for pathologic study and for culture
    D. Skin tests for tuberculosis and candida

A needle aspirate of the lung stained with Gomori's silver methenamine revealed the presence of 7 - 10 mu cysts (Fig. 37. 2) with a morphology consistent with Pneumocystis carinii.

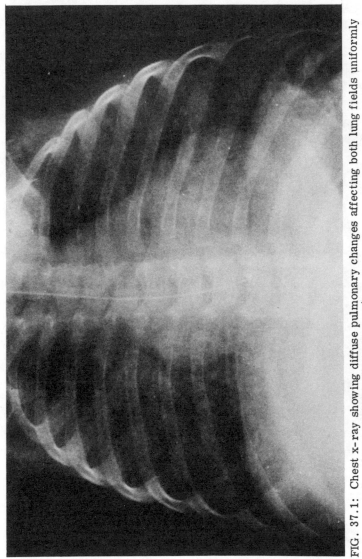

FIG. 37.1: Chest x-ray showing diffuse pulmonary changes affecting both lung fields uniformly (hazy "ground-glass" appearance).

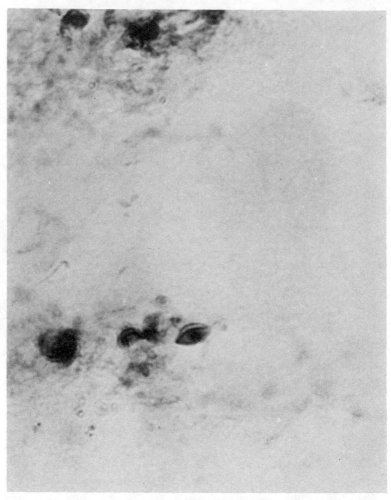

FIG. 37. 2: Cyst of Pneumocystis carinii from lung aspirate preparation (Gomori silver methenamine stain).

QUESTIONS:

3. Successful treatment of Pneumocystis carinii infection can
   include which of the following antimicrobials? If you find
   more than one effective regimen, which is the drug of choice?
   A. No treatment has been found to be successful and none is
      warranted
   B. Tetracycline
   C. Pentamidine isethionate
   D. Sulfadiazine and pyremethamine
   E. Trimethoprim-sulfamethoxazole
   F. Corticosteroids

4. Which one or more of the following forms of supportive therapy
   will you employ?
   A. Small transfusions of fresh blood
   B. Vitamins
   C. Regular injections of immunoglobulin

ANSWERS:

1. (A-C)

Although mycoplasma can cause interstitial pulmonary disease and
constitute a threat to patients with sickle cell disease, there are no
reports substantiating this risk to other immunocompromised hosts. It
is unlikely that this child's lung infection has been caused by bacteria
since the blood gases clearly indicate the presence of an interstitial
process. Although the leukopenia might reduce the severity of a
visible pulmonary infiltrate, there is no reason to suppose that this
would result in an altered blood-gas pattern. It is likely that an infectious agent capable of inducing an interstitial pneumonia is responsible for the pulmonary infection. This might include viruses or
protozoa. In the face of immunodeficiency, common infectious agents,
ordinarily harmless, may become opportunistic invaders [4,5].

2. (C, B, D)

Specimens of nose and throat secretions and a tracheal aspirate
should be obtained for bacterial, fungal and viral culture.

Although it is unlikely that a bacterial infection is responsible for the
present pulmonary condition, the spread of secondary invaders must
be monitored and anticipated.

Virus cultures must be requested, especially for CMV and common
respiratory pathogens such as adenoviruses, RSV, and parainfluenzae.
The specimens may also be cultivated in appropriate culture systems
for mycoplasma. Immunofluorescent studies, if available, will en-
able the rapid identification (one to two hours) of a number of respiratory pathogens.

Brush and transtracheal biopsy have been successful means of evaluating patients for the presence of Pneumocystis carinii, but examination of a tracheal aspirate is not reliable. A recent report describes
identification of pneumocystic by toluidine blue stain of gastric as-
pirates. It is generally considered most reliable to obtain a diagnosis by open lung biopsy or needle aspiration. Unfortunately, the infected lungs are frequently inelastic and a pneumothorax may occur
with attempted needle aspiration. For this reason, open biopsy is
often the procedure of choice.

Work in progress gives encouragement that the in vitro cultivation of
Pneumocystis may soon be successfully accomplished. If this is the
case, the usefulness of a lung biopsy or aspirate will be expanded.

If material such as the biopsy or aspirate is to be sent for special
culture, it is important to consult the responsible laboratories in
advance. It is also useful for the responsible physician or consultant
to be in attendance at the procedure. It can thus be assured that the
samples are handled in the optimal manner. Samples for virus culture should be transported promptly to the virus diagnostic laboratory
either in virus transport medium (a balanced salt solution containing
antibiotics and a source of protein) or, failing this, the specimen
should be moistened or immersed in saline or broth. The optimal
transport temperature is that of wet ice (4°C). Contact with the responsible laboratory prior to the procedure will insure that the material is handled in the best possible manner for recovery of the suspected infectious agents.

Answer A is incorrect since treatment is available for Pneumocystis
carinii as well as for many mycoplasma infections. In addition, some
modes of effective anti-viral therapy have begun to emerge.

In order to help substantiate loss of delayed hypersensitivity, an antigen to which 90% of infants of this age will respond (i. e. Candida), as
well as an IPPD, would be appropriate in this infant with pulmonary
disease.

3. (C, D, E)

Neither tetracycline nor steroid therapy is appropriate treatment as
the former is ineffective and the latter may exacerbate the infection.
The administration of steroids should be discontinued or the dosage
reduced if possible in the face of proven Pneumocystis infection.

Pentamidine isethionate has been found to be an effective form of
therapy. The combination of sulfadiazine and pyrimethamine (one form
of therapy recommended for treatment of Toxoplasma gondii) may
also be useful, but this drug combination has not been used extensively
in man.

Trimethoprim-sulfamethoxazole has been compared in a careful study to pentamidine isethionate. The drugs were equally efficacious and TMP-SMX was considerably less toxic. For this reason, TMP-SMX may prove to be the first choice for therapy of pneumocystic infection. Should any one drug fail to be effective, an alternative should be tried.

4. (C)

Transfusion of whole blood may be very hazardous when administered to an individual with a severe combined immunodeficiency. The viable transfused lymphocytes may replicate in the recipient and initiate a graft-vs-host (GVH) reaction. Measures must be taken, (irradiation) to remove lymphocytes from peripheral blood when transfusion is essential.

Vitamins are of no specific or supportive value provided that the general diet is adequate.

The administration of immune serum immunoglobulins is of specific benefit in the case of a child with a severe immunodeficiency. Plasma infusions from a single donor have also been utilized to replace absent immunoglobulins. Immune serum globulin should be administered at regular intervals of approximately 4 weeks.

FINAL NOTES: Further laboratory studies of lymphocyte function substantiated the presumptive diagnosis of severe combined immunodeficiency. In a case such as this one, more than one opportunistic microbe may be invasive. For example, Pneumocystis frequently co-exists with CMV as do other members of the commensal microbial flora. The recovery of one agent should not deter the search for others. [8]

We have not mentioned the potential and controversy surrounding the therapeutic use of Transfer Factor. Nor have we made reference to the effectiveness or problems associated with marrow transplantation as a means to reconstitute the immune capability of deficient individuals.

REFERENCES

GENERAL:

1. Symposium on Pneumocystis Carinii Infection. Natl. Ca. Inst. Monograph, No. 43, In Press, 1977.

2. Robbins, J. B.: Pneumocystic carinii pneumonitis: a review Pediat. Res. 1:131-158, 1967.

3. Walzer, P. D., et al.: Pneumocystis carinii pneumonia in the United States. Ann. Int. Med. 80:83-93, 1974.

SPECIFIC:

4. Feigin, R. D. , Shearer, W. T. : Opportunistic infection in children.
    II. In the immunocompromised host. J. Pediat. 87:677-694, 1975.

5. Rosen, F. S. : Primary immunodeficiency. Pediat. Clin. N. A.
    Pediat. Clin. N. A. 21:533-549, 1974.

6. Hughes, W. T. : Treatment of Pneumocystis carinii pneumonitis.
    NEJM 295:726-727, 1976.

7. Lipsom, A. , et al. : Treatment of Pneumocystic carinii pneumonia.
    Arch. Dis. Child. No. 52, In Press, 1977.

8. Abdallah, P. S. , et al. : Diagnosis of cytomegalovirus pneumonia
    in compromised hosts. Am. J. Med. 61:326-332, 1976.

9. Chan, Helen, et al. : Comparison of gastric contents to pulmonary
    aspirates for cytologic diagnosis of Pneumocystis carinii pneu-
    monia. J. Pediat. 90:243, 1977.

::

CASE 38: ACUTE SWELLING OF ONE EYE, FEVER, AND NASAL
          DISCHARGE

HISTORY: This 4-9/12-year-old black boy was in excellent health
until 24 hours prior to admission when he began to complain of fever
and a headache. He was begun on oral penicillin V by his physician
who also noted that the conjunctivae of his left eye was red. The following morning his left conjunctiva was red and weeping and the tissue surrounding the eye was swollen so that he was unable to open
the eye. The child had had no recent trauma to head, face or eye
and had no bug bites to the area. He had not had frequent respiratory
tract infections or known sinus disease.

At admission he was a toxic-appearing child. His temperature was
39°C, pulse 120, respirations 30. Height and weight were within the
50th percentile for age. Significant physical findings were as follows:
Pupils were reactive and equal, extraocular movement was intact.
Fundi were unremarkable and vision was intact. Both tympanic membranes were bulging and myringotomies produced a small amount of
bloody purulent drainage.

The left side of the face was edematous. There was a boggy swelling
which was maximal to the left of the nose and extended from just below the lacrimal duct. The involved area was neither warm nor tender. There was bloody purulent discharge in moderate amounts from
the left nostril, which on Gram stain revealed profuse polymorphonuclear leukocytes but few microorganisms which were irregular
gram-negative filamentous rods.

LABORATORY FINDINGS: Hemoglobin was 10. 4 gm%, WBC count
was 14,950 with 83% polymorphonuclear leukocytes, 2% stabs, 14%
lymphocytes and 1% mononuclear cells. Sickle cell preparation was
negative. Serum electrolytes were within normal limits but he exhibited a mild metabolic acidosis. Roentgenographic studies revealed
advanced opacification of the left maxillary and ethmoid sinuses.
Blood cultures and cultures of the nasal discharge were taken and
yielded no growth. The child was begun on therapy with nafcillin and
ampicillin. For the next few days the child continued to have unre-
mittant fever of 38-39°C and he underwent a surgical drainage of the
abscess of the left cheek and left nasal antrostomy. His course improved thereafter and he had rapid decrease in ocular findings.

Aerobic cultures of the material from the abscess revealed no growth.
Anaerobic cultures yielded growth of Peptostreptococci, Fusobacterium sp. and Bacteroides sp. On the sixth hospital day he had recurrence of fever of 38. 6°C and increased swelling with tenderness
over the left lacrimal duct. Repeated surgical exploration revealed
recurrent ethmoidal abscess formation. Ethmoidectomy was performed, he was begun on penicillin G, and thereafter made an uneventful recovery.

QUESTIONS:

1. The statement: "The majority of orbital inflammatory disease is
    secondary to sinus disease" is:
    A. True
    B. False

2. Commonly reported complications of acute sinusitis include:
    A. Brain abscess and meningitis
    B. Orbital cellulitis or abscess
    C. Cavernous sinus thrombosis
    D. Osteomyelitis of adjacent structures

3. The organisms which would likely have caused this child's disease
    would initially have been expected to have been:
    A. Hemophilus influenzae type B
    B. Streptococcus pneumoniae
    C. Anaerobic streptococci (peptostreptococcus)
    D. Bacteroides sp.
    E. A combination of highly pathogenic aerobic species plus
        anaerobic flora
    F. Staphylococcus aureus

4. Appropriate therapy of this child's illness at the time of admis-
    sion might have included the following regimens:
    A. A cephalosporin administered parenterally
    B. Penicillin G with chloramphenicol administered parenterally
    C. Erythromycin administered orally
    D. Nafcillin plus clindamycin administered parenterally

5. In the interpretation of the significance of the opacification of
   the left maxillary and ethmoid sinuses, the following statements
   pertain:
   A. The proportion of children of this age who have an opacified
      sinus or sinuses during an attack of sinusitis is similar to
      the proportion of children with opacified sinus(es) during an
      uncomplicated upper respiratory tract infection
   B. Unilateral opacification of a paranasal sinus is highly indica-
      tive of a diseased condition of that sinus
   C. The statement: "The reaction of the maxillary sinus to chronic
      inflammation and its reaction to allergy cannot be differen-
      tiated on the basis of roentgenographic findings alone" is
      true
   D. The statement: "The reaction of the maxillary sinus to chronic
      inflammation and its reaction to allergy cannot be differen-
      tiated on the basis of roentgenographic findings alone" is
      false

ANSWERS:

1. (A)

Although there is some variation in estimated etiologies of orbital
inflammatory edema, orbital cellulitis, and orbital abscess formation, many reports indicate that underlying sinus disease is most
frequent. See, for example, the report by Chandler et al. Other
prominent causes include trauma, thyrotoxicosis and tumors.

2. (A, B, C, D)

Extension of the infectious process from the sinus to any adjacent
structure may result in a variety of complications. Meningitis is
most commonly associated with infection of the frontal sinuses and
with infections of the mastoid areas. Many cases are hematogenous
in origin and are secondary to the bacteremia which may accompany
acute sinus disease with highly pathogenic organisms such as H. influenzae type B and encapsulated pneumococci. Other infections may
cause a brain abscess or a parameningeal abscess by direct extension of the infectious process. Thrombosis of small veins is thought
to be a major mechanism in the pathogenesis of this form of spread.
In most series on the etiologies of brain abscesses, acute and chronic
infections of the middle ear, mastoid, and nasal sinuses represent
a large proportion of the known underlying causes.

Orbital cellulitis is most commonly secondary to disease of the ethmoid or sphenoid sinuses. Disease may range from edema of the
periorbital structures to suppurative cellulitis, subperiosteal abscess, and orbital abscess. In the preantibiotic era approximately
17% of patients with orbital cellulitis died of meningitis and 20% became blind. In the report by Haynes et al. comprising the experience of 26 children with acute ethmoiditis, three developed orbital

abscesses, one developed periosteal, epidural, and subdural abscesses of the right hemisphere of the brain, and one developed
aseptic meningitis. The complication rate in this series was, therefore, 5 of 26, 20%.

Osteomyelitis of the orbital bones is not rare and may lead to chronic
disease, orbital displacement, and blindness. Cavernous sinus thrombosis, likewise, is probably due to direct extension of the infectious
process and is a rare complication of acute sinusitis.

3. (A-F)

The microbial flora of the diseased sinuses appears to depend upon
whether the child has an acute infection with rapid spread, as in
this case, or chronic disease limited to the sinuses. In patients with
chronic disease, anaerobic organisms, especially Peptostreptococcus
and Bacteroides sp, predominate, and even when aerobic species are
present it is usually in association with anaerobic species. In contrast, in patients with acute sinus disease with rapid extension, high-
grade aerobic pathogens, such as encapsulated S. pneumoniae, H.
influenzae type B, and group A Streptococcus pyogenes, are present,
often as the only organisms, from surgical material. In addition,
children with acute sinus infection and orbital cellulitis are bactere-
mic in approximately one third of untreated instances. This child
had received penicillin before admission and parenteral ampicillin
and nafcillin before the first procedure. This may have obscured
the presence of aerobic organisms. It would have been appropriate
to examine material from this child by counter immunoelectrophoresis for the presence of H. influenzae type B antigen or S. pneumoniae
antigens, but the technique was not available at this patient's hospital
at the time of his illness.

4. (B)

Both erythromycin and the cephalosporins have been shown to penetrate the secretions of diseased sinuses very poorly. In addition,
both drugs are inherently marginally efficacious in the therapy of
Hemophilus sp., which was a likely pathogen and also of questionable
efficacy in the therapy of many anaerobic flora, which were also expected to be likely causes of his disease. It was subsequently shown
that this patient had a sinus infection with a variety of anaerobic
species of bacteria.

Penicillin and chloramphenicol have a good distribution to the sinuses
and to the central nervous system. Their spectrum of activity includes
the anaerobic upper respiratory flora, H. influenzae, S. pneumoniae,
group A Streptococcus pyogenes, and many Staphylococcus sp. If an
untreated bacterial species had been present, such as S. aureus, it
would have been expected that they would have been visualized on
Gram stain of the nasal discharge. This does not rule this out, however.

5. (A, C)

In a study of children who had roentgenographic studies of their sinuses for a variety of reasons, Shopfner at al. demonstrated that
the proportion of children with abnormalities of the sinuses correlates
very poorly with the clinical course. Children with sinusitis demonstrated mucosal thickening in 28% of instances and opacity in 38% of
instances. Among children with upper respiratory infection but not
suspected of sinus disease, 33% had mucosal thickening and 48% had
opacity. It should be noted that the majority of children who were
less than 2 years of age had sinus films which were interpreted to be
abnormal (including 90% of children who had no clinical evidence for
any upper respiratory or sinus disease). In older age groups, the
proportion of sinus studies which were interpreted to be abnormal
declined.

Unilateral opacification of a sinus, particularly in young children,
may be caused by a number of conditions, such as cellulitis of overlying tissues, asymmetrical development of the sinuses, redundant
normal mucous membranes, which is a normal condition in young
children, and tears caused by crying. In none of the above conditions
would unilateral opacification have been caused by an acute or chronic
inflammatory response.

The response of sinuses to chronic inflammation resembles the response to allergy. Thickened mucosal membranes and walls muco-
celes, and a local sclerosing of the bony walls of the sinus are typical of both conditions.

REFERENCES

1. Alexsson, A. , Brorson, J. E. : The concentration of antibiotics
   in sinus secretions. Ann. Otol. Rhinol. and Laryngol. 83:323-331,
   1974.

2. Chandler, J. R. , et al. : The pathogenesis or orbital complications in acute sinusitis. Laryngoscope 80:1414-1428, 1970.

3. Frederick, J. , Braude, A. I. : Anaerobic infection of the paranasal sinuses. NEJM 290:135-137, 1974.

4. Haynes, R. E. , Cramblett, H. G. : Acute ethmoiditis. Am. J.
   Dis. Child. 114:261-267, 1967.

5. Quick, C. A. , Payne, E. : Complicated acute sinusitis. Laryngoscope 82:1248-1963, 1972.

6. Watters, E. C., et al. : Acute orbital cellulitis. Arch. Ophth.
   94:785-788, 1976.

7. Shopfner, C. E. , Rossi, J. O. : Roentgen evaluation of the para-
    nasal sinuses in children. Am. J. Roent. Radium Ther. Nucl.
    Med. 118:176-86, 1973.

::

CASE 39: RECURRENT FEVER, SPLENOMEGALY, AND RASH

HISTORY: The patient is a 13-year-old, white male who had been
in his usual state of vigorous good health until he developed the sudden onset of chills, prostration, fever to 40°C, and headache. He
had had no pulmonary complaints or rash, and his family members
were in good health. He was brought to his local emergency room
where he was examined.

The patient was the second of three sons in his family who had recently visited their cabin in a remote lake in the Sierra Nevada of
California for the first time that spring. They had not noted unusual
evidence of death of local wild life and their cabin had not apparently
been inhabited by animals the previous winter.

PHYSICAL EXAMINATION: Physical findings included normal ears,
no conjunctivitis, no evidence of pharyngitis, and supple neck. There
were no meningeal findings, and he was alert and oriented. He had
generalized adenopathy with epitrochlear, inguinal, cervical, axil-
lary, and suboccipital nodes which were soft, nontender, approximately 1 inch in diameter, non-erythematous and not fixed to the
tissues. The spleen was not palpable and there was no abdominal
organomegaly. He was having minimal arthralgia of both knees but
there was no evidence of effusion. Neurological examination was
within normal limits.

LABORATORY DATA: The patient's white count was 8, 000 with 42%
polymorphonuclear leukocytes, 37% lymphocytes, and 11% monocytes.
Platelet count was 175, 000. His hemoglobin was 13. 5 gm% and hematocrit was 40. Liver function tests were within normal limits and
blood culture was taken and failed to reveal bacterial growth. A mono
spot test was non-reactive as was a cold agglutinin titer, ASO titer,
rheumatoid factor, antinuclear antibody and lupus erythematosus
preparation. Westergren sedimentation rate was 49 mm/hr.

A diagnosis was not made. He gradually defervesced and was afebrile and again in good health by 7 days after the onset of the illness.

Eight days after he became afebrile and 15 days after the onset of
initial illness he again experienced the sudden onset of headache,
chills, fever to 39°C and prostration. He was again examined and,
in addition to the previous findings, was noted to have hepatosplenomegaly and a macular rash over the trunk. Repeated hemoglobin was

13 gm%. and white blood cell count was 7,300 with 48% polymorphonuclear leukocytes. He had tachypnea of 42/minute but no other pulmonary findings. There was mild conjunctival suffusion which had
not been previously noted, and he was mildly nauseated. His fever
persisted at 39°C. Two days later he developed a sudden drenching
sweat, intense thirst and tachycardia and became afebrile.

He had been admitted during a holiday weekend, and a thick blood
smear for malaria which had been taken and stained with Giemsa
stain on the day of admission was not seen by an experienced observer until the day of his defervescence. At that time the presence of
coarse, irregularly coiled spirochetes were first noted. Five such
organisms were seen on the film, which were subsequently identified to be Borrelia sp.

The patient did not have further relapses and his brothers never experienced clinically apparent disease. Further questioning revealed
that the patient had slept in the cabin on the first night, while his
brothers slept in the back of the station wagon.

QUESTIONS:

1. Which of the following statements concerning human borreliosis
    are true?
    A. The disease is acquired by humans from direct contact with
        infected mammals
    B. The disease in humans in the Western hemisphere at this
        time is almost always acquired from the bite of a tick
    C. Borrelia sp. cause a disease called "undulant fever"
    D. Borrelia sp. cause a disease called "relapsing fever"
    E. Some cases of borreliosis of humans are transmitted by
        infected body lice

2. Which of the following taxonomy for borreliosis is currently
    accepted?
    A. The etiologic agent of louse-borne relapsing fever is
        Borrelia recurrentis
    B. Each species of tick-borne borreliosis is identified by
        serologic characteristics
    C. Each species of tick-borne borreliosis is identified by mor-
        phologic characteristics
    D. Each species of tick-borne borreliosis is identified by the
        species of tick vector

3. Which of the following epidemiologic characteristic of human
    borreliosis in the U.S. pertain?
    A. The disease is transmitted by a wide variety of tick genuses
    B. The disease is transmitted solely by the bite of Argasidae ticks
    C. Patients with borreliosis are usually aware of having experi-
        enced a painful tick bite
    D. The disease in humans in the U.S. is restricted to the Western
        states

4. Human tick-borne relapsing fever is characterized by:
    A. The diagnosis may be made by examining the peripheral
        blood, since Borrelia sp are the only pathogenic spirochetes
        which are sufficiently large to be seen by a direct stain
    B. The incubation period is usually over 14 days
    C. The duration of the afebrile interval between attacks is usu-
        ally about 7 days, and the duration of relapse is about $2\frac{1}{2}$
        days
    D. Nontreponemal tests for syphilis are occasionally reactive

ANSWERS:

1. (B, D, E)

Borreliosis is a natural infection of many animals, including squirrels,
gerbilles, rats, rabbits, mice, woodchucks and weasels. However,
transmission to humans by direct contact has not been documented,
but rather occurs following the bite of a tick or of a human body
louse. Disease due to lice does not now occur in the U.S., and all
cases in the present time are due to tick bites.

The disease is usually called "relapsing fever", while "undulant
fever" usually refers to brucellosis.

Cases of borreliosis which are transmitted by body lice occur in
Ethiopia at the present time, and in that setting may cause rapidly
spreading disease of epidemic proportions.

2. (A, D)

Borreliosis is divided in two major categories. All louse-borne
cases are arbitrarily identified to be Borrelia recurrentis. The
speciation of tick-borne cases of disease depends upon the vector,
and are named for the infecting tick. For example, Borrelia hermsii
is associated with the tick Ornithodoros hermsi. In many instances,
in which the vector is not known, speciation is not possible. Borrelia
sp are similar morphologically and, aside from identifying the genus,
morphological criteria have not been helpful in determining species,
nor have serologic characteristics.

3. (B, D)

Tick-borne borreliosis appears to be transmitted solely by many
members of Argasidae (soft shelled) ticks which belong to the genus
Ornithodoros. In the U.S. there are primarily O. parkeri, O. hermsi,
and O. turicata which are primarily distributed in the Western states
of the U.S. The geographic distribution of the ticks probably accounts
for the fact that almost all cases are contracted in the Western U.S.

Ornithodoros species of ticks have two characteristics which make
it unlikely that the patient will recognize that he has been bitten.
First, the bite is painless. Secondly, the tick very often feeds at
night and drops off after feeding. Therefore, unless the site of the
bite becomes infected, no bite may be recognized. In the present
case, no local lesion was identified and so the disease was not initially considered.

Borreliosis in the U. S. is recognized solely among persons who
live or have traveled in the Western States. However, the range of
both vectors and naturally infected animals is very much wider than
is the area of distribution of recognized human cases.

4. (A, C, D)

The pathogenic genuses of the family Spirochaetaceae include Borrelia, Leptospira, and Treponema. Only Borrelia sp. may be directly
visualized in smears of the peripheral blood, and this is the usual
basis for diagnosis.

The usual incubation period is 7 days but the range is wide, from 4
to over 18 days.

Attacks and relapses usually occur at rather short intervals with an
afebrile interval of about a week between attacks which last about
2-3 days each. However, afebrile periods of over 2 months may occur, and relapses may be very short, measured in hours, or may
be prolonged. The number of relapses is usually 2-3, but may also
be considerably more numerous.

The incidence of reactive nontreponemal tests for syphilis, VDRL
or Khan tests, has been reported to be as high as 30% in cases of
borreliosis but the reaction is usually transient. Reports of more
recent cases suggest that FTA-ABS tests are usually nonreactive in
patients with tick-borne borreliosis, but this question needs further
study.

REFERENCES

1. Bryceson, A. D. M. , et al. : Louse-borne relapsing fever. A
    clinical and laboratory study of 62 cases in Ethiopia and a re-
    consideration of the literature. Quart. J. Med. 39:129-170,
    1970.

2. Coffey, E. M. , Eveland, W. C. : Experimental relapsing fever
    initiated by Borrelia hermsi. I. Identification of major serotypes
    in the rat. J. Infect. Dis. 117:23-28; 29-34, 1971.

3. Felsenfeld, O.: Borrelia strains, vectors, human and animal Borreliosis: Warren H. Green, Inc., St. Louis, 1971.

4. Moulton, F. R.: Relapsing Fever in the Americas. The Science Press Printing Co., Lancaster, 1942.

5. Pickett, J., Kelly, R.: Lipid catabolism of relapsing fever Borreliae. Inf. and Imm. 9:279-285, 1974.

6. Southern, P. M., Sandford, J. P.: Relapsing fever. A clinical and microbiological review. Medicine 48:129-149, 1969.

7. Thompson, R. S., et al.: Outbreak of tick-borne relapsing fever in Spokane County, Washington. JAMA 210:1945-1950, 1969.

8. Warrell, D. A., et al.: Cardiorespiratory disturbances associated with infective fever in man. Studies of Ethiopian louse-borne relapsing fever. Clin. Sci. 39:123-145, 1970.

::

CASE 40: VAGINAL DISCHARGE, PERINEAL LESIONS, AND INGUINAL ADENOPATHY

HISTORY: This 4-year-old, black girl was well until 3 months prior to admission when her mother noted that she was having a creamy-white, slightly frothy vaginal discharge. She was otherwise in good health and received no medical care for this problem which subsided spontaneously. She was afebrile then and subsequently.

The child was admitted on the date that the mother first noted raised perianal patches. The perianal lesions were painless and not pruritic. A Sitz bath had appeared to worsen the condition. The child had had a slight stomach ache for 3 days prior to admission but was otherwise asymptomatic.

The child lived with her mother and stepfather and only sibling, a 7-year-old boy, in a large housing project. The mother had had gonorrhea four months before the initial onset of the child's symptoms. She had been treated appropriately, did not have repeated cultures, and had been free of symptoms since then. Other members of the family were well. The child spent her days with a grandmother who lived in an adjacent apartment. During a large part of her day she played in the neighborhood without supervision since the grandmother was unable to negotiate the stairs in order to accompany her. Her parents were both employed, her mother a clerk, and her father a construction worker. There had not been reported to be syphilis or lymphogranuloma venereum in the neighborhood during that year.

PHYSICAL EXAMINATION: She was a well-nourished and cheerful child in no apparent distress, in the 50th percentile for height and weight for her age. Her temperature was 37. 0°C. Significant physical findings included the following: Head, neck, chest examination was unremarkable. The abdomen was soft and without organomegaly.

Gynecological examination revealed a dried discharge over the vulva. There were numerous papillomatous, moist, raised plaques centered over the posterior forchette and anus. On the left labia was a healing chancre. On the right anterior labia was a $\frac{1}{2}$ cm. vesicular lesion with several 1-2 mm. circular lesions. There were no other cutaneous lesions.

The inguinal nodes were rubbery, non-tender, and grossly enlarged to 4-5 cm. bilaterally. Gram stain of endocervical material revealed numerous polymorphonuclear leukocytes with Gram negative intracellular and extracellular diplococci. No trichomonas were found and viral cultures were negative.

The WBC on admission was 6, 500 with 39% neutrophils, 46% lymphocytes, 4% monocytes, and 11% eosinophils. Platelets appeared adequate. Sickle cell preparation was negative. Hemoglobin was 12. 3 grams% and hematocrit was 38%.

Culture from endocervical material yielded Neisseria gonorrhoeae. The VDRL test was reactive at a dilution of 1:64, as was the Army slide test. The Reiter protein CF test was non-reactive. The FTA-ABS test was reactive. The LGV complement fixation test was reactive at a 1:256 dilution.

The child received 1. 2 million units of procaine penicillin every 6 hours for four doses. One hour after the first dose was given, material from a perianal lesion was examined by dark field microscopy and no motile treponemal forms were found. Six hours after the first dose of penicillin her temperature rose from 37°C to 39.2°C and her white blood cell count increased to 13, 900 with 66% neutrophils and 2% stabs, 23% lymphocytes, 7% monocytes, and 2% eosinophils. She defervesced within 4 hours and did not experience further fever.

The following day she received 1. 5 million units bicillin I. M. and an intradermal Frei test was applied which was subsequently non-reactive. She was discharged to receive a three-week course of sulfonamide therapy. Repeated LGV CF titer at the end of two months was 1:128. She was subsequently followed by her county health department.

Evaluation of her contacts for a source of her disease was not thoroughly satisfying. The probable source of syphilis and LGV was a young male prostitute who had been visiting a friend, lived in the complex, and had left the complex four months previously.

QUESTIONS:

1. Characteristics of the Jarisch-Herxheimer reaction during the treatment of syphilis include:
   A. Neutropenia
   B. Leukocytosis
   C. Exacerbation of local lesions
   D. Peak increase in temperature within 2 hours of initiation of penicillin
   E. Increased metabolic rate
   F. Eosinopenia is frequent

2. Diagnosis of lymphogranuloma venereum in this child:
   A. Was ruled out by a non-reactive Frei intradermal test
   B. Was confirmed by the LGV complement fixation titer which was reactive at 1:256 dilution
   C. Was unlikely because the LGV CF titer probably represented a false positive reaction, commonly seen in patients with syphilis
   D. Was justified because of the compatible physical findings, serological findings, and epidemiology

3. The following statements concerning Chlamydiaceae are true:
   A. Strains of Chlamydia trachomatis cause lymphogranuloma venereum, trachoma, and inclusion conjunctivitis
   B. There are two species of the genus Chlamydia, C. trachomatis and C. psittaci
   C. Characteristics which distinguish C. trachomatis from C. psittaci include the formation of glycogen-containing inclusions, sensitivity of the organisms to sulfonamides, and the formation of compact or dispersed intracellular microcolonies
   D. Chlamydiaceae have an obligate intracellular growth cycle and are bacteria; in these characteristics they resemble the family Rickettsiaceae
   E. Typing of specific strains of Chlamydia trachomatis may be accomplished by the microimmunofluorescent test

4. By the fact that this child had a constellation of gonorrhea, syphilis, and lymphogranuloma venereum the physician may conclude that:
   A. She had had sexual contact with several persons
   B. She had been sexually molested
   C. She probably had an underlying defect in cell-mediated immunity
   D. Diagnostic studies for other venerally-transmitted diseases should be completed

5. Acceptable regimens for treatment of this child's syphilis and
    gonorrhea could include:
    A. Procaine penicillin G. , 100,000 u/kg/I. M. plus Probenecid
        25 mg/kg/orally plus 1.2 million units benzathine penicillin
        G. I. M.
    B. Erythromycin 40 mg/kg/day for 7 days
    C. Erythromycin, 40 mg/kg/day for 15 days
    D. 1.2 million units benzathine penicillin G. I. M.

ANSWERS:

1. (B, C, E, F)

The Jarisch-Herxheimer reaction is a dramatic response to the treatment of several infections and has occurred very frequently in patients with syphilis and other spirochetoses, such as relapsing fever.
Although neutropenia is a common occurrence in the severe reaction
which may accompany the treatment of relapsing fever, it is very
uncommon during the treatment of patients with early forms of syphilis. See, for example, Warrell et al. In several other respects the
reaction during the relapsing fever is more severe than that of syphilitic patients, and there is an appreciable mortality following treatment of patients with relapsing fever. Although there may be exacerbation of local lesions during treatment of patients with syphilis, the
mortality rate is very low.

The peak increase in temperature elevation, as well as of leukocytosis following institution of therapy for syphilis occurs approximately
4 to 8 hours later, as exemplified by this child. There is a more
rapid onset of fever and earlier peak temperature in most patients
with relapsing fever. In the Jarisch-Herxheimer reaction following
both diseases there is usually an impressive increase in metabolic
rate, as evidenced by increase in arterial glucose, lactate and pyru-
vate concentrations.

Eosinopenia during a Jarisch-Herxheimer reaction has been reported
by many authors. This child demonstrated a dramatic decline in absolute eosinophils count from $715/mm^3$ to $278 mm^3$.

2. (D)

The Frei test is manufactured from prepared egg yolk material which
has been infected with C. trachomatis. In previous eras it was prepared directly from lymph node material of suspected cases. The
Frei test is neither specific, since it may be reactive in patients with
Chlamydia infections other than strains causing LGV, nor very sensitive. For example, in Abrams' report the Frei test was reactive in
only 12 of 20 patients at the time of presentation. This child, as other
patients, may have been reactive if she had retested later.

The material used for the LGV complement fixation test is also prepared from infected egg yolks. Antigen common to all Chlamydiaceae
is present, and hence patients with other chlamydial diseases such
as psittacosis, may have a reactive LGV CF titer. This reaction is
not frequently reactive in syphilitic patients who do not have Chlamydiae diseases, and positive reactions should not be ascribed to
concommitant syphilis.

In the U.S., LGV has been recognized around military installations
and in male homosexuals. The most likely contact for this child for
syphilis was from a person who was a male homosexual from a large
military base. This provided a plausible source for LGV as well as
for syphilis. In addition, she had physical findings compatible with
LGV. The small vesiculated labial lesion may have been the primary,
and the inguinal nodes were very extensively enlarged. The unusual
LGV elevation of CF titer although not specific for LGV again ren-
dered the diagnosis very likely.

3.   (A, B, C, D, E)

There are two species of the genus Chlamydia, C. trachomatis and
C. psittaci. Strains of C. trachomatis cause the human diseases
trachoma, inclusion conjunctivitis, lymphogranuloma venereum, and
probably many cases of nongonococcal urethritis of men. For a particularly excellent review of the characteristics of these organisms,
see the review of Grayston, and for a summary of serological differentiation of the strains which cause the various human diseases, see
Wang et al.

4.   (D)

One of the characteristics of persons with sexually transmitted disease is that it is common to have acquired more than one disease
with a single exposure. This is presumably because the contact may
have been promiscuous and have accrued many of the infections currently in his or her community. As an example, Brown, in 1968, found
a prevalence rate of 8% for infectious syphilis among patients with
acute gonorrhea. Similarly, herpes progenitalis has been reported to
be far more common in patients with gonorrhea than in patients without, but who were attending the same veneral disease clinic. For
these reasons, any patient with a venereally acquired disease should
be thoroughly examined for other similarly acquired infections. In
this instance, the child was found to be free of veneral warts, Trichomonas vaginalis, Herpes progenitalis, and cytomegalovirus infections.

Children are thought to acquire venereal diseases both by sexual molestation and indirect contact through fomites. One of the largest outbreaks of neonatal gonococcal arthritis occurred in a hospital in which
the infection was thought to have been transmitted via rectal thermometers which had not been adequately sterilized (see, in addition,

Shore et al.). The fact that a child is infected therefore, is not reason in itself of conclude that he or she has been abused. Nevertheless, these children should have their care and environment evaluated for sources of abuse.

There is no evidence that acquisition of these diseases is a sign of altered host defense mechanisms.

5. (A, C)

The therapy of this child's gonorrhea requires therapy which achieves an immediate peak of antibiotic which is sustained for at least 6 hours. Procaine penicillin at these doses plus Probenecid would accomplish this, as would the Erythromycin course. The majority of clinical experience has been obtained with the penicillin regimen, and alternate regimens should be used only if the penicillin regimens are specifically contraindicated.

Therapy of active syphilis requires, in contrast to therapy of gonorrhea, a sustained level of antimicrobial agent but an initial high peak is not necessary. This may be achieved by benzathine penicillin or by prolonged oral administration of therapy. A course of 7 days of oral therapy which would usually be expected to be sufficient for therapy of gonorrhea would be inadequate for syphilis in some cases.

In all of these instances it is necessary to re-examine the child to ensure adequate clinical and serological response.

ADDENDUM: A follow-up examination three years after the onset of her illness revealed that she had remained within the 50% for height and weight, was doing well in school, and was in every way asymptomatic. Serological studies were as follows:

    LGV CF titer: 1:8
    VDRL: Non-reactive
    FTA-ABS: Borderline

REFERENCES

1. Abrams, A. J. : Lymphogranuloma venereum. JAMA 205:199-202, 1968.

2. Ackerman, A. B. , et al. : Acquired syphilis in early childhood. Arch. Derm. 106:92-93, 1972.

3. Barrett-Connor, E. : Gonorrhea and the pediatrician. Am. J. Dis. Child. 125:233-238, 1973.

4. Brown, R. C. : The prevalence of infectious syphilis in patients with acute gonorrhea. South. Med. J. 61:98-100, 1968.

5. Grayston, J. T. , Wang, S. P. : New knowledge of Chlamydiae
   and the diseases they cause. J. Infect. Dis. 132:87-105, 1975.

6. Levy, H. : Lymphogranuloma venereum in childhood. J. Pediat.
   11:812-823, 1937.

7. Nelson, J. D. , et al. : Gonorrhea in preschool and school-aged
   children. Report of the Prepubertal Gonorrhea Cooperative
   Study Group. JAMA 236:1359-1364, 1976.

8. Shore, W. B. , Winkelstein, J. A. : Non-venereal transmission of
   gonococcal infections to children. J. Pediat. 79:661-663, 1971.

9. Wang, S. P. , Grayston, J. T. : Human serology in Chlamydia
   trachomatis infection with microimmunofluorescence. J. Infect.
   Dis. 130:388-397, 1974.

::

CASE 41: DIARRHEA, ABDOMINAL PAIN, AND FEVER

HISTORY: This 4-year-old, black boy was admitted in March to his
community hospital with a 4-day history of fever and lower abdominal pain. For 3 days prior to admission he had had infrequent loose
stools and had received 2 days of oral therapy with ampicillin. His
fever continued and at admission he was unable to stand because of
abdominal pain. His temperature was 39°C, he had point right lower
quadrant tenderness, but he had neither guarding nor rebound tenderness. Bowel tones were hyparactive, rectal exam was painful, but
no anterior pelvic induration was noted. Roentgenogram of the chest
showed minimal pneumonitis and of the abdomen showed marked gas
throughout the small and large bowel without areas of distention. His
WBC count was 13,900 with 89% polymorphonuclear leukocytes. The
patient lived with his parents, an older male sibling and a younger
female sibling. Their home was without running water. They had
their own well which was protected from ground water. It had been
examined by the County Health Department 8 years previously and
found to be clean. The child's two siblings had had a mild febrile
illness with one loose stool per day which lasted for one week and
ended two weeks before the onset of the child's initial symptoms.

The child was suspected of having acute appendicitis. At surgical
exploration the appendix was found to be intact and apparently normal and was resected. There was no free peritoneal fluid. Further
exploration revealed a markedly edematous and thickened terminal
ileum which extended to the patent ileocecal valve. The regional
mesenteric lymph nodes were markedly enlarged to 1 cm, discrete,
and one was excised. The child tolerated the procedure well with the
exception of a tachycardia of 160/min.

Microscopic examination of the resected appendix was unremarkable. The mesenteric node, however, contained medullary sinuses which were prominent and contained reticuloendothelial cells and increased number of plasma cells.

Following surgery the patient had daily temperatures of 39°C, total WBC count increased to 14,700, and he continued to have abdominal pain with diarrhea. Examination of his stool for leukocytes demonstrated profuse number of polymorphonuclear leukocytes. Blood cultures and urine cultures failed to yield growth of microorganisms. Because of his poor course, he was transferred to a tertiary care center.

QUESTIONS:

1. Likely diagnoses at the time of admission to his community hospital include:
   A. Appendicitis
   B. Typhoid fever
   C. Mesenteric lymphadenitis
   D. Salmonella enteritis
   E. All of the above

2. Appropriate further studies at the time of admission to the tertiary care center may have included the following:
   A. Salmonella agglutinins
   B. Intradermal PPD with 5 TU and careful family history for tbc exposure
   C. Scikle cell preparation
   D. Stool and blood culture
   E. Repeat roentgenogram of chest and upright of the abdomen
   F. Upper G. I. series with small bowel follow through
   G. All of the above

3. Bacteria which cause intestinal disease which is characterized by invasion of the intestinal wall or lymphatic system include:
   A. Vibrio cholera
   B. Shigella sp.
   C. Clostridia perfringens
   D. Yersinia enterocolitica
   E. Salmonella sp.

4. Characteristics of entero-invasive E. coli are:
   A. Production of a toxin which is similar in many respects to the toxin produced by Vibrio cholera
   B. Accurately identified by agglutination with pooled antisera to somatic antigens from several specific E. coli serotypes
   C. Ability to produce keratoconjunctivitis when inoculated into a guinea pig (the Sereny test)
   D. Presence of cross-reacting antigens with one or another Shigella serotype

5. Characteristics of Yersinia enterocolitica include:
    A. A member of the same bacterial genus as is the organism
        causing plague
    B. Poor growth on most routinely used laboratory media
    C. A zoonotic disease which occurs throughout the world
    D. The mode of spread to humans remains largely unknown
    E. Frequent asymptomatic carriers are common, and it is part
        of the normal human intestinal flora

COURSE IN HOSPITAL: The third day of hospitalization cultures
from the stool were identified as Yersinia enterocolitica.

The patient was begun on therapy with parenteral gentamicin, 5 mg/
kg/day. He continued to be febrile to 38. 5°C daily for the first 5
days after therapy and then defervesced. During this time, his Westergren sedimentation rate decreased from 66 mm/hour to 26 mm/
hour, total WBC count decreased from 22,500 with 67% polymorphonuclear leukocytes to 7,150 with 55% PMN's. His hemoglobin remained stable but serum albumin decreased to 2. 4 gm%. The Y.
enterocolitica isolate was found to be resistant to ampicillin and
carbenicillin and sensitive to gentamicin, sulphamethoxazole-tri-
methoprim, chloramphenicol, tetracycline and cephalosporins. Repeated stool culture one week after initiation of therapy failed to
yield Yersinia sp. The child was discharged in good condition.

QUESTION:

6. Further obligations to this patient include:
    A. Examination of his water supply for cleanliness
    B. Determination of the health of his sibs and parents
    C. Search for other sources of disease, such as his pets
    D. Evaluation for underlying disease which would have predis-
        posed him to this unusual infection
    E. Provision of long-term follow-up for the development of
        chronic infection

ANSWERS:

1. (E)

Physical findings, which did not indicate a typical discrete mass, led
his physician to consider it likely that the appendix was retrocecal
and had ruptured. Because of the continued febrile course with pain,
he underwent appendectomy on the day following admission. However,
his physicians also considered the possibility of salmonellosis and
of mesenteric lymphadenitis.

2. (G)

The patient presented with physical signs of continued inflammation
of the lower abdomen. Sickle cell preparation was negative. There
were no findings to support tuberculosis. Febrile agglutinins and
blood and urine cultures were negative. The upper G. I. series revealed a normal stomach and duodenum. The distal several centimeters of the ileums were markedly abnormal with loss of mucosal
appearance, some thickening, and dilation. These changes were
interpreted to be compatible with an inflammatory process of the
terminal ileum. These changes may be seen in Fig. 41. 1 at the end
of case 41.

3. (B, D, E)

The pathogenesis of the intestinal disease caused by Vibrio cholera
is the production of a soluble toxin which stimulates mucosal adenyl-
cyclase production. Clostridia perfringens causes a food poisoning
which is also dependent upon toxin production but not upon bacterial
invasion of the intestinal mucosa. Salmonella species both produce
soluble toxin and also may invade intestinal epithelium, as do Shigella species and Yersinia enterocolitica (see Grady, 1971).

4. (C, D)

E. coli may produce human disease by at least two separate mechanisms. Many strains produce soluble toxins which effect the mucosal
physiology but do not result in mucosal invasion. These strains are
frequently called "toxigenic" or "enterotoxigenic" E. coli. The alternative pathogenetic mechanism is direct adherence and invasion
of mucosal tissue. This form of disease is clinically similar to
dysentery caused by Shigella sp. or by Yersinia enterocolitica. There
is no evidence to suggest that entero-invasive E. coli regularly produce enterotoxins.

Identification of E. coli which were pathogenic for man was for many
years attempted by means of agglutination with antisera to serotypes
which had caused known disease. Production of enterotoxin is controlled by a plasmid which may be lost and transmitted to other strains.
Therefore, identification of pathogenic strains by serogroups is both
insensitive and not specific, and is particularly inadequate in identifying enteroinvasive strains (see, for example, Goldschmidt and
Tullock's articles). Enterotoxin production may currently be determined by suckling mouse assay, adrenal cell assay, and rabbit loop.
One of several standard tests used to identify E. coli with enteroinvasive potential is the Sereny test. This test is also used to identify
invasive Shigella sp. Enteroinvasive E. coli commonly share somatic antigens with Shigella sp.

5. (A, C, D)

There are three members of the genus Yersinia: Y. enterocolitica,
Y. pseudotuberculosis and Y. pestis, the causitive agent or plague.
These organisms are not fastidious and grow on most commonly used
media. Y. enterocolitica may be found in a wide range of wild and
domestic animals throughout the world. The method by which humans
acquire disease is largely unknown, but have probably included infection by contaminated water supply, direct fecal-oral spread from
the human and pets, and through contaminated food supplies. Asymptomatic carriers are probably uncommon, and there is a high ratio
of infection to clinical disease. It is not considered to be part of
the normal flora.

6. (A, B, C)

The epidemiology of Y. enterocolitica in the U. S. is not yet well-
established. Several cases and outbreaks have been associated with
contaminated water supplies, ill pets and apparent person-to-person
spread. In this case, no other infected persons or animals were dis-
covered, and their water supply was clean. However, the illness in
the child's sibs were compatible with disease due to Y. entero. and
may have been the primary cases for this family. It is particularly
important to determine that young children in affected families are
well, since disease in the very young may be especially severe.

This child did not have septicemia, and had a very classical enteric
presentation. Persons with Y. entero. sepsis frequently have associated conditions such as hemoglobulinopathies, liver disease and
malignancies. This does not appear to be the case when disease is
mild or moderate and is restricted to the intestinal tract.

Enteric disease due to Y. entero. appears to be an acute disease
which causes mesenteric adenitis and dysentery. It cannot be clinically distinguished from other causes of dysentery such as shigello-
sis or enteroinvasive E. coli. Recovery is complete and sequelae
have not been reported.

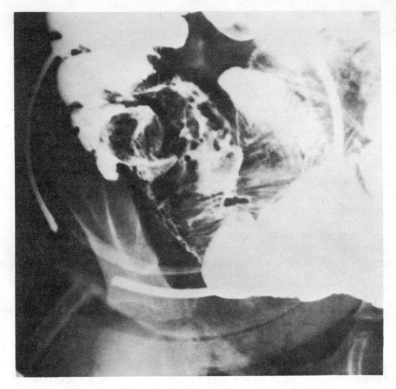

FIG. 41.1

REFERENCES

1. Ahvonen, P.: Human Yersiniosis in Finland. II Clinical features.
    Clin. Res. 4:39-48, 1972.

2. Goldschmidt, M. C., DuPont, A. L.: Enteropathogenic Escherichia
    coli. Lack of correlation of serotype with pathogenicity. J. Infect.
    Dis. 133:153-156, 1976.

3. Grady, G. F., Keusch, G. T.: Pathogenesis of bacterial diarrheas.
    NEJM 285:831-841, 1971.

4. Gutman, L. T., et al.: An interfamilial outbreak of Yersinia
    enterocolitica enteritis. NEHM 288:1372-1377, 1973.

5. Harris, J. C., et al.: Fecal leukocytes in diarrheal illness. Ann.
    Int. Med. 76:697-703, 1973.

6. Nelson, J. D., Haltalin, K. C.: Accuracy of diagnosis of bacterial
    diarrheal disease by clinical features. J. Pediat. 78:519-522, 1971.

7. Tulloch, E. F. , et al. : Invasive enteropathic Escherichia coli
    dysentery. Ann. Int. Med. 79:13-17, 1973.

::

CASE 42: ASPIRATION OF A FOREIGN BODY

HISTORY: The patient was a 4-year-old previously healthy girl
who was living with her physician parents in a medically remote
area of the world. The day of her accident the child was vigorously
rocking a rocking chair, sucking a piece of hard candy and chatting.
The chair tipped backward, and she inhaled the candy with her gasp.
She developed instantly severe right chest pain, became cyanotic,
and respirations became labored. Immediate attempts to dislodge
the candy were unsuccessful and within 30 minutes she had regained
normal color, the pain began to subside and respirations were normal. Roentgenographic examination of the chest that day was unremarkable and without evidence of pulmonary airway obstruction.
Because the aspirated object was known to be soluble and facilities
for bronchoscopy marginal, no attempt was made to remove the
candy. The child resumed usual activities.

Six days later the child developed a mild cough. The following day
her temperature rose to 38°C and the cough worsened. No sputum
was produced and there was no hemoptysis. She complained of chest
pain, fatigue, and lack of appetite. Her white blood cell count was
12,400 with 74% polymorphonuclear leukocytes and 26% lymphocytes.
Roentgenogram of the chest revealed right middle lobe pneumonia.
Blood cultures were taken. The child was begun on a course of physical therapy and oral penicillin, 250 mg qid. There was a defervescence for $1\frac{1}{2}$ days which was followed by recurrence of fever to 39°C,
decreased cough, anorexia and marked weakness. Blood cultured
from 2 days previously yielded growth of a small gram-negative rod
at the bottom of Castaneda's medium and in thioglycolate broth, but
not on a direct agar pour plate. The organism was subsequently identified to be Bacteroides melanogenicus.

The child was begun on intravenous aqueous penicillin, 200,000 units/
kg/day administered in four doses. Repeated roentgenogram of the
chest now revealed progression of pneumonia with a large area of
dense consolidation within which was a 4 x 6 cm. cavity containing
an air-fluid level.

The child continued to be acutely ill and toxic for 2 days with respiratory rate of 43, pulse 100, temperature 39. 4°C. During the following evening she developed a sudden, severe cough, vomited once,
and began to produce copious amounts of blood tinged, foul smelling
sputum, and thereafter had rapid relief of her toxic symptoms. She
made an uneventful recovery. Three months later roentgenographic
examination showed a persistent scar in the right middle lobe.

QUESTIONS:

1. To diagnose the etiology of pneumonia, the following methods of obtaining or evaluating material yield results which if positive reliably indicate the infecting organism:
   A. Blood culture
   B. Throat culture
   C. Transtracheal needle aspiration
   D. Percutaneous aspiration of the lung
   E. Counter immunoelectrophoresis for bacterial antigens
   F. Endotracheal aspiration via naso-tracheal intubation

2. The common etiologic agents from lung abscesses secondary to aspiration in previously well patients are:
   A. Gram-negative anaerobic bacilli including Fusobacterium sp. and Bacteroides sp.
   B. Staphylococcus aureus
   C. Streptococcus pneumoniae
   D. Anaerobic gram-positive cocci including Peptostreptococcus sp and Peptococcus sp.
   E. Multiple isolates, usually including anaerobic species of bacteria
   F. E. coli

3. Prior to recognition of the positive blood culture in this child, appropriate antimicrobial therapy could have consisted of:
   A. Erythromycin estolate, 40 mg/kg/day
   B. Clindamycin, 20 mg/kg/day IV
   C. Penicillin G, 50,000 U/kg/day IV
   D. Keflex with kanamycin

4. Characteristics of disease caused by inhaled foreign bodies include:
   A. Commonly lodge in the right main stem bronchus if patient is in upright position
   B. Presenting findings frequently include wheezing, hemoptysis, and recurrent pneumonia
   C. Accumulation of bronchial secretions with subsequent infection distal to the inflammatory response provoked by the foreign body may progress to chronic bronchiectasis with residual pulmonary disease

ANSWERS:

1. (A, C, D, E)

Although only approximately 5 to 10% of children with pneumonia yield the infecting organism from a blood culture, when the blood culture is positive it is a very reliable indication of the cause of the pneumonia. On the contrary, a throat culture from both children and adults yields information which cannot be interpreted. The organisms

which commonly cause pneumonia are normal flora of the upper
respiratory tract. Similarly, one may fail to isolate the causative
agent from the upper respiratory tract (see, for example, Barrett-
Connor).

Transtracheal aspiration to obtain tracheal secretions has been
widely used in adult patients with severe pneumonia, but with far
less frequently in children. The procedure is not without hazard,
and in a child the problem of immobilization and control may require anesthesia. For these reasons this procedure, although it
may yield valuable information, has not been widely employed. On
the other hand, percutaneous needle aspiration of material from an
involved segment has been found to be very valuable, technically
easy, and the hazards are minimal (see discussion by Hyde, et al.).

Endotracheal aspiration via naso-tracheal intubation may yield material revealing the infecting organism. This procedure has the dis-
advantage of frequent contamination from upper respiratory flora.
However, if the material is carefully collected, purulent material
is present, and the culture results conform to the distribution of
organisms seen by direct Gram stain, valuable information may
have been gained. In all of the above instances, it is particularly
important that the materials for culture be obtained before antimicrobial therapy is initiated.

Counter immunoelectrophoresis is a technique for determining the
presence of bacterial antigens in body fluids. It has been most widely
used to assist in the diagnosis of disseminated infection with H.
influenzae type B, which is a rare cause of pulmonary disease. Progress is being made in rendering the assay appropriate for the diagnosis of pneumococcal, staphylococcal, meningococcal and streptococcal disease. The multiple serotypes of penumococci limit the
test at the present time. Positive results are reliable, but negative
assays do not rule out the pathogen for the diagnosis of etiology of
most cases of pneumonia.

2.   (A, D, E)

Etiologic agents for aspiration pneumonia and lung abscesses usually
include the normal flora of the upper respiratory passages. Major
exceptions to this occur in the children who have hematogenously
disseminated bacterial disease which involves the lung secondarily.
The primary example of this is Staphylococcus aureus.

Although lung abscesses which follow aspiration are caused by a
wide variety of anaerobic flora, usually more than one organism
participates. Consequently a blood culture may yield only one species, while percutaneous aspiration or transtracheal aspiration may
yield a variety of strains, often two or three.

The etiology of aspiration pneumonia which is acquired outside the hospital differs from that of hospital-acquired disease. Aerobic enteric flora such as E. coli, Pseudomonas sp. and Proteus sp. play a very small role in community acquired disease, but are more frequently causes of lung abscess in hospitalized patients.

3. (C)

Erythromycin estolate has been reported to cause cholestatic hepatitis. It has an occasional role in the treatment of uncomplicated pneumonia in previously well persons, but since it is poorly effective in the treatment of anaerobic infections, it should not be relied upon in this instance.

Clindamycin has only recently been used for the therapy of severe systemic pediatric infections. Although it may be expected to be effective in the treatment of pulmonary abscesses of children, experience is still inadequate to recommend it for general use in this condition. It may be viewed as a desirable alternative to penicillin and for instances in which the patient is infected with a penicillin-resistant Bacteroides sp.

Penicillin G remains the treatment of choice for patients with aspiration pneumonia outside of the hospital setting. The normal flora of the upper respiratory tract, aerobic as well as anaerobic, are usually sensitive to penicillin and the clinical experience with this form of therapy is satisfactory. In contrast, the cephalosporins are only variably effective or ineffective for the therapy of most anaerobic organisms of the upper respiratory tract, and kanamycin would be ineffective for common Gram (+) cocci and for bacteroides.

4.   (A, B, C)

The foreign object tends to follow the more direct path which leads to the right lower lobe. In this child the object lodged in the right middle lobe.

Presenting findings may depend upon whether obstruction and its accompanying inflammation is complete, in which case atelectasis is likely to occur. Hemoptysis in a child is most commonly caused by mucosal damage due to aspirated foreign body. Other findings include wheezing, localized hyperinflation, and systemic signs of abscess formation with or without sepsis.

If the foreign body is not removed promptly, the patient runs a risk of developing chronic destructive pulmonary disease which may include bronchiectasis, obstructive pulmonary disease, and recurrent pneumonia. Physical therapy and efforts to obtain excellent drainage either via bronchial drainage or effected surgically is essential in the prevention and treatment of these complications. Bronchoscopy may aid in establishing drainage, even in the absence of a foreign body.

REFERENCES

1. Barrett-Connor, E. : The nonvalue of sputum culture in the diag-
    nosis of pneumococcal pneumonia. Am. Rev. Resp. Dis. 103:845,
    1971.

2. Bartlett, J. G. , et al. : Bacteriology and treatment of primary
    lung abscess. Am. Rev. Resp. Dis. 109:510-518, 1974.

3. Bartlett, J.G. , et al. : The bacteriology of aspiration pneumonia.
    Am. J. Med. 56:202-207, 1974.

4. Bartlett, J. G. , Gorbach, S. L. : Treatment of aspiration pneu-
    monia and primary lung abscess. Penicillin G vs Clindamycin.
    JAMA 234:935-937, 1975.

5. Hyde, R. W. , et al. : New pulmonary diagnostic procedures. Are
    they practical alternatives to open-lung biopsy? Am. J. Dis.
    Child. 126:292-295, 1973.

6. Lorber, G. , Swenson, R. M. : Bacteriology of aspiration pneu-
    monia. A prospective study of community-and hospital-acquired
    cases. Ann. Int. Med. 81:329-351, 1974.

7. Pyman, C. : Inhaled foreign bodies in childhood. A review of
    230 cases. Med. J. Austr. 1:62-68, 1971.

::

CASE 43: STAPHYLOCOCCAL DISEASE IN A NEWBORN NURSERY

HISTORY: A county hospital reported that 5% of their newborn infants had been experiencing staphylococcal disease for two months.

The nursery admitted approximately 250 babies delivered at the
hospital each month and had a daily census of approximately 30-45
babies. The nursery had 5 rooms each of which could receive 10-12
babies. There was a nursing station between each 2 rooms and a
separate procedure room. Infants were admitted to one room until
it was full. That room then received no new admissions until it had
emptied which occurred every 3-4 days. Babies spent most of their
time in the nursery as there was no rooming in. There was an attempt to cohort nursing personnel, but this was not rigidly enforced.
The nursery had a large number of rotating personnel, including
nursing students from three nursing schools who rotated monthly.
Fathers but no other relatives were welcomed into the nursery. There
was an adequate scrub area for visitors and their scrub and gowning
was supervised. Infants were washed daily with 3% hexachlorophene
soap and had Betadine applied daily to the cord. Nursery personnel
used Betadine for hand washing.

In the most recent three months, 24 infants had had overt signs of staphylococcal disease. Three had mastitis, one had staphylococcal sepsis, two had Ritter's Disease, and six had omphalitis, and 10 had pustules over the diaper area. Ten of these illnesses had occurred prior to discharge after routine deliveries and the remaining 14 had occurred within three weeks of discharge and had been noted by their private pediatrician.

Initial evaluations included the following:

1. All current nursery personnel were questioned concerning active staphylococcal disease and none was found.

2. Discharge cultures of the anterior nares for S. aureus of all infants was begun.

3. All S. aureus from colonized or infected infants were stocked in order to provide phage type identification.

4. Environmental settle plates were placed in each room of the nursery complex and selected swabs were made of common areas.

5. The importance of hand washing between handling infants was re-emphasized.

6. All infants who developed any sign of inflammation were isolated in a single room.

7. Attention was given to the cleaning of areas in which there was indirect contact between babies, such as the procedure room.

The results of the above measures demonstrated that both the settle plates and the swabs from the procedure room yielded heavy growth of S. aureus. The circumcision board was heavily contaminated, as were the outsides of large bottles containing antiseptic solutions. Other areas of the nursery were not overtly contaminated. The rate of colonization of the anterior nares was 69% at the beginning of the surgery, but had declined to 5% at the end of the next 2 months. Cleaning between procedures in the procedure room was facilitated, for which a 1:500 aqueous quarternary ammonium solution was used. Attention to hand washing was emphasized.

Clinically apparent disease occurred in 3 of the next 300 births, and 1 of the subsequent 400 births. Colonization rates remained below 15% for the next 6 months, after which surveillance one week of every four was instituted. Forty S. aureus isolates were phage typed. Six were from infants with clinically apparent disease. Phage types 80/81, 71+, nonreactive, D-11, 96, 94/96, and 29/52/52 A were identified. There was not a predominant type for ill children, colonized children or environmental isolates.

QUESTIONS:

1. Evidence for toxicity of 3% hexachlorophene when used for daily body bathing of infants rests upon the following data:
   A. The mean blood hexachlorophene concentration of low birth weight infants after this regimen is approximately 0.5 ugm/ml
   B. Metabolism of hexachlorophene by the liver is immature in the newborn and therefore the half-line is prolonged
   C. CSF hexachlorophene concentrations have been found to correlate with clinical signs of CNS irritation in humans
   D. Studies showing a significant statistical association of the whole-body bathing of premature infants with vacuolar encephalopathy of the brain stem reticular formation in these infants has been reported
   E. There is similarity between serum hexachlorophene concentrations which lead to experimental encephalopathy in rats and serum hexachlorophene concentrations observed in newborn infants

2. In December, 1971 the FDA recommended that hexachlorophene be discontinued for routine bathing of newborn infants. Prior to that time routine bathing of newborn infants with hexachlorophene had been definitely demonstrated to:
   A. Decrease the rates of staphylococcal colonization of newborns
   B. Retard the progression of staphylococcal disease during nursery epidemics
   C. Increase the rate of disease caused by gram-negative enteric bacteria
   D. Prevent the outbreak of serious staphylococcal disease if colonization rates are maintained at 10% or less

3. Current recommended regimens for care of the cord of the newborn include:
   A. Use of triple dye
   B. Betadine solution applied locally
   C. Use of hexachlorophene applied locally
   D. Soap and water baths
   E. All of the above

4. The epidemiologic results of this outbreak support the following mechanisms of spread of disease:
   A. A single source of contamination of diseased and colonized infants, probably from infected personnel
   B. Multiple introduction of strains of S. aureus with indirect spread via common-source contamination
   C. Multiple introduction into the nursery from infected fathers and nursing students, leading to direct inoculation of infants

ANSWERS:

1. (A, D, E)

Hexachlorophene serum concentrations following daily bathings of
low birth weight infants is variable, and is generally higher in the
smaller infants. In one study of full-term infants, the mean concentration was 0.11 ugm/ml. In another study of low-birth weight infants it was 0.5 ugm/ml. Concentrations of hexachlorophene in plasma
of rats which have manifested brain lesions have been 1.2 to 1.5
ugm/ml. The concentrations in humans are, therefore, approximately
$\frac{1}{2}$ to 1/3 that of a toxic range for experimental animals, ranges which
may be considered similar.

The metabolism of hexachlorophene is primarily by the liver with
excretion by the liver and kidney. The half-life of hexachlorophene
may be expected to be prolonged in the small infant but has not been
determined. Neither have CSF levels been determined to correlate
with overt clinical disease.

One of the primary studies supporting the concept of human toxicity
of hexachlorophene was performed by Alford et al. He examined
autopsies on infants who were 1400 grams or less and survived at
least 4 days.

Analysis was made without knowledge of whether or not the infant
had received hexachlorophene bathing. Results strongly supported
an association between exposure to hexachlorophene and development
of vacuolar encephalopathy in deceased premature infants.

2. (A)

Numerous studies have demonstrated the efficacy of hexachlorophene
bathing in decreasing staphylococcal colonization of the newborn.
Routine use was stimulated by the assumption that low colonization
rates would be associated with low rates of disease. This was true
in some instances but in many nurseries virulent stains of S. aureus
have led to the emergence of disease when colonization rates are low
or moderate. Hexachlororphene bathing has not been demonstrated
to alter the course of an established epidemic (see, for example,
Gehlbach). For a discussion of the efficacy of hexachlorophene, see
the review by Kensit. Several studies have demonstrated a moderate
increase in colonization with gram-negative enteric flora of infants
who are bathed with hexachlorophene compared with infants not so
bathed. The question of whether or not a significant increase in disease due to these organisms occurs is not definitely settled but it is
doubtful (see, for example, Light et al.).

3. (A, D)

Triple dye contains brilliant green, proflavine hemisulfate, and crystal violet. It has been demonstrated to decrease rates of colonization with S. aureus and group B beta hemolytic streptococci. Disadvantages include retardation of cord dessication. Toxicity where used locally is unknown but not well studied.

Betadine solution is used in some new series, but lack of information concerning absorption renders this an undesirable form of local care. Hexachlorophene is still used in some area, but because of possible absorption in small infants, even from a small area, it should be avoided.

Many nurseries currently use only soap and water with careful attention to the cord.

The current recommendations concerning care of the cord and skin of newborn infants gives the opportunity for each hospital to choose one of several regimens. See the statement on "skin care of newborns".

4. (B)

The critical information in this outbreak was that diseased and colonized infants harbored S. aureus with a variety of phage types, obviating a single introduction from an infected person. Failure to recognize disease in any personnel further decreased the likelihood that an individual member of the personnel would be found to be the source. The fact that the procedure room was highly contaminated and other areas of the nursery were not renders it likely that that area was not receiving adequate cleaning between each infant, the area had become highly contaminated with several strains, and infants entering the area were then contaminated. After meticulous cleansing of the area between each infant and emphasis of the importance of hand washing between handling infants was begun, the epidemic subsided.

REFERENCES

1. Gehlbach, S. H. , et al. : Recurrence of skin disease in a nursery: Ineffectuality of hexachlorophene bathing. Pediatrics 55:422-424, 1975.

2. Kensit, J. G. : Hexachlorophene: Toxicity and effectiveness in prevention of sepsis in neonatal units. J. Antimic. Chemother. 1:263-672, 1975.

3. Light, I. J. , et al. : Ecologic relation between Staphylococcus aureus and pseudomonas in a nursery population: Another example of bacterial interference. NEJM 278:1243-1247, 1968.

4. Shuman, R. M., et al.: Neurotoxicity of hexachlorophene in humans, II: A clinicopathological study of 46 premature infants. Arch. Neurol. 32:320-5, 1975.

5. Symposium: Hexachlorophene - Its usage in the nursery. Pediatrics 51, No. 2, Part 2 (supplement) February, 1973.

6. Editorial: Skin Care of Newborns. Pediatrics 54:682-3, 1974.

::

CASE 44: FEVER, SHOULDER PAIN AND JAUNDICE IN A BLACK CHILD

HISTORY: This 6-year-old, black male was admitted for the second time on 6-18-72 with a complaint of fever and jaundice of one week's duration. He had been well until the onset of jaundice and a slight decrease in appetite. Four days prior to admission he developed fever and pain in his left shoulder. He had no diarrhea, no skin rash, had been receiving no medications, and there was no known illness in other members of his family.

The child's first admission was at the age of 3 years when he developed a spinal epidural abscess at T6 due to Staphylococcus aureus. During that admission he was diagnosed to have sickle cell disease and treatment of his acute infection led to full recovery. He developed normally, was in the 30% for height and weight, and was doing well in school.

On admission the child had a temperature of 40. 4 degrees C, was icteric and in apparent distress. Significant findings included the following: There was marked scleral icterus. There was a Grade 3/6 systolic ejection murmur which was best heard over the sternal border. The pulse was bounding. There was right upper quadrant with tenderness over the liver. The liver was 4 cm. below the right costal margin. The spleen was not palpable. The anterior capsule of the left shoulder was slightly swollen and with limitation of range of motion.

LAB TESTS: Total white blood cell count was 26,500 with 64% polymorphonuclear leukocytes, 16% stabs, and 20% lymphocytes. Hematocrit was 24% and the reticulocyte count was 10%. Hemoglobin was 8. 6 gm%. Target and sickle forms were apparent. Howell-Jolly bodies were not seen. The sickle cell preparation showed 20% immediate sickling. The mono spot test was non-reactive. The HBsAg test was negative. Liver function tests showed LDH=436 IU (26-186 nl); SGOT=66 IU (10-26 nl); SGPT = 33 IU (10-26 nl); alkaline phosphatase = 114 IU (20-67 nl). Repeat studies in 3 days showed marked increases in LDH to 699 IU and alkaline phosphatase to 261 IU. Serum

bilirubin - at admission was 6. 6 gm% with 5. 3 gm% direct, which
rose during the next 3 days to a total of 29. 6 with 16. 6 gm% direct.
Other serum chemistries were within normal limits with the exception of serum albumin which was 1. 7 gm% at admission and was subsequently ≤ 1 gm%. Heterophile antibody and agglutinins to S. typhi
"O", S. para A "O", and S. para B "O" antigens were negative.

ROENTGENOGRAPHIC FINDINGS: Chest - cardiomegaly with prom-
inence of pulmonary vasculature, compatible with the patient's chronic
anemia. Left Shoulder - No soft tissue changes. Irregularity and
destruction of the metaphyseal cortex and of the medullary area of
the humerus was seen and interpreted to be indicative of osetomye-
litis. Subsequent films demonstrated involvement of the proximal
diaphysis in addition and extension of the process. Liver - Spleen
Scan - Technetium scan of the liver and spleen demonstrated an
enlarged liver whose lower edge was approximately 10 cm. below
the costal margin and there was not any evidence of areas of localized decrease in tracer concentration. The spleen was normal in
position, size and function.

Cultures were taken of throat, stool, urine and blood. On the second
hospital day blood cultures yielded growth of a non-lactose ferment-
ing gram-negative rod which was subsequently identified to be Salmonella enteritidis. The MIC to trimethoprim was 0. 15 ugm/ml, to
sulfamethoxazole was 24. 5 ugm/ml, and to both in a combination
of 1:20 was 0. 05/0. 95 ugm/ml. The MIC's to other antimicrobial
agents were: chloramphenicol 2. 5 ugm/ml; ampicillin 0. 15 ugm/ml;
gentamicin 1. 25 ugm/ml; tetracycline 1 ugm/ml. The stool and throat
cultures did not yield significant pathogens. Therapy with 300 mg/kg/
day ampicillin had been initiated and the patient defervesced within
36 hours. At the third day his temperature rose to 40. 3 degrees C. ,
he continued to be irritable, and his shoulder was markedly tender.
Serum bactericidal and bacteriostatic concentrations of his serum to
his Salmonella enteritidis revealed the following results taken just
before and one hour after infusion of ampicillin were:

	Bacteriostatic	Bactericidal
Pre dose	None	None
1 hr. after dose	1:8	None

These data were interpreted to indicate a poor response due to an
inadequate concentration of drug and he was begun on 100 mg/kg/day
of chloramphenicol. His clinical course did not improve, and repeated
serum studies indicated failure to achieve bacteriostatic concentrations in serum either before or following medication.

Fifteen days after admission he had developed signs of septic arthritis in the involved shoulder. The joint was drained surgically and no
organisms were seen or cultured from the synovial pus. Following
this procedure he began therapy with trimethoprim-sulfamethoxazole,

200 mg. TMP/m^2/day p. o. Peak serum concentrations were 20 times the MIC of the organism, and nadir concentrations were 4 times the MIC.

The patient subsequently did well. Although roentgenographic evidence of extensive bony destruction of the shoulder persisted through four years of follow-up, return of function was excellent.

QUESTIONS:

1. For evaluation of antimicrobial therapy of patients with septicemia due to Salmonella sp. , the following considerations pertain:
   A. It is good practice to administer that antimicrobial agent to which the organism is most highly sensitive
   B. Treatment of enteric fever due to Salmonella sp. decreases the incidence of chronic carrier status
   C. The clinical response to chloramphenicol in enteric fever due to Salmonella sp. is superior to ampicillin in achieving a more rapid defervescence and a decreased incidence of relapse
   D. Administration of chloramphenicol by mouth is a common cause of inadequate therapy; intramuscular administration is indicated for therapy of enteric fever due to Salmonella sp.
   E. None of the above

2. Characteristics of Salmonella infection in patients with sickle cell disease include:
   A. There is frequent involvement of multiple sites with osteomyelitis, many of which are symmetrical diaphyseal areas
   B. Salmonella sp. is the most common cause of osteomyelitis in sicklers
   C. These patients share the propensity for developing Salmonella sp. septicemia with patients with schistosomiasis, with other conditions which cause chronic hemolysis, and with malignancies
   D. The relative risk of developing salmonellosis in patients with sickle cell disease is similar to the risk of developing pneumococcal meningitis

3. Normal splenic size and function in this patient, which was demonstrated by technetium scan of liver and spleen may indicate:
   A. Tuftsin deficiency would not be expected
   B. Functional asplenia may be present, although the spleen is apparently normal in size and Howell-Jolly bodies were not seen

4. There are numerous characteristics of children with sickle cell disease which may participate in their especial susceptibility to bacterial infections. Included are:
   A. Chronic hemolysis which results in reticulo-endothelial blockade and subsequent less effective reticulo-endothelial function
   B. Abnormal phagocytosis of gram $\oplus$ organisms by polymorphonuclear leukocytes in the presence of low concentrations of specific opsonin
   C. Deficient ability to produce specific opsonin
   D. Functional asplenia
   E. Infarction of tissue leading to increased incidence of bacteremia from enteric organisms and seeding of areas of infarcted bone
   F. Altered ability initiate phagocytosis by the alternate pathway of complement

ANSWERS:

1. (E)

Human disease due to Salmonella sp. is an example of divergence of results of in vitro sensitivity tests with those of clinical experience. Although demonstration of resistance to an antimicrobial agent probably indicates it will be inefficacious, demonstration of in vitro sensitivity does not necessarily correlate with efficacy. The aminoglycoside antimicrobial agents, for example, are effective in inhibiting bacterial growth at low concentrations in vitro, but are ineffective in altering the course of disease (see, for example, Dawkins et al.). Chloramphenicol and ampicillin remain the most commonly efficacious agents and therapy may be chosen on the basis of the MIC data for these two agents. Recent experiences with chloramphenicol-resistant strains of Salmonella sp. are alarming but mainly restricted to travelers.

Rather than decreasing the incidence of chronic carrier states, treatment of salmonellosis with antimicrobial agents is highly associated with an increased incidence of prolonged excretion from the gastrointestinal tract.

Numerous studies have compared the response achieved by chloramphenicol therapy with that of ampicillin (see, for example, Robertson et al.). Small differences may be found in rate of defervescence, but significant and consistent differences have not been apparent.

Chloramphenicol is absorbed from the gastrointestinal tract with a high degree of reliability, even in patients with gastrointestinal disease. Oral administration achieves serum concentrations which approximate those of intravenous administrations. Intramuscular administration, on the contrary, produces serum concentrations which are highly variable and this route should be avoided.

2. (A, B, C)

The differential diagnosis of osteomyelitis versus aseptic infarction
in a patient with sickle cell disease is often difficult. Areas of bone
which have undergone infarction are highly predisposed to the development of osteomyelitis following bacteremia. Children with
sickle cell disease commonly present with painful symmetrical
swelling of the hands and feet together with fever and leukocytes,
the "hand-foot syndrome". Similar disease may be caused by salmonella osteomyelitis.

Although organisms other than Salmonella sp. cause osteomyelitis
in patients with sickle cell disease, Salmonella sp. are the most
common.

Numerous diseases appear to predispose the patient to salmonella
sepsis. Common denominators of these conditions appear to be
chronic hemolysis and depression of reticulo-endothelial function
such as occurs in chronic disease of the liver and in many malignancies. See, for example, data concerning the effect of hemolysis
on the susceptibility to salmonella infections by Kaye and Hook.

While the relative risk of sicklers developing salmonellosis has been
estimated to be approximately 25 times that of the general population,
the relative risk of developing pneumococcal meningitis is estimated
by Barrett-Connor to be very much greater, approximately 579 times
that of the general population.

3. (A)

Production of Tuftsin, a tetrapeptide which stimulates phagocytic
activity of polymorphonuclear leukocytes, appears to be dependent
upon normal splenic function. Tuftsin is important in phagocytosis
of gram $\oplus$ organisms but less well substantiated for gram $\ominus$ where
lysis with complement is mediated via IgM. This child's spleen was
normal in size and function by techneticum scan, and Howell-Jolly
bodies were not seen on peripheral smear. It would be surprising,
therefore, if there were a major defect of host response on the basis
of abnormal splenic function. Many patient's with sickle cell disease
do not have normal splenic function. Although methods of evaluating
splenic function are imprecise, this patient appears to be exceptional
by having normal function.

4. (A, B, D, E, F)

The role of hemolysis in facilitating bacterial infections has been
demonstrated in animal models and in numerous human diseases.
Likely mechanisms include increased free iron in the circulation,
and decreased reticuloendothelial function.

Patients with sickle cell disease produce polymorphonuclear leukocytes with a normal ability to phagocytose organisms in the presence
of optimal amounts of opsonin. They have a normal ability to produce
specific opsonin following challenge although the rate of production
of antibody may be delayed with first exposure.

On the contrary, in sickle cell disease patients who have suboptimal
concentrations of specific opsonin, phagocytosis of pneumococci is
depressed when compared with that of non-sickle cell disease patients. This may be due to a deficient use of the alternate pathway
of complement, which requires properdin, for the fixation of C3.

Many of these children have infarcted spleens or spleens which are
nonfunctional, as described above. Infarction of other tissues is
common, especially early in the infectious process, and commonly
leads to pulmonary infarcts, gastrointestinal malfunction and bacterial invasion, and localization of infection to areas of bone (see
studies by Johnson et al.).

REFERENCES

1. Barrett-Connor, E.: Bacterial infection in sickle cell anemia
    Medicine 50:97-112, 1971.

2. Constant, E., et al.: Salmonella osteomyelitis of both hands and
    the hand-foot syndrome. Arch. Surg. 102:148-151, 1971.

3. Dawkins, A. T., Hornick, R. B.: Evaluation of antibiotics in a
    typhoid model. Antimic. Agts. & Chemoth., 1966. pp. 6-10.

4. Engh, C. A., et al.: Osteomyelitis in the patient with sickle cell
    disease. J. Bone and J. Surg. 53-A: 1-15, 1971.

5. Johnson, R. B., et al.: An abnormality of the alternate pathway
    of complement activation in sickle cell disease. NEJM 288:803-
    808, 1973.

6. Johnson, R. B.: Increased susceptibility to infection in sickle
    cell disease: Review of its occurrence and possible causes. South.
    Med. J. 67:1342-1348, 1974.

7. Kaye, D., et al.: Factors influencing host resistance to Salmo-
    nella infections: The effects of hemolysis and erythrophagocytosis.
    Am. J. Med. Sci. 254:205-215, 1967.

8. Robertson, R. P., et al.: Evaluation of chloramphenicol and
    ampicillin in Salmonella enteric fever. NEJM 278:171-176, 1968.

CASE 45: STAPHYLOCOCCAL PNEUMONIA

HISTORY: This 2-9/12-year-old, white boy was transferred in July
from his community hospital to a medical center with a two day history of fever, pneumonia and irrational behavior. When he had ar-
rived at his community hospital he had been found to have left lower
lobe pneumonia and was treated with 1,000,000 units aqueous penicillin per day. Twenty-four hours after admission he had experienced
a generalized seizure. The following morning he had developed shrill
cries, began to bite himself, and failed to recognize his parents.
His white blood cell count was 2,900 with 64% lymphocytes and 36%
polymorphonuclear leukocytes. Examination of the cerebrospinal
fluid revealed 4 WBC, protein 13 mg%, and sugar 58%. Opening
pressure was not measured but was not thought to be elevated.

The child had two older siblings who are well. Other members of
the family were in good health. There was no history of tuberculosis.

At admission, following transfer to the medical center, he was a
pale, distressed child. Respiratory rate was 100/min, pulse 160/min,
temp. 39. 7°C. Height and weight were on the 25th% for age. Blood
pressure was 120/90. Significant physical findings were as follows:
No papilledema, PERRLA; ears normal. Lungs revealed decreased
breath sounds across the left lung field with rales in the upper and
lower lobes. Examination of the heart was normal. The liver was
palpable 2 cm. below the right costal margin, and the spleen was not
palpable. The neurological examination was unremarkable. His skin
was unremarkable except for scattered insect bites and impetigenous
lesions over both pretibia.

LABORATORY FINDINGS: Hemoglobin 10. 8 gm%, WBC 4,200 with
47% neutrophils, 20% lymphocytes, 19% stabs. There were 7% early
and abnormal lymphocytes. PO_2 was 70, sedimentation rate was
113/mm/hr. , serum salicylate level 7. 3 mg%. Serum chemistries
were unremarkable with the exception of a serum sodium of 127
meq. /L. Roentgenography of the chest revealed the left hemithorax
to be homogenously opacified and with a shift of the mediastinum to
the right, demonstrating increased volume of left pleural cavity
consistent with a large pleural effusion or soft tissue mass. Blood,
throat, sputum, urine cultures were taken, and the child was begun
on 200 mg nafcillin/kg/day I. V.

HOSPITAL COURSE: The patient remained disoriented and in acute
distress. The following day he demonstrated cyanosis of his finger-
beds. Pleural tap yielded 400 cc. of dark blood tinged fluid with a
protein of 6 gm%, Gram (+) cocci in clusters, and profuse polymorphonuclear leukocytes. The mediastinum returned to midline position
and an Argyle chest tube was placed which drained 130 cc/day for
the next 2 days. The patient gradually regained his orientation, and
mild restriction of free water was accompanied by a gradual rise of
his serum sodium to a normal range.

On the 3rd hospital day he developed a confluent macular pruritic rash over his thighs and had loose bowel movements. Benadryl was added to his regimen and the rash resolved during the next 2 days, as did his diarrhea.

The patient continued febrile to $39^{\circ}C$ and leukocytosis slowly increased to 26,000 with 9% stabs and 59% neutrophils on the 10th hospital day. Multiple areas of abscess formation became apparent on roentgenography. Drainage from the chest tube continued to yield growth of S. aureus.

The MIC of his S. aureus to nafcillin was 1.25 ugm/ml, to penicillin G was 0.31 ugm/ml, and to gentamicin was 1.25 ugm/ml. Serum Schlicter determinations on the 9th hospital day revealed:

	Serum bacteriostatic dilution	Serum bactericidal dilution
Pre therapy	none	none
2 hours post therapy	1:2	none

The dose of nafcillin was therefore increased from 200 mg/kg/day to 300 mg/kg/day, and gentamicin, 5 mg/kg/day was added. Two days later the child began defervescence, appetite began to improve, and he became more responsive. Chest tube drainage on the 14th hospital day, however, continued to yield growth of S. aureus.

On the 21st hospital day the patient underwent bronchoscopy to rule out obstruction of bronchus (e. g. with foreign body), for which there was no evidence. Repeated Schlicters which were taken 2 hours after medication showed a bacteriostatic and bactericidal concentration in the serum at 1:128 dilution.

On the 25th hospital day the chest film was thought to be showing minimal but definite signs of beginning resolution. The patient was becoming playful. He continued to be afebrile and pleural fluid failed to yield S. aureus on culture.

On the 31st hospital day, the patient was begun on 750 mg. penicillin p. o. q4h plus 40 mg/kg/day probenecid. Serum Schlicters before and after this course yielded no bacteriostatic or bactericidal concentrations. The patient was discharged on this regimen and continued to make an uneventful recovery.

QUESTIONS:

1. Characteristics of children with staphylococcal pneumonia include:
   A. Age less than 2 years
   B. Underlying disease is uncommon
   C. Recent hospitalization or contact with a hospital is common
   D. Pulmonary findings are almost always apparent initially
   E. Disease is most common during the summer

2. The in vitro MIC data concerning his Staphylococcus aureus isolate indicated that it was:
   A. Sensitive to penicillin G, nafcillin, and gentamicin
   B. Sensitive to penicillin G and gentamicin but resistant to nafcillin
   C. Sensitive to penicillin G but resistant to nafcillin and gentamicin
   D. Resistant to penicillin G but sensitive to nafcillin and gentamicin

3. The evidence supplied by MIC and serum Schlicter determinations in this case indicate that the slow response which he exhibited for the first 10 days of hospitalization:
   A. Was probably a reflection of the slow response of most children with staphylococcal pneumonia, even when therapy is optimal
   B. May have been due to the use of nafcillin, to which his organism was resistant in vitro
   C. May have been due to inadequate doses of nafcillin, to which his organism was sensitive in vitro
   D. May have been due to difficulty in achieving adequate pleural drainage
   E. May have been due to the failure to use an aminoglycoside in the initial therapeutic regimen

4. Studies of the distribution of antimicrobial agents into bronchial secretions indicate that:
   A. There is often a direct correlation between concentrations of gentamicin in serum and bronchial secretions
   B. There is a general correlation between concentrations of penicillin in serum and in bronchial secretions, although the penicillin concentrations in bronchial secretions are usually lower than in serum
   C. Concentrations of ampicillin and cephalosporins in bronchial secretions are usually very much lower than in serum and are also highly variable

5. The child's serum sodium was 127 meq/L at the time of transfer
    to the medical center. Likely interpretations of this finding
    include:
    A. Excessive free water had been infused during the initial
        hospitalization
    B. This reflected the syndrome of inappropriate antidiuretic
        hormone secretion
    C. The child probably had Rocky Mountain spotted fever
    D. May be associated with the cerebral dysfunction which this
        child manifested

ANSWERS:

1. (A, B, C)

Children with staphylococcal pneumonia are, in most series, primarily infants or in early childhood. In Rebhan's experience, for
example, 68% of cases were less than 1 year of age. In addition,
the majority of the fatal cases occur in the youngest children, and
there is a predominance of males over females.

Although staphylococcal pneumonia may occur with any debilitating
illness, such as measles, influenza and prematurity, the majority
of children do not have known predisposing factors. Exceptions include skin pustules which precede disease in approximately 15% of
cases, as in this child, and recent hospitalization in approximately
35% of cases, both of which presumably represent a source of infection rather than an underlying disease state.

This child presented with fever and confusion as major signs of
disease and initial considerations included encephalitis. It is not
uncommon for manifestations of the pulmonary focus to be delayed.
Fever, convulsions, acidosis, bacteremia, neutropenia, and nausea
or vomiting may precede overt pulmonary findings by hours or days.
In Hendren's experience in 1958, 11% of children with staphylococcal
pneumonia had no pulmonary findings when they were first seen. As
in other cases, this child also presented without leukocytosis and
also had a slightly depressed serum sodium.

Staphylococcal pneumonia has usually occurred in the fall and winter
months. This child was an exception and presented in the spring.

2. (D)

The determination of sensitivity or resistance of Staphylococcus
aureus isolates to penicillin G was a subject of some confusion in
the 1960's when the organism was first being studied. Although
serum concentrations greatly exceeding 0. 31 ugm/ml (the MIC of
this isolate) can be achieved, clinical and animal studies have indicated that response of such an isolate to penicillin G is frequently
poor. In 1961, Finland's laboratory demonstrated that pencillinase

producing S. aureus strains had a range of MIC to penicillins of
0. 4 to greater than 100 ugm/ml. In contrast, the ranges of MIC's
of non-penicillinase producing S. aureus to a variety of β-lactamase
susceptible penicillins was between 0. 005-0. 04 ugm/ml. Therefore,
it is usually accepted that the MIC of a strain of S. aureus should be
0.1 ugm/ml or less to be considered sensitive to β-lactamase
susceptible penicillins. Organisms with higher MIC's should be assumed to be penicillinase producers and therefore potentially resistant to these antimicrobial agents.

3. (C, D, E)

The response of children with staphylococcal pneumonia is indeed
often alarmingly slow, and frequent evaluation of the patient may
fail to reveal a cause for continued fever and toxicity other than the
basic disease. In this case, however, the child failed to receive
adequate evaluation of his antimicrobial regimen until the 10th day
of hospitalization. At that time his organism, which had an in vitro
MIC to nafcillin 1. 25 ugm/ml (sensitive) was neither inhibited nor
killed by his pretherapy serum and only inhibited at a 1:2 dilution
of his post-therapy serum. Although he was receiving the standard
recommended dose (200 mg/kg/day), he was therefore not achieving
a satisfactory therapeutic serum concentration of drug. This information could and should have been obtained at a much earlier time
in the course of this critically ill child.

Adding to the difficulties in the treatment of this child was the problem of achieving adequate pleural drainage. His care required frequent evaluation and manipulation by skilled thoracic surgeons.

Recent evidence, based on in vitro data and on experimental animal
models, indicates that an aminoglycoside with a β-lactamase resistant penicillin is more rapidly effective in arresting the growth
and viability of penicillinase producing S. aureus. See, for example,
studies by Watanakunakorn and Steigbigel. Such a combination may
be desirable in the management of critically ill children or in children with inadequate host defenses. In this instance, the dose of
nafcillin was increased concomitantly with the addition of gentamicin. The result of the combined alterations in therapy was that serum
Schlicter determinations then were both bactericidal and bacteriostatic at 1:128 dilutions. This improvement in apparent efficacy was
accompanied by a clinical response which cannot be attributed to
either change alone.

4.   (A, B, C)

The concentration of gentamicin in bronchial secretions appears to
be parallel to that of serum in the majority of studied patients (see,
for example, Wong et al.). This may also partially account for the
efficacy of the gentamicin which was added to the regimen of this
child on the 10th day of hospitalization.

In contrast, the concentration of penicillin is considerably lower in bronchial secretions than in blood, and that of both ampicillin and cephalosporins may be undetectable when serum concentrations are otherwise adequate. These studies have been performed on adult patients and similar data on children with pulmonary disease are very sparse, as are data concerning the pulmonary distribution of β-lactamase resistant penicillins.

5. (A, B, D)

Children as well as adults frequently manifest acute hyponatremia during infectious diseases. The finding appears to be most common during infections in which a vasculitis is a prominent finding, such as Rocky Mountain spotted fever, but also occurs in numerous other conditions including severe pneumonia. Inappropriate secretion of antidiuretic hormone has been noted in some instances and is characterized by an inappropriate excretion of sodium in the urine during hyponatremia. This was not determined in this child, and so this etiology could not be confirmed or denied. It is also common to over-hydrate children during initial fluid therapy, and it is equally possible that this would explain the finding. In this instance, the rapid recovery of normal cerebral function was associated with correction of the hyponatremia, which can be expected to have played a major role in his confusion and obtundation.

ADDENDUM: In Fig. 45.1 is shown the roentgenogram of the chest on the 10th hospital day, demonstrating widespread areas of abscess formation with pleural exudate.

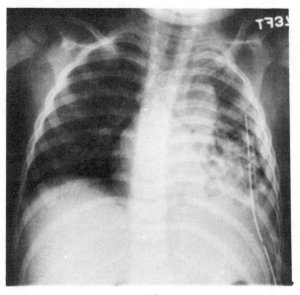

FIG. 45. 1

REFERENCES

1. Finberg, L. , Gonzales, C. : Experimental studies on the hypo-natremia of acute infections. Metabolism 14:693-8, 1965.

2. Hafez, F. F. , et al. : Penicillin levels in sputum. Thorax 21: 219-225, 1965.

3. McCarthy, C. G. , et al. : In vitro activity of various penicillins. Am. J. Med. Sci. 241:143-159, 1961.

4. Rebhan, A. W. , Edwards, H. E. : Staphylococcal pneumonia: A review of 329 cases. Canad. Med. Assn. J. 82:513-517, 1960.

5. Sabiston, D. C. , et al. : Surgical management of complications of staphylococcal pneumonia in infancy and childhood. J. Thoracic Cardiovas. Surg. 38:421-34, 1959.

6. Steigbigel, R. T. , et al. : Antibiotic combinations in the treatment of experimental Staphylococcus aureus J. Infect. Dis. 131:245-251, 1975.

7. Watanakunakorn, C. , Glotzbecker, C. : Enhancement of the ef-fects of antistaphylococcal antibiotics by aminoglycosides. Antimic. Agts. & Chemother. 6:802-806, 1974.

8. Wong, G. A. , et al. : Penetration of antimicrobial agents into bronchial secretions. Am. J. Med. 59:219-223, 1975.

::

CASE 46: POSTOPERATIVE INFECTION

HISTORY: This 20-month-old white male was admitted for repair of secundum atrial septal defect and valvular pulmonic stenosis. The child had had normal growth and development. At the age of 6 months he had begun to experience frequent URI's and middle ear infections. His cardiac disease was otherwise asymptomatic.

Pertinent physical findings at admission were restricted to the chest. There was a palpable thrill over the base with a grade IV/VI systolic ejection murmur which radiated from the precordium to the back and left sternal border. No diastolic murmurs were heard. He was acy-anotic, not in failure, and in excellent general health. His level of activity was comparable to that of his peers.

His hemoglobin was 12. 8 grams%, WBC count was 11,200 with 24% neutrophils, 53% lymphocytes, 6% monocytes, 16% eosinophils, and 1% basophils.

On the 2nd hospital day he underwent cardiac surgery. Cephaloridine was administered just prior to surgery and for the subsequent 6 days. The operative site was prepared with tincture of Zephirin. He was on cardiac pump for 50 minutes and was in pulmonary edema when removed from the pump. In the recovery room the patient's vital signs were stable but frothy blood-tinged material was obtained from the endotracheal tube.

His first postoperative day was complicated by continued tracheal seepage of blood which subsequently subsided. The next day he developed oral thrush and received oral mycostatin. His temperature rose to 39. 0 C. , and he developed right middle and lower lobe pneumonia and oliguria. Foreign bodies in place at that time included a Foley catheter, endotracheal tube, internal jugular line to monitor central venous pressure, arterial line in the left radial artery, a venous line in the left arm, and two chest tubes for drainage. By the 8th hospital day his serum creatinine was 2. 6%, oliguria was continuing and potassium was within normal limits. He was unable to maintain a satisfactory PO_2, repeat cardiac catheterization demonstrated recurrence of an atrial septal defect with 63% right-to-left shunt, and the patient returned to surgery. A small residual ASD was found and repaired, and postoperatively he sustained a PO_2 of approximately 40 mm Hg. with 45% inspired oxygen.

On the 12th day after reoperation he was noted to be febrile and draining purulent material through his chest tube. Serratia marcescens was recovered which had a MIC to gentamicin of 1. 25 ugm/ml. His serum creatinine was 1. 8 mg%, his weight 12 kg, and he was given 16 mg. of gentamicin at 16 hour intervals. Serum gentamicin concentrations 30 minutes after an infusion was 7. 5 ugm/ml and just before the next dose was 5 ugm/ml. The response to therapy included decrease in fever, decrease in thoracotomy drainage, and increased responsiveness. Renal function improved temporarily and the Foley was removed, to be reinserted on the 24th reoperative day because of transient hyperkalemia. Clindamycin was added to his regimen.

On the 26th reoperative day, while the patient was continuing to receive gentamicin and clindamycin, his temperature rose to 39.5°C. His affect became irritable and inappropriate and drainage from the thoracotomy site increased significantly. He complained of blurred vision. He was also found to have 50-100 wbc/hpf in the urine and profuse Gram (-) rods on an unstained sample. Cultures from both sites yielded Serratia marcescens, with an MIC to gentamicin of 5. 0 ugm/ml. The patient developed shock and died the following day.

Autopsy findings included positive cultures for Serratia sp. from blood, lungs, spleen and urine, and positive cultures for Candida sp. from the lungs and kidneys. There was severe acute left ureteritis with ureteral obstruction, and acute hydronephrosis with pyelonephritis of the left kidney.

There was extensive destruction of lung parenchyma with acute and chronic pneumonitis, thickened alveolar septi, and purulent pleural fluid. Focal cerebral microabscesses which revealed candida fungal spores were found.

QUESTIONS:

1. Zephiran is a compound of the following class:
    A. Phenolic
    B. Quarternary ammonium
    C. Alcohol
    D. Biguanide
    E. Iodophor

2. Quarternary ammonium compounds have the following characteristics:
    A. May fail to inhibit or may support growth of Pseudomonas sp. at 1:1000 dilutions
    B. Non-irritating when used for dermal antisepsis
    C. Rapid inactivation by soap and anionics
    D. Greater effectiveness in general against gram-positive than against gram-negative bacteria
    E. Low penetrating power
    F. All of the above

3. Medical management which might have prevented the onset or decreased the severity of this child's urinary tract infection might have included:
    A. Decreased duration of catheterization
    B. Meticulous perineal care
    C. Prophylactic administration of parenteral sulfonamide
    D. Replacement of catheter alternate days or whenever a urine culture is taken
    E. Manipulation of catheter only by a "catheter team"

4. Characteristics of Serratia marcescens which are isolated from clinically significant infections include:
    A. Are usually pigmented
    B. Produce extracellular DNase
    C. Produce lipase
    D. Are most commonly acquired from the normal flora of the patient's gastrointestinal tract
    E. Development of antibiotic resistance is rare

5. Candida albicans:
   A. May be identified by growth on blood agar plates after 24
      hours incubation
   B. Causes septicemia which is frequently associated with ocular
      disease
   C. Is normal flora of the gastrointestinal tract of the majority
      of well persons
   D. Causes septicemia mainly in persons who have had prolonged
      antimicrobial therapy following surgical procedures especial-
      ly of the gastrointestinal tract

6. The original serum concentrations of gentamicin would indicate
   that his serratia infection:
   A. Would probably be erradicated if surgical drainage of the
      area was adequate
   B. Would have less than a 50% likelihood of being controlled
      even if surgical drainage was adequate

ANSWERS:

1. (B)

Zephiran is a trade name for a quarternary ammonium which has
been widely used for dermal disinfection.

2. (F)

Quarternary ammonium compounds are currently used at dilutions
of the approximately 1:750 in U. S. hospitals. At this concentration
they are probably adequate for dermal cleaning of a non-critical
nature, such as hand washing. They are most effective against gram-
positive organisms and have been shown to support growth of such
gram-negative bacteria as Serratia, Alkaligenes, Enterobacter and
Pseudomonas species. Their use for dermal antisepsis of operative
sites is therefore not desirable. Iodine or iodophors remain the
single most effective skin disinfectant for this purpose (see, for
example, Topley and Wilson, and Spaulding).

3. (A, B)

Meticulous aseptic insertion of the catheter, maintenance of a closed
system, and perineal care will greatly decrease the incidence of
early catheter-associated infections. Nevertheless, catheterization
for greater than 2 weeks is associated with significant number of
bacteriuria. Kunin and McCormack, for example, were able to maintain sterile urine in 50% of catheterized males for 13. 5 days using
excellent catheter care. Similarly, maintenance of excellent perineal care in bedridden catheterized patients decreases the incidence
of catheter-associated infections. Although prophylactic use of antimicrobial agents may decrease the incidence of urinary tract infection following certain postoperative situations, it has not been shown

to be efficacious during prolonged catheterization. Frequent recatheterization unless concretions occur is equally inefficacious.

Maintenance of catheters is a technical skill which may be taught to any member of the hospital personnel. Some hospitals have found it to be most convenient to have a "catheter team". Other hospitals rely on instruction of all nursing personnel. The most essential factor is that whoever cares for the catheterized patient be well motivated and instructed.

4. (B, C)

The majority of Serratia marcescens isolated from clinical specimens are non-pigmented. Outstanding biochemical characteristics of Serratia marcescens are production of lipase and of extracellular DNase. The only Enterobacteriaceae that produce detectable lipase are S. marcescens, E. liquefaciens, P. vulgaris and P. mirabilis, and the only ones that produce extracellular DNase are S. marcescens, E. liquefaciens, some Proteus sp., and Providencia.

Serratia sp. are seldom found in the gastrointestinal tract of persons unless they have been hospitalized and been receiving antimicrobial therapy. They are commonly acquired by transmission in hospital settings, and are prominent nosocomial infection of the urinary tract. In the study by Maki, et al., for example, the hands of hospital personnel harbored organisms during an outbreak. These organisms, like pseudomonads and other members of the Klebsiella - Enterobacter - Serratia group, are frequently multiply-resistant to antimicrobial agents. Development of resistance during therapy is not rare.

5. (A, B, C, D)

Candida sp. are rapidly-growing and are frequently identified by growth on bacteriological media such as blood agar. Candida sepsis may have many manifestations, but ocular disease is common and may often by recognized by careful direct physical examinations. Prominent ocular manifestations include white fluffy exudates, hemorrhagic exudates, hypopion with or without inflammation of the anterior chamber, iritis, and conjunctivitis. The patient frequently complains of pain in the eye and of decreased vision, as occurred for this patient.

Candida albicans is part of the normal human intestinal flora. Clinical infection usually occurs in patients who have had antimicrobial therapy, major surgical procedures, are debilitated, and/or have indwelling foreign bodies. This child satisfies all of the above situations. The death rate for candida sepsis, even when recognized, is approximately 50% of cases.

6. (B)

The MIC of the isolated Serratia marcescens was 1. 25 ugm/ml to gentamicin. His peak serum gentamicin concentration was 7. 5 ugm/ ml. Therefore, the ratio of his MIC to serum concentration was 1:5. Where this ratio is less than 1:8 in patients with parenchymal infections, current experience suggests that the likelihood of therapeutic success not optimal (see, for example, Klastersky et al.).

REFERENCES

1. Edwards, J. E. , et al. : Ocular manifestations of candida septicemia: Review of seventy-six cases of hematogenous candida end-ophthalmitis. Medicine 53:47-75, 1974.

2. Klastersky, J. , et al. : Antibacterial activity in serum and urine as a therapeutic guide in bacterial infections. J. Infect. Dis. 129:187-193, 1974.

3. Kunin, C. M. , McCormack, R. C. : Prevention of catheter-induced urinary tract infections by sterile closed drainage. NEJM 274:1155-1162, 1966.

4. Maki, D. G. , et al. : Nosocomial urinary tract infection with Serratia marcescens: An epidemiologic study. J. Infect. Dis. 128:579-587, 1973.

5. Spaulding, E. H. : Role of chemical disinfection in the prevention of nosocomial infections. P. 247 in: Proceedings of the International Conference on nosocomial infections. Center For Disease Control, August 3-6, 1970. Published by American Hospital Assn. , Chicago, 1971.

6. Stamm, E. W. : Guidelines for prevention of catheter-associated urinary tract infections. Ann. Int. Med. 82:386-390, 1975.

7. Wilson, G. S. and Miles, A. editors: Principles of Bacteriology, Virology, and Immunology. Williams and Wilkins Co. Publishers, Baltimore, Md. , pp. 144-186, 1975.

::

CASE 47: PNEUMONIA IN A CHILD WITH SICKLE CELL DISEASE

HISTORY: This was the 4th admission for a 6-year-old, black female child with known sickle cell disease. Previous admissions were at the time of a normal delivery, at the age of 13 months for sickle cell crisis and pneumonia, and at the age of 4 years for pneumonia. The child had been in her usual state of fair health until 3 days prior to admission when she developed rhinorrhea and a non-productive cough. She continued to eat well and to be active until the evening prior to admission when she developed a fever of 39 degrees C, chills, intense coughing spells with production of frothy sputum, and disoriented behavior.

PHYSICAL EXAMINATION: Physical examination revealed an acutely ill child. Temperature was 39 degrees C, Pulse 120, Respirations 25. Pertinent physical findings included moist rales at the right base of the lung and in the right axilla. Breath sounds were decreased on the right. The liver was palpable 2 cm. below the right costal margin and the spleen was not palpable. There were no rashes and no joint abnormalities.

The patient's 12-year-old brother had had a moderately severe cough with an initial slight fever for the preceding 7 weeks. The child had not seen a physician and aside from the cough was in good general health. Other members of the family had had no illness. There was no known tuberculosis within the household.

LABORATORY DATA: Admission hgb was 6. 5 grams, hct 20, WBC 27,500 with 64% segs, 9% bands, 18% lymphs, 7% monos, and 2% eosinophils, Retic. count was 40. 3% and platelets were adequate. Serum bilirubin was 1. 1 mg.%. Roentgenogram of the chest revealed a dense infiltrate of the right upper lobe. There was no demonstrable pleural fluid. Cultures of blood, tracheal aspirate and urine were taken, and the child was started on I. V. penicillin, 100,000 units per kilogram.

QUESTIONS:

1. Likely diagnoses(is) include(s):
   A. Pneumococcal pneumonia
   B. Mycoplasma pneumoniae pneumonia
   C. Pulmonary infarct
   D. Adenoviral pneumonia
   E. Hemophilus influenzae pneumonia

2. Appropriate diagnostic measures may include:
   A. A serum counter immunoelectrophoresis (CIE) for Hemophilus influenzae B antigen
   B. A serum counter immunoelectrophoresis for pneumococcal antigen
   C. A percutaneous aspiration of the lung
   D. Throat culture for Mycoplasma pneumoniae, and M. pneumoniae CF titer
   E. Direct examination of sputum for culture and Gram stain
   F. Blood culture
   G. Throat culture for pneumococci and staphylococci

The patient failed to respond to therapy and on the 3rd day was continuing to have daily fever to 39. 3 degrees C. Physical therapy was
instituted. Frothy and nonpurulent sputum production was moderate
and Gram stain revealed a predominance of polymorphonuclear leukocytes and occasional epithelial cells. Approximately one large
mononuclear cell per high power field were also seen with sparse
mixed organisms. The patient's WBC rose to 45,000. Initial cultures
of blood and sputum had not yielded growth of significant bacteria.
Sera for cold agglutinins and mycoplasma CF titer were lost on the
way to the laboratory. The serum counter-immunoelectrophoresis
for Hemophilus influenzae B and pneumococcal antigen were non-
reactive. Percutaneous aspiration of the lung on the 6th day yielded
0. 5 cc. of serous fluid with no bacterial growth and no organisms
seen on Gram's stain. There were three large mononuclear cells.

QUESTION:

3. Appropriate management may include:
    A. Continued current therapy without major alteration
    B. Review of the diagnostic results and repeated physical exami-
        nation
    C. Initiation of gentamicin therapy to prevent pneumonia due to
        gram-negative bacteria
    D. Change to erythromycin therapy because Mycoplasma pneu-
        moniae may be a pathogen

The patient continued to have daily fever to 40. 0 degrees C through
the 9th day of hospitalization, when she began to defervesce. The
roentgenograms of the chest remained unchanged through the hospitalization. The child was discharged in good condition on the 15th
day after admission. On that day a CF titer to M. pneumoniae was
reported to be 1:1024, and the cold agglutinin titer was 1:160.

QUESTIONS:

4. The physician may conclude that:
    A. These titers are not unusual in healthy persons and probably
        do not indicate a recent infection
    B. It is characteristic of many healthy children with sickle cell
        disease to have an antibody response to mycoplasmal anti-
        gens, and it is often similar in magnitude to the response
        found in this child
    C. This is a very unusually high CF titer and, although a single
        titer does not prove a diagnosis, it is presumptive evidence
        that the child had mycoplasma pneumonia. A repeated titer
        would be helpful if there were a decline in titer over the next
        few months

5. Cold hemagglutination of the patient's red blood cells by his serum:
   A. Is a specific test for Mycoplasma pneumoniae pneumonia if the titer is 1:40 or greater
   B. Most commonly is associated with Mycoplasma pneumoniae pneumonia but occasionally occurs in patients with other conditions
   C. Occasionally occurs in patients with cirrhosis of the liver, Hodgkin's disease, trypanosomiasis, and lymphosarcoma

6. Characteristics of infection with M. pneumoniae in children include:
   A. Disease in early childhood is usually asymptomatic
   B. After infection, complement fixing antibody persists for over 1 year in 75% of children who are 6 months to 3 years of age
   C. There is a strong seasonal occurrence of M. pneumoniae infections with a peak in the fall and early winter
   D. Peripheral lymphocyte culture response to M. pneumoniae antigen demonstrates that there is a greater proportion of significant stimulation in older children and adults than in younger children
   E. Repeated episodes of infection with M. pneumoniae in healthy children is probably very rare

ANSWERS:

1. (All of these)

This patient presented with the acute onset of pulmonary disease which is consistent with pneumococcal pneumonia. However, the differential diagnosis of pulmonary disease in children with sickle cell disease is very difficult and etiology often cannot be determined when the patient is first seen. Any of these diagnoses are likely. Because progression of pneumococcal bacteremia in children with sickle cell disease may be rapid or fulminant, it is appropriate to treat sickle cell patients who have pneumonia of uncertain etiology for pneumococcal disease. The low serum bilirubin concentration renders a pulmonary infarct unlikely.

2. (All of these except G)

Children with sickle cell disease may have severe infections with encapsulated bacteria other than pneumococci. H. influenzae type B also cause severe disease in these children, and evidence of such infection may be obtained from the presence of bacterial antigen. This method is technically excellent for H. influenzae type B antigen.

A percutaneous aspiration of pulmonary material for culture may yield valuable information concerning etiology. This procedure should be performed before therapy is begun for children with severe pneumonias, and may be expected to indicate if the patient is infected with

an organism for which the antimicrobial therapy is inadequate.
Other conservative methods of obtaining a diagnosis should be followed including continued search for evidence of M. pneumoniae
infection.

Blood culture yields growth of the infecting organisms in only approximately 7. 5% of children with pneumonia, but when positive gives
very reliable information on the etiology of the pneumonia and should
therefore be performed.

A throat culture seldom yields reliable information concerning the
etiology of pneumonias because the normal flora of the pharynx reflects the common causes of pneumonia.

3.   (A, B, D)

A decision to continue the present management is consistent with an
understanding of the natural history of pneumonia in children with
sickle cell disease. Resolution of fever and infiltrate is very delayed
in spite of appropriate therapy.

Review of the diagnostic findings should include a repeated effort to
obtain a CF titer to M. pneumoniae, which in this case had been initially
lost. Notice should also be taken of the persistent pulmonary disease in
the patient's older sibling. Prolonged but mild pulmonary disease
with spread to other family members is characteristic of M. pneumoniae. If there is confirmatory evidence for this infection in either
the patient or her brother, changing the antimicrobial therapy to
erythromycin would be appropriate.

This patient has no evidence of pneumonia due to gram-negative organisms and prophylactic therapy is not indicated.

4.   (C)

Although it has been reported that many children with sickle cell
disease have cold hemagglutinins, there is no evidence to suggest that
children with sickle cell disease have an increased incidence of CF
antibody to mycoplasma antigens unless they are infected with mycoplasma. This titer of 1:1024 is unusually high and may, therefore,
represent a peak titer during an acute illness. A repeat in several
months would support the diagnosis if the titer were falling, since
CF antibody to mycoplasma antigens declines rapidly following infection.

5.   (B, C)

Determination of the presence of cold hemagglutination is not technically difficult. This finding is present in the majority of patients with
mycoplasma pneumonia but is not specific for this disease.

6. (A, C, D)

In recent studies of children in a day-care center, only 7 of 24 instances in which M. pneumoniae was isolated from the respiratory tract were associated with symptoms of respiratory tract disease. From this and other experience, it appears that younger children may acquire M. pneumoniae but seldom manifest clinically apparent disease. In addition, the serologic response of young children to M. pneumoniae infection wanes rapidly following infection, and numerous children have been shown to have recurrent M. pneumoniae infections separated by intervals of a year or more. Lymphocyte culture response to M. pneumoniae antigen in persons who are not known to be infected is significantly more active in older children and adults than in younger children (see, for example, Fernald, et al.).

ADDENDUM: A repeated mycoplasma CF titer three months later was 1:32, completing the serological evidence that she had an acute infection with that organism during her illness.

REFERENCES

1. Barrett-Connor, E.: Bacterial infection and sickle cell anemia. Medicine 50:97-112, 1971.

2. Collier, A. M., Clyde, W. A.: Appearance of Mycoplasma pneumoniae in lungs of experimentally infected hamsters and sputum from patients with natural disease. Am. Rev. Resp. Dis. 110: 765-773, 1974.

3. Denny, F. W., et al.: Mycoplasma pneumoniae disease: Clinical spectrum, pathophysiology, epidemiology, and control. J. Infect. Dis. 123:74-92, 1971.

4. Ferrald, G. W., et al.: Respiratory infections due to Mycoplasma pneumoniae in infants and children. Pediatrics 55:327-335, 1975.

5. Kabins, S. A., Lerner, C.: Fulminant pneumococcemia in sickle cell anemia. JAMA 211:467-471, 1970.

6. Petch, M. C., Sergeant, G. R.: Clinical features of pulmonary lesions in sickle cell anaemia. Brit. Med. J. 3:31, 1970.

7. Shulman, S. T., et al.: The unusual severity of mycoplasma pneumonia in children with sickle cell disease. NEJM 287:164-167, 1972.

CASE 48: DOG BITE WITH SECONDARY INFECTION

HISTORY: The patient was a healthy 11-year-old girl who was at-
tacked by the neighbor's German shepherd when she entered her
neighbor's back yard to return a bottle of milk. The two families
had lived next to each other for one year, and the dog was kept in
a small pen when the family was not at home. At the time of the
attack the family was away, and the dog was able to knock a board
loose from the cage. The dog inflicted three lacerations on the
girl's cheek and one of her arms with his teeth, and seven deep
scratches on her abdomen and chest with his claws before her
screams brought a neighboring boy to her rescue. The child was
taken to the local emergency room where the wounds were cleaned
with a quarternary ammonium solution and washed vigorously. It
was not known whether the dog had received rabies vaccination, and
he was confined for observation.

QUESTIONS:

1. The major considerations which will determine whether or not a
    child who has suffered an animal bite should receive human ra-
    bies immune globulin (HRIG) are:
    A. Was the biting animal a dog or cat, wild carnivore, bat,
        rodent, or opossum?
    B. If the animal was a dog, was that bite provoked?
    C. Has the animal, if dog or cat, been vaccinated against rabies?
    D. Is rabies endemic in the area?
    E. If the biting animal is a wild carnivore, and the animal has
        been captured, are there signs of disease within 10 days?

2. Appropriate prevention of tetanus for this child would include:
    A. Tetanus toxoid and tetanus human immune globulin should be
        administered
    B. If she had her primary series of immunizations, and has
        received a tetanus booster within 2 years, no specific tetanus
        therapy is required
    C. If she had her primary series of immunizations, and has re-
        ceived a tetanus booster within 5 years, no specific antiteta-
        nus therapy is required

3. Other appropriate therapy for this child would include:
    A. Human rabies immune globulin (IG) injected into the sites of
        the wounds
    B. A discussion of her case with the State Rabies Control Officer
    C. Suture the facial laceration to decrease the possible disfig-
        urement
    D. Institute penicillin therapy
    E. Flush profusely with water and clean with quarternary ammo-
        nium compound

Sixteen hours later the child developed swelling, bluish discoloration, pain, and a blood tinged serous discharge from one of the facial lesions, two of the abdominal, and one of the arm lesions. She was afebrile but moderately uncomfortable. Her heart rate was 100, respirations 24, blood pressure 100/60. Her WBC was 11,200 with 64% polys, 12% stabs, and 24% lymphocytes. Gram stain of the discharge showed few WBC's, moderate numbers of small and regular gram (-) rods and coccobacilli, moderate numbers of RBC's, and cellular debris.

QUESTIONS:

4. This infection is most likely due to the following organism(s):
   A. Clostridium welchii
   B. Pasteurella multocida
   C. Escherichia coli
   D. Bacteroides melaninogenicus
   E. Pseudomonas pseudomallei

5. Appropriate therapy would consist of:
   A. Penicillin, 1.2 million units I. M. plus gentamicin, 5 mg/kg/day I. M.
   B. Tetracycline, 1 gram q. i. d. p. o.
   C. Cephalexin, 50 mg/kg/day p. o.
   D. Penicillin G, 250 mg q. i. d. p. o.
   E. Clindamycin, 15 mg/kg/day p. o.

6. Characteristics of P. multocida and the infections caused by this organism include:
   A. Fails to grow on media containing bile salts, usually is oxidase positive, produces indole, and reduces nitrates
   B. Inhabits an ecologic niche in the nasopharynx of dogs similar to that of Streptococcus viridans in man
   C. Grows on MacConkey's media
   D. Is a prominent cause of veterinary diseases, including cholera of wild fowl and hemorrhagic septicemia of cattle
   E. Most strains causing dog or cat bite infections in human are type B

Pasteurella multocida was recovered as expected from cultures of the wound and her lesions responded within 12 hours to penicillin therapy. She recovered without further incident.

ANSWERS:

1. (A, B, C, D)

The epidemiology of rabies in each of the groups of animals listed in A is unique, and hence, the type of biting animal is very important in determining the risk of acquiring rabies following a bite. A dog or

cat may excrete rabies in the saliva for no more than five days
prior to onset of signs of disease, and hence observation of a cap-
tured animal for 10 days allows assurance that the animal was not
rabid at the time of the bite. In the U. S. at the present time, rabies
in dogs is a very unusual problem. Other areas of the wound continue
to harbor rabies in dogs, however. On the contrary, wild carnivores
(foxes, skunks, raccoons) excrete virus in the saliva for a highly
variable and often unknown period of time before onset of signs of
disease. Therefore, these animals should be caught and sacrificed
following a bite. If they escape, serious consideration should be
given to vaccination plus serum administration. Bats have become
a source of human rabies and if the bats in a community are known
to be rabid, a bite from one should be vigorously treated. Signs of
rabies in bats are variable and many rabid bats are asymptomatic.

Rodents and opossums rarely transmit rabies to humans, and rodent
bites seldom if ever require specific anti-rabic treatment.

In this instance, the bite should be considered to be provoked, since
the child entered the yard which he was protecting. This is an important question when deciding whether or not to confine the animal
for observation. If the dog or cat has been vaccinated, the chance of
transmitting rabies is vanishingly small. In this instance, the dog
had not been vaccinated. Nevertheless, in this area there was virtually no canine rabies and it had not occurred for 25 years. The dog
was urban and confined, so chances of acquiring disease from a
rabid carnivore were also minimal.

2. (C)

The child has had a traumatic injury with soil contamination of the
wounds. A careful history should be taken to insure that her primary
vaccination series were completed. If that has been ascertained, she
need not receive a tetanus toxoid booster more frequently than every 10
years if the wound is clean, and every 5 years if the wound is contaminated
according to the current recommendations of the American Academy of
Pediatrics.

3. (B, E)

Cleansing a wound with quarternary ammonium compound is especially
effective in preventing rabies following a bite of a rabid animal. Although the animal that bit this child is almost surely not rabid, it is
still a good policy to apply appropriate local preventive therapy (see,
for example, Kaplan). If the physician is not up-to-date with the
rabies epidemiology of his area, the State Rabies Control Officer
will assist in the evaluation of the patient's exposure. In this instance,
HRIG was not indicated. The incidence of serious infectious disease
following an animal bite increases if the lesion is sutured. For these
reasons no animal bite should be sutured if it can be avoided.

The prophylactic use of penicillin following an animal bite is con-
troversial, but should not be routinely administered. See further
discussion below.

4. (B)

The evidence of Gram stain is that a gram-negative coccobacillus
will be present in pure growth and that the cellular inflammatory
response has been minimal. Clostridia sp. are gram-positive rods.
Pseudomonas pseudomallei is the etiologic agent of meliodosis, a
very rare disease in the U. S. which is primarily pulmonary and one
which is unlikely to present in this fashion. Neither Bacteroides sp.
nor E. coli are likely to cause an infection of the skin which leads
to this acute invasive edematous response.

Pasteurella multocida is the classical and still most common agent
to infect dog or cat bites. In a report by Lee and Buhr, 29% of dog
bites become infected and P. multocida was the causative agent in
half of these cases. This is the basis for the occasional use of penicillin in the initial care of a dog bite. It was noted here, as elsewhere, that wounds which are sutured are more likely to become infected than are wounds not sutured. These infections may be local
as in this instance, and confined to the area of the injury, but it is
not unusual for the infection to extend to subjacent bone or joints,
or disseminate hematogenously.

5. (D)

This organism has almost always been found to be sensitive to penicillin and patients have responded well to this form of therapy if the
infection has not disseminated. Follow-up examination should ensure
that underlying bony structures have not been involved.

6. (A, B, D)

The organism is not a member of the family Enterobacteriaceae. The
eighth edition of "Bergey's Manual of Determinative Bacteriology"
identifies it as a genus of uncertain affiliation. Most members of the
Enterobacteriaceae may grow on media containing bile salts, such as
MacConkey's agar, but Pasteurella sp. will not.

These organisms represent the majority of the normal flora of the
nasopharynx of dogs and cats. In addition, cats are more likely to
harbor these organisms in their claws than are dogs.

The P. multocida is a relatively minor cause of human disease but
has a major role in veterinary medicine. Most strains causing human
disease are not typeable, whereas most causing animal disease may
be typed by their capsular material as types A, B, C, or D.

REFERENCES

1. Corey, L. , Hattwick, M. A. W. : Treatment of persons exposed to rabies. JAMA 232:272-276, 1975.

2. Plotkin, S. A. , Clark, H. F. : Prevention of rabies in man. J. Infect. Dis. 123:227-240, 1971.

3. Kaplan, M. M. , et al. : Studies on the local treatment of wounds for the prevention of rabies. Bull. W. H. O. 26:767-775, 1962.

4. Steele, J. H. : The epidemiology and control of rabies. Scand. J. Infect. Dis. 5:299-312, 1973.

5. Hubbert, W. T. , Rosen, M. N. : Pasteurella multocida infection due to animal bite. Am. J. Pub. Health 60:1103-1108, 1970.

6. Heddleston, K. L. , Wessman, G. : Characteristics of Pasteurella multocida of human origin. J. Clin. Micro. 1:377-83, 1975.

7. Tindall, J. P. , Harrison, C. M. : Pasteurella multocida infections following animal injuries, especially cat bites. Arch. Derm. 105:412-416, 1972.

::

CASE 49: CERVICAL ADENITIS IN A PREVIOUSLY WELL CHILD

HISTORY: The patient was a 22-month-old, white female from the southeastern U. S. who presented with the complaint of a "swelling in the jaw". She had been well until $2\frac{1}{2}$ months prior to her visit when one evening her parents thought she felt warm. The following morning they first noted a swelling in the superior cervical submandibular area which was approximately 4 x 2 cm. , non-tender, and without warmth or erythema. Her fever subsided spontaneously and did not recur. She had no other systemic signs of disease, including no loss of weight. She had had no trauma to the area, and had not had dental disease. The swelling persisted, and one month prior to visit she received a three day course of daily penicillin injections from her physician. The condition did not improve, and she was referred to a medical center for further evaluation.

PHYSICAL EXAMINATION: Examination at that time revealed a well-nourished, cheerful child in no distress. She was afebrile. Physical examination was unremarkable with the exception of a 5 x 3 cm. firm, non-tender, non-movable mass in the area of the left mandibular angle. The overlying skin was not adherent. There were several adjacent smaller nodes in both the left and the right submandibular areas.

Other physical findings were noncontributory. A Tine test produced 2 x 2 mm. areas of induration at each prong. The roentgenogram of the chest, AP and lateral revealed neither hilar nor parenchymal infiltrates or masses. The hemoglobin was 10. 8 grams. WBC 10,900 with 67% segs, 4% bands, 27% lymphs and 2% monos. Total protein was 7. 4 gm%. Albumin was 4. 7 gm%. ASO titer 66 Todd units and culture of the throat did not reveal group A beta hemolytic streptococci.

QUESTION:

1. Appropriate diagnostic steps might include the following:
   A. A careful family history for Tbc
   B. Intradermal PPD
   C. Intradermal PPD-S, PPD-B, PPD-G, and PPD-Y
   D. A trial of dicloxacillin therapy
   E. A 3-month course of isoniazid
   F. A family history for contact with kittens

The intradermal PPD-S, intermediate strength, provoked an area of induration of 5 x 5 mm at 48 hours. The family history revealed no evidence of recent active disease, and their county health department reported that there had been no recent active disease in her community. The family owned one cat who was 4 years old.

The child then received intradermal tests with PPD-Y, PPD-G, and PPD-B which produced the following zones of induration at 48 hours.

    PPD-Y: 10 x 6 mm
    PPD-G: 10 x 8 mm
    PPD-B: 10 x 12 mm

QUESTIONS:

2. The most likely diagnosis, based on the results of all skin tests and clinical findings is:
   A. Infection with Runyon Group III mycobacteria, represented by PPD-B
   B. Infection with any of the organisms from Runyon Groups I, II, or III, since the size of the reaction does not accurately indicate the etiology
   C. Asymptomatic tuberculosis, since the Tine test was reactive
   D. Staphylococcal lymphadenitis

3. If the patient continued to have a very large, hard mass which was not decreasing in size, appropriate therapeutic measures might include:
   A. Treatment with INH
   B. Treatment with INH plus rifampin
   C. Incision and drainage of the mass
   D. Excision of the node
   E. Continue expectant observation

ANSWERS:

1. (A, B)

Although cervical tuberculosis (scrofula) was common when bovine
tuberculosis was transmitted by infected milk, it is now a rare
presentation of disease. Nevertheless, Tbc continues to be an important disease in children and the reactive Tine test result should
stimulate a careful history for Tbc in the family, which is the most
likely source of disease for a young child.

The Tine test is not specific for M. tuberculosis since there is cross
reactivity with other Mycobacteriaceae. The Tine test also fails to
provide a quantative evaluation of reactivity for tuberculoprotein.
Therefore, when a patient is being evaluated for possible tuberculous
disease, a PPD-S, 5TU, should always be applied.

The evidence in favor of a diagnosis of tuberculosis at this point does
not support a decision to begin INH therapy.

Common causes of cervical adenitis in children include infection
with atypical mycobacteria, cat scratch disease, streptococci and
staphylococci. A history of contact with a kitten is not very helpful
since the majority of all children handle these animals. A trial of
dicloxicillin is expensive, but is used by some physicians under
these conditions. Intradermal application of PPD-Y, -B, and -G
is not indicated until PPD-S has been evaluated.

2. (A)

The size of the PPD-S reaction may not be a definitive indication of
the presence or absence of tuberculous infection; for example, there
is a substantial degree of cross reactivity between the reaction stimulated by M. tuberculosis and the other atypical mycobacteria.
Therefore, a borderline reaction to PPD-S may represent tuberculous infection or may represent infection with atypical mycobacteria
of the Runyon groups. In this instance the 5 x 5 mm reaction to the
PPD-S indicated that tuberculous disease was unlikely.

While the area of induration with the atypical mycobacterial antigens
does not necessarily indicate which one represents the infecting organism, there is a general correlation between causitive agent and
antigen causing largest area of induration. In addition, cervical adenitis in children from the southeastern U.S. due to atypical mycobacteria are most likely to be Runyon Group III strains.

The terminology of the atypical mycobacteria of the Runyon groups
is shown in Table 49.1.

TABLE 49. 1		
RUNYON GROUP	CHARACTERISTICS	ANTIGEN
I	Photochromogenic	PPD-Y (Yellow)
II	Scotochromogenic	PPD-G (Gause strain)
III	Nonchromogenic	PPD-B (Battey strain)
IV	Rapid Growers	PPD-F (Fortuitum strain)

3. (D)

Antimicrobial therapy for cervical adenitis due to atypical mycobacteria has not been successful. These organisms are only moderately sensitive to most forms of drug therapy, and the response is usually poor.

Incision has frequently resulted in chronically draining sinuses. Continued expectant observation may be appropriate if the node is small and unlikely to drain spontaneously. However, in this child there is a risk that she will develop a disfiguring area of drainage if the node is allowed to continue to enlarge. Total excision of the localized infection of a single node is the therapy of choice.

ADDENDUM: The node was excised. Areas of granulomas with central necrosis were widespread within the node. Auramine-rhodamine fluorescent stains revealed acid-fast organisms. Culture for acid-fast organisms yielded growth of atypical mycobacteria of Runyon Group III, the Avian-Battey strains. The patient had an uneventful postoperative course, received no antimicrobial therapy, and has remained well for 2 years of follow-up. Histopathology of the excised node revealed noncaseating granulomata, which are shown in Fig. 49.1.

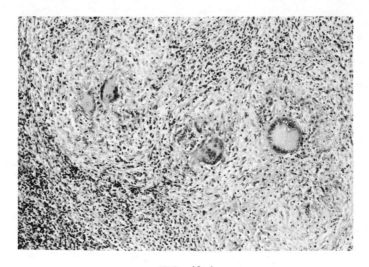

FIG. 49. 1

REFERENCES

1. Arnold, J. H. , et al. : Specificity of PPD skin tests in childhood tuberculin converters, Compairson with mycobacterial species from tissue and secretions. J. Pediat. 76:512-522, 1970.

2. Fogan, L.: Atypical mycobacteria. Medicine 49:243-255, 1940.

3. Manorstein, B. L. , et al. : The role of nontuberculous mycobacterial skin test antigens in the diagnosis of mycobacterial infection. Chest 67:320-324, 1975.

4. Margileth, A. M. : Cat scratch disease: Nonbacterial regional lymphadenitis. Pediatrics 42:803-818, 1968.

5. Salyer, K. E. , et al. : Surgical management of cervical adenitis due to atypical mycobacteria in children. JAMA 204:103, 1968.

6. Smith, D. T.: Diagnostic and prognostic significance of the quantitative tuberculin tests. The influence of subclinical infection with atypical mycobacteria. Ann. Int. Med. 67:919-946, 1967.

:::

CASE 50: WEIGHT LOSS WITH PERSISTENT PULMONARY CONSOLIDATION

HISTORY: This 6-year, 10-month-old, black female was in her usual state of health until 2 weeks prior to admission when she developed chest pain, a cough, and nasal congestion without fever. She was given symptomatic treatment, but she developed fever of 38°C. two or three days later. She was taken to her local doctor who gave her an antibiotic and iron which was without effect on the fever, although the cough improved during the first part of the antibiotic therapy. When she did not improve, she returned to her private doctor who changed her antibiotic. Her symptoms persisted, she was admitted to her local hospital, and was given inhalation therapy. Chest roentgenograms showed pneumonitis in the right lung, and she had iron deficiency anemia. A Tine test was non-reactive. Throat and nose culture were without significant pathogens. Her cough had been productive but without hemoptysis and the sputum was clear, white and thick. There was no history of aspiration. She was referred to a medical center for further evaluation including bronchoscopy.

The mother stated that the child had lost 15 pounds during the month prior to admission. Other family members were in good health. There were no pets in the household. The family home was in eastern North Carolina, and they had not traveled out of that area. The family was not known to be tuberculous and had had good medical care.

PHYSICAL EXAMINATION: She was a well-developed, well-nourished, black female in no acute distress. T=38. 4, P=100, R=28, B. P. 100/70. HEENT - The eyes were normal. Fundi - clear. TM's normal. Nose - clear. The tonsils were 2+ enlarged bilaterally and otherwise normal. The lungs were clear to auscultation. There was a questionable change in the percussion note with the right greater than the left. Heart sounds were normal without murmurs. Abdomen was unremarkable. Extremities were normal. Neurological examination was normal. Skin showed some areas of depigmentation which were reported to represent healing insect bites.

LABORATORY DATA: White blood cell count was 27,400 with 85% segs, 11% lymphs, 2% monos, 1% eosinophils and 1% basophils. Morphology was normal. Hemoglobin was 8. 2 gm. % and hematocrit was 26. 5%. Serum chemistries were within normal limits as was urinalysis.

Cold agglutinins were non-reactive, blood and stool cultures were unremarkable. Bacterial cultures of the sputum revealed Streptococcus viridans. Westergren sedimentation rate was 113 mm/hr.

Serum immunoglobulins were:

     IgG 3880 mg% (nl = 597-1517)
     IgA 470 mg% (nl = 52- 329)
     Igm 124 mg% (nl = 28- 114)
     IgE 6200 mg% (nl =   5- 621)

Roentgenograms of the chest revealed consolidation of all lobes of the right lung and especially advanced involvement of the right middle lobe.

HOSPITAL COURSE: The child underwent bronchoscopy on the 3rd hospital day. The orifice of the right middle lobe was clear and without secretions. Material was washed from the bronchus for fungal, viral, bacterial cultures and for cytology. The following day she underwent percutaneous lung aspiration with retrieval of a small amount of clear fluid. Four days later these cultures remained non-contributory, as did direct examinations of the material. Blastomyces yeast phase complement fixation test was reported to be 1:160 on the 8th day while serologic tests to histoplasmin and coccidioidin were negative. Skin tests to PPD-S, histoplasmin and blastomycin were non-reactive at 48 hours, but to candida 1:100, 5 mm. of induration was produced.

On the 13th hospital day the patient was about to receive general anesthesia in order to undergo an open biopsy of the lung when the previously obtained bronchial washings yielded growth of Blastomyces dermatitidis. She was begun on amphotericin B and 1 week of therapy was receiving 1 mg/kg/day for two of every three days. The therapy was tolerated very well, and she received a total of 1,000 mg.

The roentgenographic findings subsided and at the time of discharge, after 66 days of hospitalization, there were only minimal residual infiltrates. She remained well with complete pulmonary resolution through 6 months of follow-up. Pulmonary function studies 2 months after discharge revealed mild obstructive and restrictive disease which improved during the following 2 months. Serum IgE concentration had declined to 2340 u/ml by 2 months after discharge.

QUESTIONS:

1. Characteristics of systemic human disease due to Blastomyces dermatitidis include:
   A. Broad and septate hyphae are commonly found in tissue
   B. Budding yeast forms with a broad base are visualized in tissue
   C. Blastomycosis is an indication of a serious defect in host cellular immunity
   D. The disease is most common in the central and southeastern United States

2. Characteristics of patients with primary pulmonary blastomycosis include:
   A. The blastomycin skin test is usually reactive
   B. Onset is often accompanied by chest pain
   C. The patients commonly have cross reacting precipitating antibody with Histoplasma capsulatum
   D. The treatment of choice for cavitary pulmonary blastomycosis is 2-hydroxystilbamidine

3. Aspects of the epidemiology of North American blastomycosis include:
   A. Soil surrounding the home of infected persons often yield the organism on culture
   B. The organism is probably disseminated by bird droppings, especially pigeons
   C. Several small epidemics have been reported
   D. The infection attacks children commonly, and the disease tends to be especially severe in younger patients

ANSWERS:

1. (B, D)

In tissue samples, hyphae are almost never visualized, although it is a prominent feature of in vitro growth. The yeast phase is characteristic in tissue where the organisms are seen to bud. Usually a mature cell yields one daughter; and the base between the mother and daughter cells is broad in contrast to Candida sp., in which the base is very narrow. The cell walls of B. dermatitidis are very thick.

Most patients with North American blastomycosis have a primary
infection and were previously in good health. The organism is probably acquired by inhalation and infection is not usually considered
to be an opportunistic infection (see, for example, Witorsch and
Utz).

Although the disease occurs throughout the U. S. , the vast majority
of cases occur in the central and southeastern states of the U. S. ,
and this child came from an endemic area.

2. (B, C)

As in this patient, the blastomycin skin test is very frequently non-
reactive, even in patients with active disease. The test is reactive
in persons who are apparently well, and there is very commonly a
cross-reactivity with histoplasmin (see Furcolow et al.). In addition, the blastomycin skin test is non-reactive in the majority of
proven cases of both acute and chronic blastomycosis.

Not only is there a cross reactivity of intradermal histoplasmin
with blastomycin in many patients with blastomycosis, but the
serological evidence of blastomycosis may be confused by cross
reacting humoral antibodies to histoplasmin. Complement fixation
tests to blastomycin mold phase and to blastomycin yeast phase antigens may both yield confusing reactions, and the titer to histoplasmin may be higher than the titer to blastomycin in a patient with
blastomycosis.

The serological test which is currently thought to be most specific
as well as sensitive for blastomycosis is the immunodiffusion test
with parallel use of specific reference sera. The morphology of the
precipitation bands of the test serum may be compared with those
of the reference serum, and if similar it may permit a correct diagnosis to be made in approximately 80% of cases (see Kaufman, et al.).

Early symptoms of disease include chest pain, weight loss, fever
and fatigue. This patient demonstrated all of these complaints.

Although stilbamidine is an effective form of therapy for non-cavitary
primary pulmonary blastomycosis, the therapeutic results with amphotericin B are equal. Amphotericin B is to be preferred for cavitary or severe pulmonary disease, such as this child had, or for
extrapulmonary blastomycosis. B. dermatitidis is virtually always
sensitive to clinically achievable concentrations of amphotericin B.

3. (C)

The organism causing North American blastomycosis, B. dermatitidis,
has very seldom been recovered from the soil. This may be
due in part to the observation that B. dermatitidis will not grow on
unsterilized soil, and that growth as well as sporulation is fostered

by enriching the soil with organic matter. Nevertheless, the failure to isolate organisms even in the neighborhood of multiple cases has created doubt concerning the theory that contaminated soil is the main reservoir. Similarly, the organism has not been shown to be transmitted by infected bird droppings such as occurs for crypto-coccosis. Blastomycosis is a disease of dogs but there is no evidence to suggest they are a usual source for human disease.

Several small epidemics have occurred, including one in Minnesota and two in North Carolina. The mode of transmission has been assumed to be by inhalation of air-borne spores from infected soil, but this has not been demonstrated and the means of transmission remains unknown. The infection is not unusually severe in children, in contrast to several other systemic mycoses, and the age distribution of patients also does not favor children disproportionately.

REFERENCES

1. Blastomycosis - North Carolina. Center for Disease Control Morbidity and Mortality Weekly Report 25:205-206, 1976.

2. Busey, J. R. : Blastomycosis III. A comparative study of 2-hydroxy-stilbamidine and amphotericin B therapy. Am. Rev. Resp. Dis. 105:812-818, 1972.

3. Furcolow, M. L. , Smith, C. D. : A new hypothesis on the epidemiology of blastomycosis and the ecology of Blastomyces dermititidis. Trans. N. Y. Acad Sci. 35:421-430, 1973.

4. Kaufman, L. , et al. : Specific immunodiffusion test for blastomycosis. Appl. Micro. 26:244-247, 1973.

5. Parker, J. D. , et al. : A decade of experience with blastomycosis and its treatment with amphotericin B. A national communicable disease center cooperative mycoses study. Am. Rev. Resp. Dis. 99:895-902, 1969.

6. Smith, J. G. , et al. : An epidemic of North Carolina blastomycosis. JAMA 158:641-646, 1955.

7. Sarosi, G. A. , et al. : Clinical features of acute pulmonary blastomycosis. NEJM 290:540-543, 1974.

8. Witorsch, P. , Utz, J. P. : North American Blastomycosis. A study of 40 patients. Medicine 47:169-200, 1968.

:::

CASE 51: PRIMARY ISONIAZID-RESISTANT TUBERCULOSIS

HISTORY: This 13-month-old black girl was referred from her
local pediatric clinic for evaluation of meningitis. The child had
been in her usual state of health until approximately 3 days prior
to admission when she developed a slight cough, fever, and vomited
twice. She attended her clinic for a previously scheduled routine
visit, was found to have meningismus and a bulging fontanelle and
lumbar puncture revealed 78 WBC/mm^3, all polymorphonuclear leukocytes.

The child had had a poor weight gain since birth, and was below the
3rd% for both height and weight. She had been receiving iron supplementation for the previous 4 months for anemia, and had made moderately delayed developmental progress prior to this illness. The
mother stated that she seemed to have grown and developed similarly to her other 5 children.

At the time of admission she was found to be small, irritable, jittery and apparently chronically ill.

PHYSICAL EXAMINATION: Pulse 140. Respirations 36. Temperature 39.3°C. Wt. 6.26 kg. Head circumference 44 3/4 cm., B.P.
110/80. Head: Fontanelle bulging, sutures widened. Ears: TM's
dull. Eyes: Pupils equal, reactive, extraocular movements intact.
Throat unremarkable. Neck markedly stiff, but without adenopathy.
Lungs: Clear. Heart: Unremarkable, without murmurs. Abdomen:
Soft, scaphoid. No masses. Liver, spleen normal in size. Neurological: Irritable child with a generalized fine intention tremor. No
localized findings were made. DTR's were symmetrical. Roentgenographic Findings: Hilar lymphadenopathy with streaking peripheral
parenchymal lesions of the left lower lobe were found. The cranial
sutures were widened. No bony abnormalities were visualized.

LABORATORY FINDINGS: WBC 15,300 with 37% neutrophils, 61%
lymphocytes, 1% monocytes and 1% eosinophils. Hemoglobin 10.2
grams. Hematocrit, 32%. Platelets were adequate. Cerebral spinal
fluid re-examination: Opening pressure was 330 mm H_2O, closing
pressure 210 mm H_2O. CSF glucose was 36 with blood glucose of
95. Protein was 44 mg%. There were 125 $cells/cm^3$, 96% of which
were activated monocytes. Gram stain of the CSF revealed no microorganisms.

QUESTION:

1. Immediate care and evaluation should include:
   A. Intravenous therapy with penicillin and chloramphenicol
   B. Careful evaluation of family history for tuberculosis
   C. Application of intermediate strength intradermal PPD
   D. Stain of sputum or gastric aspirate for acid-fast bacilli

The family did not volunteer information concerning tuberculosis in the household. When asked, however, they stated that the patient's paternal uncle had been hospitalized 6 months previously for tuberculosis. At the time of the diagnosis of the uncle's disease, both parents exhibited intradermal reactivity to PPD and were begun on INH preventive therapy. The patient had had a non-reactive PPD six months previously, at the time of the uncle's diagnosis, and had received no preventive therapy.

The patient had an area of induration of 17 mm. at 24 hours and of 20 mm. at 48 hours to 5TU, PPD-S.

Cerebrospinal fluid and gastric aspirate specimens were examined by fluorescence microscopy for acid-fast bacilli and none were seen. CSF yielded no growth of bacteria by day 3 and counter-immunoelectrophoresis for H. influenzae type B capsular antigen was negative.

QUESTION:

2. The following steps should be promptly taken:
    A. The local Health Department and the institution caring for the patient's uncle should be contacted to determine whether or not isolation of M. tuberculosis was achieved and, if so, the sensitivity pattern to antituberculous agents of the isolate
    B. The patient should be begun at this time, if not sooner, on INH plus streptomycin
    C. Because the risk of INH hepatotoxicity and neurotoxicity would be increased in this jittery child, preliminary therapeutic choices may best consist of streptomycin plus PAS or streptomycin plus ethambutol
    D. The Health Department nearest the family should be contacted to determine the incidence of resistant strains in that community or family
    E. Other family members should be re-evaluated for adequacy of preventive therapy and for current clinical status

Fortunately, the uncle's isolate had been tested and was found to grow uninhibitedly in the presence of 1.0 ugm/ml isoniazid. This information became known during the second hospital day, and the child, who was receiving INH plus streptomycin, had ethionamide and rifampin added to her regimen.

The duration of the child's hospital stay was 3 months and four days. Salient aspects of her course were as follows:

1. The child's irritability and jittery behavior increased during the first 3 weeks. She remained intermittently febrile, appeared to have pain in her head, and continued to have significant elevation of her CSF pressure. A 5 day course of dexamethasone failed to be of apparent benefit. A ventriculo-peritoneal shunt was inserted during the third week and her state of alertness and disposition improved markedly thereafter.

2. The child had persistently inadequate appetite. An attempt was made to provide approximately 400 calories/day and this goal was usually not achieved. The diagnosis and treatment of this condition was not achieved during her hospitalization in spite of a period of 3 weeks when provision of nutrition was the prime objective during which no studies were performed.

3. She was demonstrated during her hospitalization to have M. tuberculosis from the initial 2 cerebrospinal fluid cultures and from the initial gastric aspirate. The isolates were, as expected, INH resistant.

4. She experienced prolonged and unexpected fevers.

5. Her therapeutic regimens were as follows:
   a) Initial therapy: INH plus streptomycin with ethionamide and rifampin added on day 3
   b) DC INH on day 11
   c) DC streptomycin on day 21
   d) DC rifampin after 3 months
   e) Maintain patient following discharge on ethionamide plus paraminosalicylate for 18 months

Following discharge from hospital she began a slow gain in weight and by 1 year after diagnosis had reached the 3rd% for weight. Neurological findings included persistent weakness of the left arm and leg and delayed verbal ability. Her shunt has not been a source of medical problem.

Summary of Family History: The patient lived with her mother, father, and 3 sibs, age 5 to 13 years. One teenage sib who was PPD non-reactive was excreting M. tuberculosis from her sputum. The household of the patient's grandparents was near and in it lived the infected maternal uncle who was the source and his two teenage children. The family had been resistant to efforts to examine and treat the members, and had a history of violent life style. During the follow-up of this patient a newborn infant in the household died violently and a daughter was raped by a relative.

Rifampin was chosen for preventive prophylaxis of household contacts of these cases.

QUESTIONS:

3. Characteristics of tuberculosis due to a primary drug resistant strain include:
   A. The incidence is higher in the patients who are in the younger age groups than those in older age groups
   B. Disseminated disease is rare and the strains appear to have attenuated virulence

    C. Transmission to susceptable contacts may be prevented by
        INH even though the strain is INH resistant

    D. In the U. S. A. at the present time, INH resistance is more
        common than is streptomycin resistance and is increasing
        in incidence

4. Adverse reactions or disadvantages to use of ethionamide have
    included:

    A. Serum sickness-like reactions
    B. Optic neuritis with blindness
    C. Hepatic and gastrointestinal disturbances
    D. Ototoxicity
    E. Cross-resistance with INH

ANSWERS:

1. (A, B, C, D)

In the first hours of this child's evaluation the possibility of bacterial
meningitis was paramount and appropriate therapy may approximately
have been instituted. In the following days, the diagnosis of acute
bacterial meningitis failed to be supported, and the initial therapeutic regimen was altered.

This particular child presented with findings suggestive of tuberculous meningitis. The presence of activated monocytes in the cerebrospinal fluid should bring this consideration to the forefront. Supporting this consideration was an indolent presentation, elevated
protein with slightly decreased glucose, and significantly elevated
pressure. These findings in the presence of a pulmonary infiltrate
with hilar adenopathy should lead to further rapid evaluation of this
possibility.

In the current era, sporadic cases of tuberculosis in children from
non-familial contacts is very unusual unless the community is unusually highly involved. The great majority of tuberculous children have
adult household contacts who have active disease. An immediate
family history for tuberculous household members or for adults with
symptoms of tuberculosis is very likely to provide supportive evidence of exposure of the child to this disease.

In a child who is debilitated, and has disease consistent with tuberculosis, a non-reactive tuberculin reaction is not helpful in ruling
out tuberculosis. However, if positive at this age it would confirm
that she had had contact with the infection and would increase the
likelihood of this diagnosis. Similarly, an examination of sputum
or gastric aspirate for acid-fast bacilli is likely to be positive if
large numbers of bacilli are being excreted, and this may not be
the case in children even with active disease. Therefore, a negative
study does not rule the diagnosis out, but a positive study would make
the diagnosis of tuberculosis very likely.

2. (A, B, D, E)

A presumptive diagnosis of tuberculous meningitis had been made
and the child required prompt and effective therapy. Standard forms
of therapy which have yielded adequate results have all included
isoniazid, usually in combination with one or two other agents. Isoniazid is known to have excellent distribution into the central nervous
system, is mycobactericidal, and is presumably the agent responsible for the control of the meningeal component of this infection. It
is essential, therefore, to ensure that the isolate is likely or known
to be INH sensitive. Since the sensitivity characteristics of the child's
contact will probably reflect that of the patient, the physician should
take the earliest opportunity to ascertain the results of the isolates
from the contact. Similarly, if the patient comes from an area in
which there is known to be a high incidence of resistant organisms,
additional therapeutic decisions would have to be made. In the absence of information suggesting that a resistant strain is likely, INH
plus streptomycin would form a satisfactory initial choice. The alternative regimens mentioned (streptomycin plus PAS or ethambutol)
have neither been demonstrated to provide a rapid mycobactericidal
effect in vitro nor a satisfactory clinical response in children. The
consideration of INH neurotoxicity or hepatotoxicity should be anticipated and the patient followed appropriately, but both are rare problems in children and should not deter its use in children with tuberculous meningitis.

In any family in which a case of active Tbc has occurred, the health
of the other family members may be in jeopardy. In this instance
the opportunity to prevent disease in the children first occurred at
the time of the diagnosis of the uncle. The other family members,
including children, should now be re-examined and prophylactic
therapy begun on all members who were not previously treated.

3. (A)

There is a decreasing incidence of primary resistant strains with
increasing age (see, for example, Doster et al.). These findings
pertain to both isoniazid- and streptomycin-resistant isolates. The
explanation of these findings is not yet clear, but may reflect recent
transmission of resistant organisms to young patients, transmission
which has occurred since the use of antimycobacterial drugs became
prevalent.

There is no evidence to suggest that the transmission of primary
drug resistant strains is less frequent or disease due to these strains
is less severe than occurs with sensitive strains. Similarly, INH
preventive therapy has been repeatedly shown to fail to prevent
transmission or disease to susceptible persons if the strain is INH
resistant. Articles of Steiner et al. describe recent experiences indicating full virulence and transmission of INH resistant strains.

In spite of heightened awareness of the problems of drug-resistant strains of M. tuberculosis, the current evidence suggests that primary resistance to INH and to streptomycin has not increased in incidence during the past decades. Single streptomycin resistance is slightly more common (1. 5% of strains) than is single isoniazid resistance (0. 9% of strains). Approximately 3. 5% of all strains are resistant to one or more drugs.

These considerations highlight the importance of a vigorous effort to isolate M. tuberculosis from patients suspected of being tuberculous and of performing sensitivity tests on all isolates.

4. (A, C)

Ethionamide is a derivative of isonicotinic acid, as is isoniazid. However, the compound seldom shares cross resistance with INH and is fully active against isoniazid-resistant bacilli. It is, furthermore, mycobacteriocidal to actively multiplying organisms. It has been well tolerated in most children and has the major advantage that most serious adverse reactions to this drug may be diagnosed without the co-operation of the child which may be difficult to achieve. On the contrary, ethambutol may cause serious optic neuritis which is difficult to diagnose in the very young. Rapid development of resistance has been reported if ethionamide is used alone, and so should always be used in combination with a second antituberculous drug.

ADDENDUM: A photomicrograph of cells from this patient's cerebrospinal fluid after 1 week of therapy is shown in Fig. 51.1. Large active monocytes predominate with occasional lymphocytes also present.

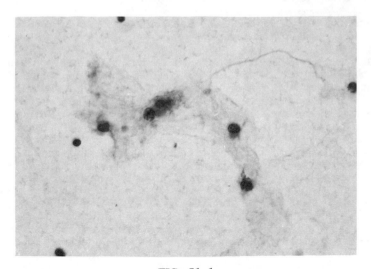

FIG. 51. 1

REFERENCES

1. Comstock, G. W. , et al. : The prognosis of a positive tuberculin reaction in children and adolescence. Am. J. Epidemiol. 99:131-136, 1974.

2. Current trends: Prevention therapy of tuberculous infection. Center For Disease Control, Morbidity and Mortality Weekly Report 24:71-78, 1975.

3. Doster, B. , et al. : A continuing survey of primary drug resistance in tuberculosis. 1961 to 1968. Am. J. Resp. Dis. 113:419-425, 1976.

4. Hughes, I. E. , et al. : Ethionamide: Its passage into the cerebrospinal fluid in man. Lancet I: 616-617, 1962.

5. Stead, W. W. : Pathogenesis of the sporadic case of tuberculosis. NEJM 277:1008-12, 1967.

6. Steiner, M. : Newer and second-line drugs in the treatment of drug-resistant tuberculosis in children. Med. Clin. N. A. 51: 1153-1167, 1967.

7. Steiner, M. , et al. : Primary drug-resistant tuberculosis in children. Am. Rev. Resp. Dis. 102:75-82, 1970.

8. Steiner, P. , Portugaleza, C. : Tuberculous meningitis in children. Amer. Rev. Resp. Dis. 107:22-29, 1973.

CASE 52: FEVER AND INGUINAL ADENOPATHY IN AN AMERICAN INDIAN

HISTORY: This 6-year-old American Indian boy was in good health until 2 days prior to admission when he had the sudden onset of a shaking chill. His fever rose to 38. 2°C, he complained of abdominal pain which was most severe in the right lower quadrant, and he then developed headache, dizziness and generalized malaise. During the next 12 hours his throat became sore, the pain in his abdomen increased, and he began to have the swelling in the right groin which finally brought him to medical attention. He was having no diarrhea or vomiting, no rash, and no signs or symptoms of disease of the genitourinary tract. He had completed his childhood immunizations and received regular medical attention. He had two younger siblings who were in good health. His home was of adobe in a village with a population of approximately 500 persons in northeastern New Mexico. He had had no known exposures to wild animals and he had not had unusual recent insect bites, although occasional bites were common at that time of the year, August. His pet dog had not been ill.

On admission he was a moderately ill, well-nourished child who was oriented and alert. His blood pressure was 110/70, pulse 130, temperature 38. 5°C. He was in moderate distress. Pertinent physical findings included the following: He had a mild palpebral and bulbar conjunctivitis, but ocular examination was otherwise unremarkable. His ears were normal. The posterior pharynx was injected but there was no exudate and only moderate slightly tender cervical lymphoadenopathy. The neck was supple and there were no meningeal findings. The child had a slight brassy cough, and there were scattered rales across the left lower lung field. Abdominal organs were not enlarged. Bowel tones were normal and he had had a recent bowel movement. He had moderate diffuse abdominal pain which was without rebound tenderness and which appeared to be a reflection of the lesion of his right inguinal area, where he had developed a 4 x 5 cm., very tender mass of lymph nodes. The overlying skin was erythematous and edematous with a bluish coloration. The area was warm to the touch. There were no lymphangitic streaks from the area. There was a small macular area on the right thigh distal to the lesion. Rectal examination was unremarkable.

LABORATORY FINDINGS: The white blood cell count was $8,700/mm^3$ with 70% polymorphonuclear leukocytes, 3% bands, 24% lymphocytes, and 3% monocytes. His hemoglobin was 12. 3 gm% and Westergren sedimentation rate was 38 mm/hr. The SGOT was 75 units and alkaline phosphatase was 58. 5 King-Armstrong units. Heterophile agglutinins were negative. Roentgenographic examination of the chest revealed a streaky and diffuse infiltrate in the left lower lobe with minimal consolidation. Flat plates and upright examination of the abdomen were unremarkable. At the time of admission the patient had three blood cultures and a throat culture taken.

QUESTIONS:

1. Initial working diagnoses should include:
    A. Bubonic plague
    B. Appendicitis
    C. Tularemia
    D. Incarcerated inguinal hernia
    E. Staphylococcal lymphadenopathy
    F. Streptococcal lymphadenopathy
    G. Yersinia enterocolitica

2. Further immediate measures which should be taken in the care of this child at the time of admission include:
    A. Barium enema with abdominal compression to determine appendiceal patency
    B. Gram stain of the buffy coat of his peripheral blood
    C. Transfer to the surgical service for exploration of the inguinal area
    D. Aspiration of an involved inguinal node for Gram stain
    E. Institution of streptomycin with or without tetracycline therapy
    F. Order initial respiratory isolation for the patient
    G. Repeat heterophile antibody determination, order antistreptolysin 0 titer, and await culture results

3. Characteristics of plague in the U. S. at the present time are:
   A. Streptomycin-resistant strains of Y. pestis are becoming increasingly common
   B. The disease is transmitted by a wide variety of insect vectors
   C. The disease is restricted to areas west of the 100th meridian
   D. The majority of persons who acquire plague have had contact with wild mammals, especially prairie dogs, squirrels, and chipmunks; this contact may be direct, as with hunters and campers, or indirect, as when a pet dog brings home an infected animal

4. Major virulence factors for Yersinia pestis include:
   A. Fraction 1 antigen
   B. Pesticin I
   C. Pigmentation
   D. Purine independence
   E. V and W antigens
   F. Murine toxin

ANSWERS:

1. (A-F)

The two primary diagnostic considerations should be bubonic plague and tularemia. This child lived in a plague endemic area, became ill during the summer, the season at which most cases occur, and was from a rural community. His presenting acute symptoms, which include conjunctivitis, pneumonitis, fever, and marked inguinal adenopathy were highly compatible with these two diseases. In addition, two other more generally common causes of acute infections lymphadenopathy should have been considered, streptococcal and staphylococcal lymphoadenopathy. Yersinia enterocolitica would be an unlikely but possible cause of this boy's disease.

The continued excellent bowel function and the acute febrile onset of the symptoms, as well as the pharyngitis and conjunctivitis, render the diagnosis of appendicitis and inguinal hernia unlikely. Nevertheless, these conditions should have been considered initially.

2. (B, D, E, F)

It is critically important to the patient that he be rapidly evaluated when there is the likelihood of plague. In this instance, two sources of material for Gram stain were available. An aspirate of material from an affected inguinal node, taken prior to institution of therapy, is likely to yield material showing typical bipolar pleomorphic gram-negative rods. This would be adequate information to make a presumptive diagnosis prior to completion of cultures or serology.

A second source of rapid diagnostic material is the peripheral blood. In a study of 25 patients with plague in Vietnam, Butler et al. demonstrated that 11 had greater than 10^2 colonies/ml in the peripheral blood. In the 4 patients who had 10^6 colonies/ml, organisms were readily seen on direct peripheral smear. Furthermore, there is a general correlation between increased numbers of bacteria in the peripheral blood and increased mortality rate. Since it is unusual to be able to determine the presence of fewer than 10^5 organisms/ml by direct examination, the procedure may assist in assessing the severity of the patient's illness and his ability to contain the infection.

Patients with bubonic plague may present with apparently mild or slowly progressive disease and thereafter have a rapid decompensation with the onset of shock and disseminated intravascular coagulation. It is, therefore, recommended that appropriate cultures be taken, examinations made, and the patient with suspected plague then be begun on appropriate therapy. Therapy should not be delayed until a definitive diagnosis is made.

This child had early findings of pulmonary involvement. Although the pulmonary findings were minimal, he may have had the capacity to spread disease via infected droplets. All such patients should have respiratory isolation, since spread of plague via droplets is highly contagious.

3.   (C, D)

Although streptomycin-resistant strains of Y. pestis have been isolated in the Far East, they are virtually unknown in the U.S. It may be assumed, therefore, that victims of plague in the U.S. have disease with streptomycin-sensitive organisms.

One of the major differences between plague and tularemia in the U.S. is their modes of transmission. Plague is transmitted predominately by the bite of wild rodent fleas or by direct contact with infected wild mammals. Tularemia, in contrast, may be transmitted by the bite of an unusual variety of insect vectors including deer flies, ticks, fleas and mosquitoes, and by direct contact with a wide variety of naturally infected mammals.

Another major difference between the epidemiology of tularemia and plague in the U.S. is that tularemia may be acquired in almost any area, whereas plague is restricted to the territory approximately west of a line extending from the middle of North Dakota through the middle of Texas. This happens to coincide with the area in which there are dense populations of colonizing rodents, who appear to be of great importance in the perpetuation of the sylvatic cycle of plague.

Plague in the U. S. is now almost solely acquired through inadvertent contact with a sylvatic cycle. Thus, hunters may kill an infected animal, campers may camp in an area in which rodent deaths due to plague has released unusual numbers of infected fleas, and human pets may catch a diseased animal, bring it into human proximity, and thus populate the area with infected fleas (for example, see Rust et al.).

4. (A-E)

Fraction 1 antigen is found on the bacterial envelope, is best produced at 37°C compared with lower temperatures, is highly immunogenic, and antibody to fraction 1 is protective in both humans and experimental animals. It is used for several diagnostic tests for plague.

Pesticin I is produced concomitantly with coagulase and fibrinolysin and strains lacking these three components are fully infectious for the mouse or guinea pig but lethality is attenuated.

Pigmentation enables cells to absorb exogenous hemin to form colored colonies, and mutation to non-pigmentation leads to avirulence.

Mutational loss of the ability to synthesize adenine or guanine de novo is correlated with loss of virulence.

V and W antigens were the first virulence factors to be identified. They are selectively produced during periods of stasis of bacterial growth, are always produced concomitantly , and may be produced following phagocytosis.

The function of murine toxin as a determinant of virulence has not been elucidated.

REFERENCES

1. Brubaker, R. F.: The genus Yersinia: Biochemistry and genetics of virulence. Current Topics in Microbiology and Immunology 57:111-158, 1972.

2. Burgdorfer, W. , et al. : Zoonotic potential (Rocky Mountain spotted fever and tularemia) in the Tennessee Valley Region. II. Prevalence of Rickettsia rickettsii and Francisella tularensis in mammals and ticks from land between the lakes. Am. J. Trop. Med. Hyg. 23:109-117, 1974.

3. Butler, T.: A clinical study of bubonic plague. Observations of the 1970 Viet Nam epidemic with emphasis on coagulation studies, skin histology and electrocardiograms. Am. J. Med. 53:268-276, 1972.

4. Butler, T. , et al. : Yersinia pestis infection in Vietnam. II.
    Quantitative blood cultures and detection of endotoxin in the
    cerebrospinal fluid of patients with meningitis. J. Infect. Dis.
    133:493-499, 1976.

5. Francis, E. : Symptoms diagnosis, and pathology of tularemia.
    JAMA 91:1155-1161, 1928.

6. Kartman, L. : Historical and ecological observations on plague
    in the United States. Trop. Georgr. Med. 22:257-275, 1970.

7. Klock, L. E. , et al. : Tularemia epidemic associated with the
    deerfly. JAMA 226:149-152, 1973.

8. Reed, W. P. , et al. : Bubonic plague in the southwestern United
    States. A review of recent experience. Medicine 49:465-486,
    1970.

9. Rust, J. H. , et al. : The role of domestic animals in the epi-
    demiology of plague. II. Antibody to Yersinia pestis in sera of
    dogs and cats. J. Infect. Dis. 124:527-531, 1971.

10. Young, L. S. , et al. : Tularemia epidemic. Vermont 1968.
    NEJM 230:1253-1260, 1969.

::

CASE 53: MULTIPLE DRUG THERAPY WITH SUBSEQUENT
          CHRONIC NEUTROPENIA

HISTORY: The patient was a 13-year-old, black male who presented
with the rapid onset of fever, malaise, mucopurulent drainage from
the right nostril, right ptosis, and extreme pain of his face. He had
been previously well, had not had recurrent sinusitis, had had no
trauma to the face, and denied insertion of a foreign body. It was
known that he did not have sickle cell trait or disease. There was no
history suggestive of diabetes and there were no diabetics in his
immediate family members.

PHYSICAL EXAMINATION: Salient physical findings included the
following: Temperature was 39°C. Pulse 80. Head was normocephalic.
Ears and pharynx were unremarkable. The right eye was proptosic
grossly edematous in the periorbital tissues, and painful. Extraocular movement was present and symmetrical. Vision was difficult to
assess. Ocular fundi were benign. There was a slight serous discharge from the conjunctivae. The nose was swollen and mucopurulent drainage was found bilaterally. His neck was supple and lymphoadenopathy was minimal. There were no significant findings of the
thorax, abdomen, genitalia, or peripheral neurological examination.

LABORATORY DATA: Laboratory findings included the following: White blood cell count was 13,900 with 92% polymorphonuclear leukocytes, 4% lymphocytes and 4% monocytes. Hemoglobin was 13gm%, liver function tests were unremarkable as were serum ketone, glucose and pH. Gram stain of the nasal discharge revealed profuse leukocytes with gram-positive cocci in chains. Blood culture was negative, but culture of nasal discharge yielded Streptococcus pyogenes with anaerobic streptococci. Lumbar puncture was unremarkable and yielded no growth.

Roentgenographic examination revealed extensive pansinusitis with erosion of the right orbital plate. Surgical drainage was performed and Streptococcus pyogenes with anaerobic streptococci were recovered from an ethmoid sinus abscess. A diagnosis of orbital cellulitis and pansinusitis was made and the child was begun on intravenous therapy of chloramphenicol 75/mg/kg/day, plus methicillin which was continued for 6 days. A single serum chloramphenicol concentration was assayed one hour after a dose and was 15 ugm/ml. He appeared to make a satisfactory recovery and was discharged. Three weeks later he was readmitted for swelling of the right periorbital area. An abscess was found and drained from which untypeable Hemophilus influenzae was recovered. He was treated with clindamycin and chlorpromazine for 85 days.

At the time of his second admission he had a white cell count of 6,450 with an absolute neutrophil count of 4,200. One month later his absolute neutrophil count was 3,100 and 3 weeks later 1,300. During the subsequent nine months he maintained absolute neutrophil counts of 1,300-1,900 as determined on 14 consecutive occasions. Platelets remained adequate, hemoglobin was unchanged and the neutrophils which were present were normal in morphology. His general health remained good. He made a slow but uneventful complete recovery from his orbital osteomyelitis. During his first hospitalization he received 11 drugs including chloramphenicol, meperidine, promethazine, anectine and halothane. During his second hospitalization he received 16 drugs including diazepam, chlorpromazine, diaphenydramine, and acetaminophen.

QUESTIONS:

1. Which of the following statements concerning this patient are correct?
   A. The child received multiple drugs, several of which may have caused his neutropenia
   B. Since he received all doses of chloramphenicol parenterally, it is very unlikely that chloramphenicol caused his neutropenia
   C. The delay in onset of his neutropenia is characteristic of other cases of neutropenia, which are probably caused by chloramphenicol administration
   D. Since his serum chloramphenicol concentration was within a desired therapeutic range, it is unlikely that his neutropenia was caused by this drug

2. Further diagnostic procedures which would be appropriate include:
   A. The patient may be challenged with 10 mg/kg chloramphenicol orally and then a bone marrow examination repeated in 2 weeks
   B. The patient's serum folate concentration should be determined, and he should be treated with pyridoxine if abnormally low
   C. The patient's serum iron concentration should be assayed and treated if low
   D. The bone marrow should be examined

3. The incidence of severe chloramphenicol-induced blood dyscrasias are probably approximately 1 in 20,000 cases to 1 in 40,000 cases. Indicate which of the following conditions probably occur more frequently:
   A. Anaphylactic reactions following use of penicillin
   B. Severe thromboembolic accidents during use of oral contraceptives
   C. Sulfonamide-associated aplastic anemia
   D. Clindamycin-associated colitis

4. Major forms of adverse reaction to chloramphenicol in humans include which of the following?
   A. Optic neuritis
   B. Dose-related and reversible depression of all components of hematopoesis
   C. Suppression of immunologic function
   D. Shock and metabolic acidosis of the newborn
   E. Idiopathic development of aplastic anemia

5. Which of the following medical conditions may warrant the use of chloramphenicol?
   A. Meningococcal meningitis in a person known to be severely sensitive to penicillin
   B. Typhoid fever
   C. Otitis media in a newborn
   D. Meningitis of unknown cause in a child less than 6 years of age
   E. Brain abscess of unknown etiology
   F. Suspected Rocky Mountain spotted fever
   G. A family contact of a person with meningococcemia

ANSWERS:

1. (A, C)

This child is an example of the problem of attributing an adverse reaction to a given drug when the patient has received multiple drugs. Among the drugs which he received and which have been associated with such a reaction are aspirin, chlorpromazine and chloramphenicol. In all cases the attribution of neutropenia to the use of chloramphenicol is only based upon an epidemiologic association, such as occurred in this instance. However, other drugs could also have been responsible. For example, in Yunis's series of 94 cases of chloramphenicol-induced blood dyscrasis, 67 patients received chloramphenicol alone while the remaining 27 received an additional drug.

Although the majority of the first recognized cases of post-chloramphenicol dysplasia occurred in patients who had received oral therapy, there have been well documented cases following parenteral therapy alone.

Chloramphenicol-associated blood dyscrasias usually become apparent after the course of therapy has been completed. In the study by Best, of 284 patients, only 22% of patients were recognized to have an adverse reaction while receiving the drug. The reaction developed 10 days or less after the initial dose in 10% of patients, in 95 days or less in about 50% of patients, and 260 days or greater in 10% of patients. The present case, therefore, corresponds with a delay in presentation.

The reported cases of chloramphenicol-associated blood dyscrasias indicate that some persons develop this complication following even very short courses of therapy (less than 4 days) and even very low doses (less than 8 mg/kg/day). Therefore, there is no basis for suspecting that the moderate serum concentration which this patient achieved means that his condition is not due to the use of chloramphenicol.

2. (D)

In a patient who has had a delayed bone marrow dysplasia following the use of chloramphenicol, there is no justification for challenging with the potentially offending drug. The risk that it will further depress marrow function cannot be taken.

Evidence that he has had a deficiency of either pyridoxine or iron to account for his dysplasia is absent. First, hemoglobin synthesis is intact and would be expected to be impaired if pyridoxine or iron stores were deficient. Normal platelet counts also indicate a normal pyridoxine supply, as does the presence of morphologically normal neutrophils.

Although this child has been tolerating his condition, examination of the marrow would provide further important information concerning his current status. In addition, the possibility of leukemia, although remote at best, would be ruled out.

3. (A, D)

Anaphylactic shock probably occurs in approximately one of each
7, 000-8, 000 courses of parenteral penicillin therapy, and there is
a fatality rate of approximately 10% in these patients. Such data
come from the World Health Organization.

Severe or fatal thromboembolic events during use of oral contraceptives occurs in approximately 1 of 22, 000 women, which is similar
to the major chloramphenicol reaction.

Although the rate of granulocytopenia or aplastic anemia following
sulfonamide therapy is not definitely known, it may approach that
of chloramphenicol. Jutscher in 1954 noted granulocytopenia in 1. 5
cases/1000 treated with sulfisoxazole and found this rate to be higher
than in patients treated with chloramphenicol.

Clindamycin produces diarrhea in approximately 20% of persons and
pseudomembraneous colitis in approximately 10% of patients. Although cessation of the use of the drug usually is followed by remission, there have been numerous fatalities and remission is not always prompt.

4. (A-E)

All of the named reactions have been recognized to be potential complications of the use of chloramphenicol. Optic neuritis is a rare reaction and recent reports are particularly sparse. Little is known
of the etiology.

A pharmacologic effect of chloramphenicol involves depression of
maturation of all elements of the bone marrow. It is rarely recognized when serum concentrations are maintained below 20 ugm/ml,
being related to higher concentrations. The onset is usually within
a few days of the initiation of therapy. It is associated with a retic-
ulocytopenia and rise in serum iron concentrations. Recovery follows modification of the dose of drug or withdrawal of the drug.

Chloramphenicol is an active immunosuppressive agent. It has been
shown to prolong the life of transplanted organs and has an effect on
the course of lupus nephritis. Studies in experimental animals have
also indicated a suppressive effect on cell mediated immunity.

Compared with adults, infants and toddlers have a decreased rate of
conjugation of chloramphenicol. When given doses of chloramphenicol
which are extrapolated from adult experience, therefore, they accum-
ulate chloramphenicol and develop very high serum concentrations.
Before this fact was recognized, children who were subjected to such
high doses developed shock and metabolic acidosis, termed the "Grey
Baby Syndrome". It is now recommended that newborns should receive
chloramphenicol only if the hospital has the facilities to monitor the
infants' serum chloramphenicol concentrations.

The most feared complication of the use of chloramphenicol is probably also the most rare, aplastic anemia. It is described as idiopathic
because it is not directly related to dose or duration of therapy. The
occurrence of this complication in both members of two sets of identical twins has stimulated the idea that there may be important ge-
netically determined aspects of individual susceptibility.

5.   (A, B, D, E, F)

Both meningococcal and pneumococcal meningitis are well treated
with chloramphenicol. It is, therefore, an excellent therapeutic
choice for those patients who are known to be likely to have a major
reaction to penicillin.

Chloramphenicol remains an effective form of therapy for typhoid
fever, except for areas in which chloramphenicol resistant S. typhi
are prevalent. Other therapeutic choices are ampicillin, and under
some circumstances, trimethoprim-sulfamethoxazole.

Otitis media of the newborn is most likely to be due to S. aureus or
a member of the Enterobacteriaceae, and chloramphenicol is therefore not the best choice of therapy.

The major causes of acute bacterial meningitis in children, beyond
the newborn period, are H. influenzae, pneumococci, and meningococci. Since the advent of ampicillin - resistant H. influenzae,
chloramphenicol has become the drug of choice for initiation of
therapy.

Penicillin plus chloramphenicol comprise the usual choice for therapy
of brain abscesses of unknown etiology. Brain abscesses frequently
are caused by a combination of anaerobic bacteria plus a low grade
aerobic pathogen such as Staphylococcus albus, and chloramphenicol
would be expected to be effective for most anaerobic bacteria in
these circumstances.

Rocky Mountain spotted fever may be treated with chloramphenicol
or tetracyclines. An advanced case may be clinically indistinguishable from meningococcemia, and under those circumstances chloramphenicol is an appropriate choice.

Chloramphenicol is not an effective agent in the prophylaxis of contacts for meningococcemia.

REFERENCES

1. Best, W. R.: Chloramphenicol-associated blood dyscrasias. A review of cases submitted to the American Medical Association Registry. JAMA 201:181-188, 1967.

2. Bottiger, L. F., Westernholm, B.: Drug-induced blood dyscrasias in Sweden. Brit. Med. J. 3:339-343, 1973.

3. Craft, A. W., et al.: The "Grey Toddler". Chloramphenicol toxicity. Andrs. Dis. Child. 49:235-237, 1974.

4. Howell, A., et al.: Bone-marrow cells resistant to chloramphenicol in chloramphenicol induced aplastic anemia. Lancet I:65-69, 1975.

5. McKenzie, M. W., et al.: Adverse drug reactions leading to hospitalization in children. J. Pediat. 89:487-90, 1976.

6. Psicofitta, A. V.: Drug-induced leukopenia and aplastic anemia. Clin. Pharm. and Therapeut. 12:13-43, 1971.

7. Polak, B. C. D, et al.: Blood dyscrasias attributed to chloramphenicol. Acta. Med. Scand. 192:409-414, 1972.

::

CASE 54: EOSINOPHILIA AND PARASITES

HISTORY: CH was a 2-year-old white male who was well until October 1, 1974, when he experienced a sudden rise of temperature to 40°C, accompanied by labored breathing and wheezing. He was hospitalized and treated with an antihistamine, a decongestant and penicillin. He recovered rapidly, went home the next day, and was well until October 9th, 1974, when his fever and respiratory symptoms recurred. He was hospitalized again, and at that time a chest x-ray was reported to show left lower lobe pneumonia. From the 10th to the 25th of October white blood cell counts on seven occasions ranged from 23,000 to 60,200 per mm^3. On the 10th of October the white cell count was 30,000 per mm^3 and the differential count showed 89% "segmented forms" and 11% lymphocytes. On the 14th of October the white count was 23,800 per mm^3. There were 27% eosinophils, 32% segmented neutrophils and 41% lymphocytes. Urinalysis on the day of hospitalization revealed 4+ protein but subsequently his urine was normal. His hemoglobin was 10 g.% on the 10th of October.

After seven days of hospitalization, his fever and respiratory signs and symptoms disappeared, and he went home. He was referred to a medical center because of concern over the persistently high white count, the anemia and the eosinophilia. At the medical center on October 29, 1974, additional history of frequent dirt eating, with a preference for red dirt, was elicited.

PHYSICAL EXAMINATION: The child appeared to be a normal, white male of his stated age. His liver was easily palpable 2 cm. below the right costal margin in the midclavicular line, and his spleen was thought to be slightly enlarged. There were some punctate, red papules on his skin which were considered to be insect bites.

LABORATORY DATA: Laboratory data revealed hemoglobin 8.1 g.%, hematocrit 25%; red cells appeared to be hypochromic, microcytic; white blood cell count was 41,700 per mm^3 with 80% eosinophils. Platelets were 212,500 per mm^3, reticulocytes 1.8%. Blood group isohemagglutinin titers were strikingly elevated; anti A 1:4096 and anti B 1:1024. Serum iron was 34 ug./dL; iron binding capacity was not determined. Serum electrolytes, BUN, calcium, phosphorus, glucose, and albumin were all within normal limits. A serological test for visceral larva migrans performed at the U.S. Public Health Service Center for Disease Control was reported "positive". Three stool examinations for "O and P" were "negative".

The patient was considered to have visceral larva migrans, or toxocariasis, and was returned to his community and local physician forthwith. Additionally, the diagnosis of iron deficiency anemia was made, and oral iron was prescribed.

QUESTIONS:

1. Toxocariasis is acquired by man by:
    A. Close association with the family dog
    B. Ingestion of soil containing dog or cat ascaris eggs that have been there long enough to become infectious
    C. The bite of an arthropod bearing the dog heartworm
    D. Going without shoes

2. The diagnosis of toxocariasis is made by:
    A. The assessment of a complex of clinical signs and symptoms
    B. A positive stool examination
    C. A positive blood test
    D. Liver biopsy

3. The prognosis of toxocariasis in the individual case is:
   A. Far from completely known
   B. May be benign
   C. Chronic nonspecific asthma
   D. Blindness
   E. Seizures
   F. Cirrhosis of the liver

4. The treatment of toxocariasis involves the drug thiabendazole.
   It should be prescribed:
   A. Whenever the diagnosis is made
   B. Only in severe cases
   C. Together with steroids in severe cases

5. In parasitic disease, marked eosinophilia:
   A. Always occurs
   B. Accompanies helminthic and protozoal infection
   C. Accompanies helminthic infection only
   D. Implies close association between helminth and host tissue

6. Toxocariasis or toxocarosis or visceral larva migrans are
   synonymous and quite different from toxoplasmosis, even though
   both diseases may be transmitted by cat feces and may affect the
   eye.
   A. True
   B. False

ANSWERS:

1. (B)

Visceral larva migrans syndrome usually is caused by Toxocara sp.
It can be caused by other helminths. Toxocara eggs require several
weeks in suitable soil to become infectious. They are not infectious
as they exit the dog or cat. Infectious eggs may cling to the fur of
animals that have been in contact with contaminated soil. Thus, the
issue is the child's contact with contaminated soil, especially dirt
eating, and not contact with animals. The prevalence of toxocara in
dogs is high regardless of socioeconomic status of either dog or
owner.

2. (A, C, D)

High eosinophilia and high total white blood count; age from 1 to 4;
fever; history of dirt eating; episodes of lower respiratory tract disease, often asthmatic; hepatomegaly and less marked enlargement of
the spleen are the most common clinical features. Little else can
mimic this complex of manifestations in their entirety. Central nervous system abnormalities and skin rashes occur.

Dogs and cats are the natural hosts for the ascarid worms Toxocara canis and cati respectively. Man is an unnatural host, and in man the worms are able to progress in their life cycle only to the extent of larval migration in various body tissues. They do not complete the cycle as human ascarid worms do by migrating to the intestinal lumen and thus do not reach the adult stage with egg production that would permit detection of characteristic ova in stools. Thus, stool examinations are negative for parasites including eggs or larval forms; Charcot-Leyden crystals, however, may be seen.

There is a pronounced immunological response that is characterized by hyperglobulinemia, high titers of blood group isoagglutinins and by elevation in serum antibodies detected by a variety of techniques. The sensitivity and specificity of these serological tests are improving with new developments; the Center for Disease Control as well as other laboratories perform these tests.

Demonstration of larvae in liver biopsy specimens is the only definitive diagnostic procedure, but it is rarely justified.

3.   (A, B, D, E)

High densities of larvae on the order of up to 10 per gm. of tissue may occur, each with its transient acute inflammatory reaction. With time, the reaction subsides leaving either no trace, a scar, or an encapsulated larva that from the point of view of the host's reactivity in inert. Obviously, the location of these events is important. Retinal damage and loss of vision or CNS damage with resultant epilepsy exemplify bad locations; while larvae in the liver do not seem to result in damage sufficient to interfere with liver function probably because of the liver's vast functional reserve and the nonprogressive and relatively transient nature of the basic pathological process.

Because of the inability to detect the presence of infection in the absence of the typical clinical picture, it is likely that but a small fraction of infected persons are identified - the tip of the iceberg. This limitation frustrates attempts to assess any subtle effects of toxocara infection, such as learning disabilities. At the moment it is generally believed that once past the acute stage, which may be severe, that complete recovery is the rule. However, pathological findings of toxocaral granulomata in myocardium and CNS in children dead from other causes give one pause in this regard.

4.   (C)

Evidence for efficacy of any drug is anecdotal and uncontrolled. Generally, no treatment is considered necessary. However, the proportion of those infected who will develop involvement of eye, CNS or other tissues is not known. The possibility of adverse reaction to large numbers of larvae dying simultaneously in response to a larvacidal drug has been raised but not demonstrated. Two drugs are reported to be useful: thiabendazole (50 mg./kg. daily, divided into 2 or 3 doses, for 3 days; repeat as needed after 2 day interval) or diethylcarbamazine (10 mg./kg. daily, divided into 3 doses, for 3 weeks).

Corticosteroids have been reported to provide prompt amelioration of severe respiratory or CNS involvement.

5. (C, D)

Protozoal infections such as amebiasis or malaria are not associated with eosinophilia.

Eosinophilia in parasitic disease varies according to the intensity of the host's immunologic reaction against helminth; the more intimate or invasive the association, the higher the eosinophil count. From this general rule one can predict when eosinophilia will be pronounced; that is, greater than 30% of the white blood cell count. In human ascaris, for example, intense eosinophilia may accompany the larval migratory stage that occurs soon after infection, but later when the mature worm reposes in the fecal stream with minimal tissue contact, eosinophilia is absent. In the case of toxocarosis, however, the larval worms are unable to mature in man, an unnatural host, and are doomed to prolonged aimless wandering during which they are the object of continued immunologic attack by the host with concurrent, prolonged, intense eosinophilia. The eosinophilia ends when the larvae are decomposed or succeed in walling themselves off from the host's reaction by the process of encapsulation that is so well illustrated in trichinosis and with tape worm larvae (cysticerci and hydatids).

Hookworms hold an intermediate position. During larval migration in the tissues a marked eosinophilia may occur. When the worm is mature and in the gut, some tissue contact persists, as the worm remains attached to the intestinal mucosa as it sucks blood. This relatively modest degree of tissue invasion results in sufficient continuing reaction to invoke a constant moderate eosinophilia.

Strongyloides may cause a hookworm pattern of eosinophilia, but because of its unique life cycle that permits continuing production of immediately invasive larvae from adults in the bowel, longstanding, pronounced eosinophilia may occur.

6. (A)

Toxoplasma gondii is a protozoon. Infected cats shed infective oocysts in their feces. There is no eosinophilia in toxoplasmosis. Toxo in this instance derives from the Greek word toxon, which means "bow or arc", which describes the shape of the tachyzoite form of the parasite.

Toxocara spp. are ascarid worms. Infected cats shed eggs in their feces. Eosinophilia is the hallmark of human infection. Toxo in this instance derives from the Latin word toxicum meaning poison.

Such information is essential for inner roundsmanship.

REFERENCES

1. Beaver, P. C. , et al. : Chronic eosinophilia due to visceral larva migrans. Pediatrics 9:7-19, 1952.

2. Beshear, J. R. , Hendley, J. O. : Severe pulmonary involvement in visceral larva migrans. Am. J. Dis. Child. 125:599-600, 1973.

3. Huntley, C. C. , et al. : Visceral larva migrans syndrome: clinical characteristics and immunologic studies in 51 patients. Pediatrics 36:523-536, 1965.

4. Snyder, C. H. : Visceral larva migrans, ten years' experience. Pediatrics 28:85-91, 1961.

5. Vargo, T. A. , et al. : Myocarditis due to visceral larva migrans. J. Pediat. 90:322-323, 1977.

INDEX